MYOCARDIAL REVASCULARIZATION

MYOCARDIAL REVASCULARIZATION
Novel Percutaneous Approaches

Edited by

George S. Abela

Department of Medicine
Division of Cardiology
Michigan State University
College of Human Medicine
East Lansing, Michigan

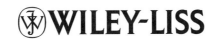

WILEY-LISS

A John Wiley & Sons, Inc., Publication

Library of Congress Cataloging-in-Publication Data:
Percutaneous transluminal endomyocardial revascularization : practical and theoretical approaches / edited by George S. Abela.
    p. ; cm.
  Includes bibliographical references and index.
  ISBN 0-471-36166-6 (cloth)
  1. Transmyocardial laser revascularization. 2. Heart catheterization.
3. Myocardial revascularization. I. Abela, George S.
  [DNLM: 1. Myocardial Revascularization—methods. 2. Heart
Catheterization. 3. Laser Surgery. WG 169 P4293 2001]
  RD598.35.T67 P47 2001
  617.4′12059—dc21
                                             2001026775

Printed in the United States of America.

10 9 8 7 6 5 4 3 2 1

This book is dedicated to the Cardiology Fellows whose commitment and efforts enrich the educational experience in Cardiovascular Medicine.

CONTENTS

Foreword

If a grandfather for myocardial revascularization were to be chosen, I would suggest the leading candidate to be Dr. P. K. Sen of Bombay, India. In October 1979, I had the pleasure of hosting a visit from Dr. Sen to our lab in Detroit. In 1965, Dr. Sen had published the first of several papers demonstrating a significant reduction in the expected mortality and in infarct size in dogs after the ligation of the left anterior descending coronary artery when the animals had been pretreated with multiple needle punctures of the left ventricular myocardium. His results were impressive regardless of the variations in the literature of expected deaths from acute LAD closure depending upon the site of ligation and other factors. Dr. Sen claimed patency of the channels at 8 weeks and stated, "There is an analogy between this mode of blood supply to the myocardium and the myocardial circulation in lower vertebrates." Following his lead, other investigators reported variations in his technique, some using larger-bore cannulas and, in one instance, heated needles. I showed Dr. Sen a film made by Dr. Mahmood (Sid) Mirhoseini, who was first to use laser energy, to create the channels. Dr. Sen agreed that this represented a definite advance in technique.

I first met Dr. Abela through our mutual interest in the activities of the American Society for Laser Medicine and Surgery. He served on the board of that organization and chaired cardiovascular sessions at several annual meetings. In 1993–1994, he was vice president and was appointed to the editorial board of the society's official journal *Lasers in Surgery and Medicine*. Dr. Abela completed a Fellowship in Cardiology at the University of Florida, where he became an Associate Professor of Medicine. He later served as an Associate Professor at Harvard and was Director of Interventional Research and The Cardiovascular Photobiology Laboratory at the New England Deaconess Hospital. He is an internationally recognized pioneer in the development and evaluation of numerous laser devices for the treatment of cardiovascular disease and was the first investigator in the United States approved for the use of laser angioplasty in the peripheral circulation. His two previous books have depicted the state of the art of laser applications for cardiovascular conditions. The first book, *Lasers in Cardiovascular Medicine and Surgery*, included one of the earliest clinical reports on successful TMR by Mirhoseini and Cayton. In a more recent book co-edited with Peter Wittaker, they took on the challenge of "direct myocardial revascularization" and succeeded in their stated objective of stimulating investigators, both clinical and basic scientific, to evaluate the role of TMR in the treatment of coronary artery disease.

Now the picture continues to change. A new, less invasive approach has emerged. A fiberoptic catheter system energized with Ho:YAG as the laser of choice is introduced percutaneously. The possibility of early denervation followed by later angiogenesis has replaced the concern about maintaining channel patency. Other forms of energy are being considered, including focused ultrasound, radio frequency, and even cryoenergy.

We are introduced to electromechanical mapping of the myocardium and the exciting potential of gene therapy including cell implantation into the myocardium.

Dr. Abela has chosen his investigators carefully. This work represents a monumental advance in the understanding of therapeutic possibilities in the management of coronary artery disease.

Ellet H. Drake, M.D., F.A.C.C.
Former Chief Division of Cardiology
Henry Ford Hospital, Detroit, Michigan

Preface

"Why abandon a belief merely because it
ceases to be true. Cling to it long enough,
and not a doubt it shall be true again, for it
so goes. Most of the change we think we see
in life is due to truths being in and out of
favor."

*Robert Frost (1874–1963). North of
Boston; 7. The Black Cottage*

The concept of myocardial revascularization
directly from the ventricular cavity is a concept that has existed for a long time. It fell
out of favor when coronary artery bypass
surgery was found to be a highly effective and
successful procedure. Recurrence of disease in
previously treated patients and patients with
diffuse coronary artery insufficiency are living
longer because of improved medical therapy.
However, once again, we face the problem
that was encountered before the advent of
coronary bypass surgery. And we must pick
up where those who started this field left off
about five decades ago. So it is that we now
are reevaluating the possibility of direct
myocardial revascularization using a variety
of techniques. These include laser, radio frequency, mechanical, cryofreezing systems and
others. Also, we have gone further to using
gene codes injected into the myocardium
to enhance neovascularization, and most

recently we have gone as far as transplanting myocytes into the myocardium to replace
dead cells. These techniques are the subject
of this text. It is expected that the reader will
encounter conflicting points of view. For,
certainly, this area of investigation has only
begun to develop, and the techniques vary
greatly.

Section I describes the background and
more recent developments in the field focusing on the work of Dr. Arthur Vineberg and
some of the impressive findings by angiography showing patent internal mammary artery
grafts over 20 years after surgery. The report
of the pioneers in this field, Mary Cayton and
Dr. Mahmood Mirhoseini, describes in their
own words the experience of the development
of transmyocadial laser revascularization.
Furthermore, the experiences of the technology are reported by Dr. Horvath, who
describes the results in the hands of those
who have critically evaluated this technique
and carried it further.

Section II describes the biological responses to direct myocardial revascularization. These include an in-depth evaluation by
Dr. Virmani and colleagues emphasizing the
important differences in the reaction of neo-
vacularization to the type of injury. Original
work from Drs. Hughes and Lowe discusses

the effect of denervation versus angiogenesis as the mechanism of action to explain the patient symptom improvements. Drs. Hage-Korban and Abela et al. list seven possible mechanisms of the potential benefit response to PMR/TMR and present arguments in favor of and against each of these mechanisms. It is likely that more than one mechanism is involved, suggesting that soon after treatment the mechanism may differ substantially from that at long-term follow-up. Supportive technologies are also reported regarding more accurate methods for targeting the laser or other therapy in the ventricular cavity. Dr. Foster and colleagues describe such a method using the NOGA™ navigation system, including the use of this approach to inject gene code into the ventricular wall.

Section III describes the clinical experience to date with use of PMR for myocardial revascularization. Drs. Eisenberg and Oesterle et al. summarize the data regarding the effectiveness of PMR. Controversial positions on the effect of placebo are discussed as well as the angina relief benefits of PMR. Much focus is placed on the importance of differences between catheter systems and laser doses and wavelengths. These are not insignificant differences, and generalizations from one study to the next can only be made with caution. Most importantly, larger randomized trials are still needed to confirm the benefits of PMR for the management of intractable angina. Other nonlaser techniques are described and compared to PMR. This is illustrated in the chapter by Drs. Abernethy and Oesterle et al. that describes a novel in situ revascularization method using stents to create channels between coronary arteries and veins to form local shunts without having to resort to open-chest procedures.

Section IV describes other methods for revascularization. These descriptions include the chapter by Drs. Kantor and Schwartz et al. on the use of radio frequency to create myocardial channels and a neovascularization response. Dr. Gallo describes a novel concept using cryofreezing to enhance the neovascularization. Dr. Verdaasdonk describes an ultrasound method to enhance neovascularization. Dr. Perin describes a method to detect the viable myocardium and help guide therapy using electromechanical mapping. Drs. Werns and Henry describe use of genes to induce neovascularization, and Dr. Boekstegers et al. provides a unique approach using retroperfusion via the coronary veins. Dr. Waxman provides a novel approach developed to use the pericardium as a reservoir for instilling gene code and other agents to enhance myocardial perfusion. Finally, Drs. Yao and Kloner describe the use of myocytes transplanted into the myocardium to provide yet another creative approach to help stabilize the patient whose heart muscle has become severely weakened. It is always important to view the technologies with respect to their market value. Will the technology be viable and survive the economic challenges? It would seem from the analysis by Dr. Woodward et al. that the likelihood for this is favorable. Only then can these concepts go beyond the realm of mere curiosity to that of clinical reality.

A great thanks is due to all the contributors. This text is a unique compilation of state-of-the-art work being done nationally and worldwide. This effort may not always be compensated, but it could make a major difference to those who suffer from debilitating angina pectoris.

George S. Abela
Editor

ACKNOWLEDGMENT

This book would not have made the deadline without the expert skills and support of Hongbao Ma and Lori Blankenship. Their efforts are deeply appreciated and recognized.

Contributors

George S. Abela, M.D., M.Sc., M.B.A., Department of Medicine, Division of Cardiology, Michigan State University, East Lansing, Michigan.

Oliver G. Abela, Department of Medicine, Division of Cardiology, Michigan State University, East Lansing, Michigan.

William B. Abernethy III, M.D., Division of Cardiology, Massachusetts General Hospital, Harvard Medical School, Boston, Massachusetts.

Rakesh C. Arora, M.D., Cardiac Surgery, Dalhousie University, Halifax, Nova Scotia, Canada.

Peter Boekstegers, M.D., Oberarzt der Med. Klinik1, Klinikum Grosshadern, LMU, München, Germany.

Charlene R. Boisjolie, R.N., Cardiology Division, Deparment of Medicine, Hennepin County Medical Center, Minneapolis, Minnesota.

Nancy Briefs, M.B.A., President and CEO, Percardia, Inc., Merrimack, New Hampshire.

Allen P. Burke, M.D., Department of Cardiovascular Pathology, Armed Forces Institute of Pathology, Washington, DC.

Mary Cayton, R.N., St. Luke's Medical Center Heart and Lung Institute of Wisconsin, Laser Research Laboratory Clement Zablocki Department of Veterans Affairs Medical Center, Milwaukee, Wisconsin.

Henk Cobelens, B.Sc., Department of Clinical Engineering and Physics, University Medical Center, Utrecht, The Netherlands.

Marc Dubuc, M.D., Department of Medicine, Montreal Heart Institute, Montreal, Quebec, Canada.

Joel D. Eisenberg, M.D., Department of Medicine, Cardiology, Michigan State University, East Lansing, Michigan.

Andrew Farb, M.D., Department of Cardiovascular Pathology, Armed Forces Institute of Pathology, Washington, DC.

Tim A. Fischell, M.D., F.A.C.C., F.S.C.A.I., Heart Institute at Borgess Medical Center, Kalamazoo, Michigan.

Peter J. Fitzgerald, M.D., Ph.D., Division of Cardiolovascular Medicine, Stanford University Medical Center, Stanford, California.

Malcolm T. Foster III, M.D., F.A.C.C., Heart Institute at Borgess Medical Center, Kalamazoo, Michigan.

Wolfgang Franz, M.D., Klinikum Grosshadern, LMU, München, Germany.

Stephen Fry, Ph.D., CardioCavitational Systems, Inc., Hanalei, Hawaii.

Richard Gallo, M.D., Department of Medicine, Montreal Heart Institute, Montreal, Quebec, Canada.

Khaled Ghosheh, M.D., Department of Medicine, Division of Cardiology, Michigan State University, East Lansing, Michigan.

Matthijs Grimbergen, B.Sc., Department of Clinical Engineering and Physics, University Medical Center, Utrecht, The Netherlands.

Paul F. Gründeman, Ph.D., Department of Clinical Engineering and Physics, Heart-Lung Institute, University Medical Center, Utrecht, The Netherlands.

Elie Hage-Korban, M.D., Department of Medicine, Division of Cardiology, Michigan State University, East Lansing, Michigan.

Timothy D. Henry, M.D., Cardiology Division, Department of Medicine, Hennepin County Medical Center, Minneapolis, Minnesota.

David R. Holmes, Jr., M.D., Division of Cardiovascular Diseases and Internal Medicine, Mayo Clinic and Foundation, Rochester, Minnesota.

Keith A. Horvath, M.D., Northwestern University Medical School, Chicago, Illinois.

Ruiping Huang, Ph.D., Department of Medicine, Division of Cardiology, Michigan State University, East Lansing, Michigan.

G. Chad Hughes, M.D., Division of Thoracic and Cardiovascular Surgery, Duke University Medical Center, Durham, North Carolina.

Birgit Kantor, M.D., Division of Cardiovascular Diseases and Internal Medicine, Mayo Clinic and Foundation, Rochester, Minnesota.

Paul C. Keelan, M.D., Fellow in Cardiovascular Medicine, Department of Medicine, Division of Cardiology, Mayo Clinic, Rochester, Minnesota.

Robert A. Kloner, M.D. Ph.D., Professor of Medicine, University of Southern California, Director of Research, Heart Institute, Good Samaritan Hospital, Los Angeles, California.

Frank D. Kolodgie, Ph.D., Department of Cardiovascular Pathology, Armed Forces Institute of Pathology, Washington, DC.

Christian Kupatt, M.D., Klinikum Grosshadern, LMU, München, Germany.

Michael A. Lauer, M.D., Heart Institute at Borgess Medical Center, Kalamazoo, Michigan.

James E. Lowe, M.D., Division of Thoracic and Cardiovascular Surgery, Duke University Medical Center, Durham, North Carolina.

Hongbao Ma, Ph.D., Department of Medicine, Division of Cardiology, Michigan State University, East Lansing, Michigan.

Mahmood Mirhoseini, M.D., Department of Cardio-Thoracic Surgery, Medical College of Wisconsin, Department of Cardiovascular and Thoracic Surgery, St. Luke's Medical Center Heart and Lung Institute of Wisconsin, Laser Research Laboratory, Clement Zablocki Department of Veterans Affairs Medical Center, Milwaukee, Wisconsin.

Stephen N. Oesterle, M.D., Department of Medicine/Cardiology, Massachusetts General Hospital, Boston, Massachusetts.

Emerson C. Perin, M.D., F.A.C.C., New Interventional Cardiovascular Technology, Texas Heart Institute, Baylor College of Medicine and University of Texas Health Science Center, Houston, Texas.

Ramon C. Raneses, Jr., M.D., F.A.C.C., Heart Institute at Borgess Medical Center, Kalamazoo, Michigan.

Rogério Sarmento-Leite, M.D., Ph.D., Cardiology Research Fellow, Texas Heart Institute, Baylor College of Medicine, Houston, Texas.

Robert S. Schwartz, M.D., Division of Cardiolovascular Diseases and Internal Medicine, Mayo Clinic and Foundation, Rochester, Minnesota.

Guilherne V. Silva, M.D., Cardiology Research Fellow, Texas Heart Institute,

Baylor College of Medicine, Houston, Texas.

On Topaz, M.D., Interventional Cardiovascular Laboratories, McGuire VA Medical Center, Division of Cardiology, Medical College of Virginia, Virginia Commonwealth University, Richmond, Virginia.

Christiaan van Swol, Ph.D., Department of Clinical Engineering and Physics, University Medical Center, Utrecht, The Netherlands.

Rudolf Verdaasdonk, Ph.D., Department of Clinical Engineering and Physics, University Medical Center, Utrecht, The Netherlands.

Renu Virmani, M.D., Department of Cardiovascular Pathology, Armed Forces Institute of Pathology, Washington, DC.

Georges von Degenfeld, M.D., Klinikum Grosshadern, LMU, München, Germany.

Sergio Waxman, M.D., Interventional Cardiology, University of Texas Medical Branch at Galveston, Galveston, Texas.

Steven W. Werns, M.D., Division of Cardiology, University of Michigan Medical School, Ann Arbor, Michigan.

Terry Woodward, Ph.D., M.B.A., Portfolio Manager, Healthcare/Biotech Venture Capital at the Ontario Teachers' Pension Plan, Ontario, Canada.

Mu Yao, M.D., Ph.D., University of Southern California, Heart Institute, Good Samaritan Hospital, Los Angeles, California.

Alan C. Yeung, M.D., Division of Cardiolovascular Medicine, Stanford University Medical Center, Stanford, California.

I

Background of Myocardial Revascularization Techniques

1

Myocardial Revascularization: The Role of the Vineberg Operation and Related Procedures

On Topaz, M.D.

Interventional Cardiovascular Laboratories
McGuire VA Medical Center
Division of Cardiology
Medical College of Virginia
Virginia Commonwealth University
Richmond, Virginia

SUMMARY

1933—Dr. Joseph Wearn demonstrated existence of vascular connections between coronary arteries and ventricular chambers of the heart.

1940s—Surgeon Claude Beck described a "trigger zone" in which revascularization would provide a blood bath of coronary blood flow and thus preserve viability of the myocardium.

1940s—Dr. Arthur Vineberg incorporated implantation of internal mammary artery into the ventricular myocardium.

1962—Dr. Mason Sones angiographically demonstrated patency of mammary implants and presence of collateral channels 5–7 years after Vineberg operation; however, later studies dismissed Vineberg operation because of high mortality. Lack of long-term data post-Vineberg operation data may be a testimony to decreased prolonged survival rate.

1990s—Resurgence of clinical interest in myocardial revascularization.

1.1. INTRODUCTION

Direct coronary artery bypass graft surgery is a well-established therapeutic modality for patients with severe coronary artery disease. This strategy was not developed all at once; rather, it was introduced after thorough scientific observations, various basic science experiments, and several small-scale clinical studies that tested hypotheses and different surgical approaches and techniques. First, the fundamental concept of myocardium rendered ischemic by obstructed epicardial coronary flow had to be assessed and then introduced to clinical management in cardio-

Myocardial Revascularization: Novel Percutaneous Approaches, Edited by George S. Abela.
ISBN 0-471-36166-6   Copyright © 2002 Wiley-Liss, Inc.

vascular medicine. The next step included exploration and development of surgical means to supply the ischemic myocardium, and only then were the most promising revascularization methods selected. Early operations paved the way to the modern surgical and percutaneous treatments of ischemic coronary artery disease used today. This chapter describes several milestones in the investigation and implementation of physiologic methodologies aimed toward improved coronary flow and myocardial perfusion. Understanding the fundamentals of "old" myocardial revascularization methods is imperative for further improvement of current approaches, for development of new concepts, and to avoid the repetition of mistakes that occurred throughout the long scientific journey leading to contemporary treatment of obstructive atherosclerotic coronary artery disease.

1.2. HISTORICAL PERSPECTIVES

Treatment of ischemic myocardium by indirect myocardial revascularization predates direct coronary bypass grafting and intracoronary balloon angioplasty. The modern era in the physiologic approach toward myocardial revascularization began in 1933 when Dr. Joseph Wearn and his colleagues demonstrated the existence of vascular communications between the coronary arteries and the chambers of the heart. These communicating vessels included "arterio-luminal" and "arterio-sinusoidal" vessels as well as "myocardial sinusoids". They postulated that gradual progression of coronary arterial occlusions allowed Thebesian veins to assume a function of supplying blood to the heart (Fig. 1-1) (Wearn et al., 1933). They also identified extra cardiac anastomoses of the epicardial coronary arteries in the form of collaterals from the pericardium and vasa vasorum leading to and from the myocardium (Hudson et al., 1932). Wearn's observations played a crucial role in the accelerated development of research and experiments aimed at new ways to enhance myocardial perfusion for patients with obstructive atherosclerotic

coronary artery disease. Several indirect myocardial revascularization operations followed and were used in the 1940s, 1950s, and 1960s (Beck et al., 1948; Glover et al., 1957; Stanton et al., 1941).

One of the first surgeons to investigate myocardial revascularization modalities of the heart was Claude S. Beck. He described a concept termed the "trigger zone," which became first the basis for his experiments and later on the target for clinical treatment. Beck postulated that the distribution of coronary blood flow was important in reference to survival and that a small increase of blood supply could, at times, make the difference between recovery and death. The purpose of surgical revascularization then was to provide a blood bath to the "trigger zone," to preserve viability of the heart muscle and prevent formation of myocardial necrosis.

1.2.1. The Beck Procedure

The surface of the heart was abraded by first using sandpaper, emery paper, and then special burs (Stanton et al., 1941). An inflammatory reaction was produced by the application of a foreign body. Among the many agents used was powered beef bone and, ultimately, asbestos. Finally, vascularized tissue such as fat, parietal pericardium, and skeletal muscle, was grafted to the surface of the heart. These grafted hearts were then investigated by several methods including selective injection of barium solution into the right and left circumflex coronary arteries followed by demonstration with X rays of the presence of vascular communications with the left anterior descending coronary artery. Another method included a comparison between normal hearts and hearts treated by abrasion after ligation of one major coronary artery. From their results, Beck and his associates concluded that intercoronary communications could be produced by the described surgical method. Then, in 1943, Beck reported additional results of experimental operations carried out over 10 years. These results were (Wearn et al., 1933) that (1) vascular

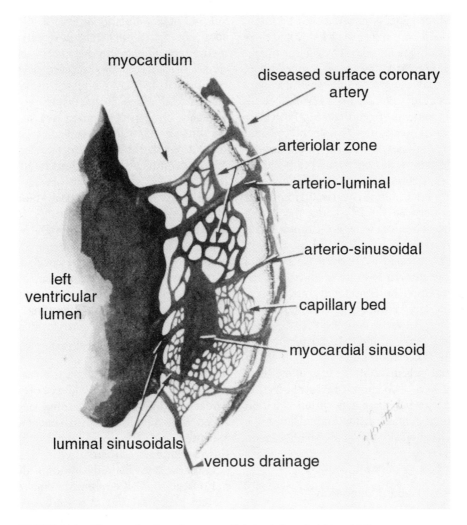

FIGURE 1-1.   Diagram showing micromyocardial circulation of right and left ventricles as described by Wearn. There is a central lakelike structure representing a sinusoid between muscle bundles. Capillaries arise from these to nourish myocardial fibers while others enter the ventricular lumen. The surface coronary arteries send branches directly into the lumen of the ventricle. Sinusoidal vessels branch from the surface coronary arteries to open into the myocardial sinusoidal spaces. In between run the arterioles. (Reprinted with permission of the publisher from Vineberg AM, *Myocardial Revascularization by Arterial/Ventricular Implants*, p.72. Boston, Massachusetts, John Wright PSG, 1982).

communications between a graft and the myocardium were established and were large enough to be seen in a clean specimen without magnification; (2) the direction and amount of flow in these channels was not ascertained; (3) no advantage could be attributed to one type of vascular graft over any other; (4) progressive, staged occlusion of the coronary artery was helpful in promoting the develop-

ment of vascular communications; and (5) the concept of the trigger zone was valid, emphasizing the importance of equal distribution of blood to the myocardium through grafts, as was the phenomenon of opening of the intercoronary channels by creation of an inflammatory reaction on the surface of the heart. Beck also reported the results of 30 operations done in humans between 1935 and 1938.

Twenty-three patients survived the operation, and fourteen were still alive in 1943. The clinical results in patients who survived the operation were reported as "satisfactory." Beck believed that the procedure was successful and efficient for several reasons (Wearn et al., 1933): (1) patients stated that they felt better as early as 1 week after the operation, and laboratory studies indicated intercoronary communications as early as 5 days after surgery; (2) examination of hearts after death demonstrated a number of vascular communications between the heart and the grafts; and (3) his colleagues were of the opinion that a similar rate of recovery and survival in patients not treated by Beck's surgery could not be expected. In 1943 Beck stated that the operation could be considered as a "procedure in therapy." However, interest in the procedure fell between 1942 and 1945, both because of the war and because of growing interest in other approaches for treatment of myocardial ischemia. Other surgical methods for improved myocardial revascularization included internal mammary artery ligation and coronary sinus ligation and anastomosis (Beck et al., 1948; Glover et al., 1957; Stanton et al., 1941).

1.2.2. The Vineberg Operation

The procedure that ultimately received the most attention was the Vineberg operation (Fig. 1-2) (Vineberg 1946, 1949; Vineberg et al., 1950, 1964). This surgery incorporated implantation of the internal mammary artery into the ventricular myocardium, presumably resulting in formation of neovascular connections between the implanted artery and the coronary circulation. Dr. Arthur Vineberg, a Canadian cardiothoracic surgeon, developed an interest in coronary artery disease as a young surgeon living at home with his parents. Because his father suffered for years from angina pectoris and congestive heart failure (Dobell, 1992), the son was determined to find a therapeutic approach for the devastating clinical condition his father and other patients were enduring. Vineberg began his experiments with the left internal mammary artery in 1946 and soon concluded that the most satisfactory method of implantation was by way of a tunnel prepared in the myocardial wall and that the left internal mammary artery had to bleed either through its distal end or its branches on implantation to remain patent. He further insisted on the merit of physiologic validation of his surgical approach relying on studies that demonstrated the existence of a vast network of vascular spaces between the myocardial muscle bundles in direct communication with the left ventricular cavity (Wearn et al., 1933). Vineberg performed laboratory studies in animals, repeatedly demonstrating patency of mammary implants into the myocardium and lack of hematoma at the anastomotic site (Vineberg et al., 1946). The first human Vineberg operation was performed in April 1950. Although the patient died 62 h later, autopsy revealed that the left internal mammary artery implant to the anterolateral wall was patent, without evidence of anterior myocardial infarction, hematoma, or hemorrhage. The second patient who underwent the Vineberg operation lived for 10 years after this revolutionary surgery.

Later on, several modifications of the original operation were developed. Vineberg ultimately expanded the procedure to include epicardioectomy and free omental grafting to the posterior aspect of the left ventricle and wrapping around the right ventricle. Effler extended the myocardial tunnel to include the posterior wall, Sewell used a vascular bundle including the internal mammary artery and vein and chest wall tissue, Bigelow left the distal end of the artery patent, and Favaloro and co-workers performed double implant procedures with the right internal mammary artery implanted into the anterolateral wall of the left ventricle and the left internal mammary artery implanted into the posterolateral and diaphragmatic walls (Bigelow et al., 1966; Effler et al., 1965; Favaloro, 1990; Favaloro et al., 1967). We encountered a patient who presented with unstable angina 21 years after a bilateral Vineberg operation (Figs. 1-3 and 1-4). We were able to obtain the

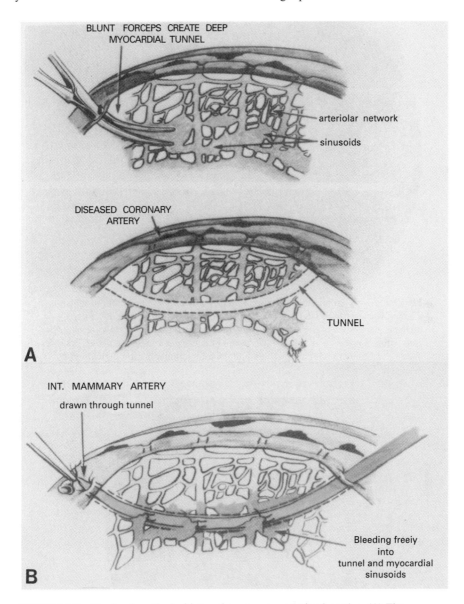

FIGURE 1-2.   Vineberg's method of internal mammary artery implantation. (A) The myocardial artery microcirculation with patent myocardial sinusoids is opened by forceps. (B) Internal mammary artery in the ventricular tunnel with bleeding intercostal arteries. (Reprinted with permission of the publisher from Vineberg AM, *Myocardial Revascularization by Arterial/Ventricular Implants*, p.16. Boston, Massachusetts, John Wright/PSG, 1982).

original surgical note from 1969, which describes a classic Vineberg operation as follows:

"With the patient supine, a median sternotomy was performed. The sternal edges were elevated in turn using the Favaloro sternal elevator and first the left and subsequently the right mammary artery pedicles were mobilized from beneath them. These are very satisfactory pedicles, containing the mammary arteries that bleed well. At the distal ends, the pedicles were ligated and divided. A conventional rib spreader was

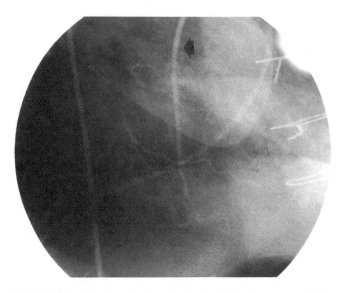

FIGURE 1-3.   Cardiac catheterization in a patient who presented with unstable angina 21 years after bilateral Vineberg operation. Angiography of a left internal mammary artery (LIMA) as utilized for Vineberg operation. The LIMA (black arrow) runs within a myocardial tunnel under the obtuse marginal branches of the circumflex artery and fills them. (Topaz et al., 1999, Published with permission by Kluwer Academic Publishers.)

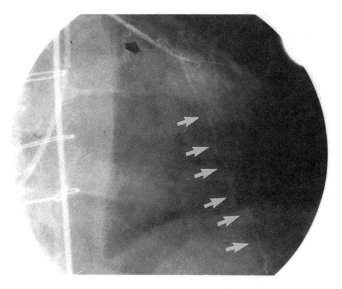

FIGURE 1-4.   Same patient with a Vineberg's right IMA (RIMA; black arrow) perfusing the left anterior descending (white arrows) and diagonal arteries. (Topaz et al., 1999, Published with permission of Kluwer Academic Publishers.)

now inserted transversely. The pericardial fat was dissected away from the front of the heart and the pericardium widely opened giving good exposure of the heart. Knowing the angiographic pattern of disease, I first made a tunnel on the posterolateral surface of the left ventricle. It is about 6 cm long and passed under most of the descending circumflex coronary artery branches. A suture was pulled back through this tunnel and, after debriding the left pedicle, the suture was tied to the end of the pedicle and it was pulled through this left posterolateral tunnel. At the distal end, a transfixion suture was placed to keep it from retracting. The heart was now allowed to fall back in its bed and a second anterior tunnel made, starting to the right of the anterior descending coronary artery and emerging on the left lateral ventricular wall, passing under all major branches of the anterior descending coronary artery. A suture was similarly pulled back through this tunnel and, after debriding the right pedicle, it was pulled through the anterior tunnel and a similar transfixion suture ,was placed at the right distal end. This was technically a very satisfactory mammary implant. The pericardial fat was pulled across the front of the heart and sutured in position. The chest was closed in layers using steel wire to approximate the sternum. The subcutaneous tissues and skin are closed with silk. The mediastinum and both pleural spaces are drained."

Interestingly, as shown 21 years later (Topaz et al., 1992), the mammary implants were still able to perfuse the myocardium and accounted for the lengthy period of clinical and hemodynamic stability of this patient.

Although there was indirect laboratory evidence and certain supportive clinical evidence as to the efficacy of the Vineberg procedure, initial acceptance was slow and criticisms were many (Boyd, 1970; Mundth et al., 1975). An analogous procedure in dogs using implantation of the femoral artery into the adductor muscle formed a significant hematoma in every case, and the implanted vessel invariably occluded. The fact that in treated patients the angina was relieved and exercise tolerance was improved was explained away on emotional rather than scientific grounds. Never the less, the lack of evidence that the procedure prolonged life or reduced the incidence of subsequent myocardial infarction did not lend support for the procedure (Takaro, 1973). The academic and clinical climate for the Vineberg operation turned positive, however, in 1962, when Dr. Mason Sones at the Cleveland Clinic

angiographically demonstrated patency of mammary implants and the presence of collateral channels communicating them to a coronary artery in two patients, 5 and 7 years after a Vineberg operation, respectively (Sones and Shirey, 1962). The fact that the implant was capable of retrograde filling of a major epicardial coronary artery was considered of paramount importance. After these landmark angiographic studies, thousands of these operations were performed (Vineberg and Walker, 1964). Cardiac catheterization became the ultimate follow-up method for proving (albeit, at random and without a systematic prospective analysis) the patency of the internal mammary implants. Analysis of pre- and postsurgery angiographic studies revealed that whenever a postsurgery angiogram demonstrated patency of the internal mammary artery and adequate opacification of the left anterior descending artery, the preoperative left anterior descending artery contained a total or subtotal obstruction. On the other hand, in most cases with a patent postoperative internal mammary artery but lacking an anastomotic connection to the left anterior descending artery or its branches, the preoperative left anterior descending artery obstruction was not critical. Nevertheless, in patients in whom the postoperative internal mammary artery was angiographically demonstrated to be occluded, no correlation could be found as to the degree of presurgical severity of left anterior descending artery disease. Proponents of the operation claimed that the mammary implant indeed perfused the myocardium. In several patients a beneficial effect on myocardial blood flow, as well as on myocardial lactate metabolism, was demonstrated (Gorlin and Taylor, 1969). Interestingly, in some patients who underwent a Vineberg procedure and years later needed a repeat cardiac operation, cardioplegic arrest during aortic cross-clamping could only be achieved by transient occlusion of the internal mammary artery implant because its antegrade flow continued during cross-clamping (Salerno et al., 1979).

In 1966, a Veterans Administration co-operative study was undertaken to finally examine the efficacy of the Vineberg procedure in a controlled prospective manner. The historical results in 146 patients clearly indicated a high operative mortality of 12% [significantly higher than previous reports of 4–5% (Vineberg and Walker, 1964)], implant patency at 1 year of only 67%, and no difference in cumulative survival (Bhayana et al., 1980). A year later, Kolessov (Kolessov, 1967) described the direct internal mammary artery grafting to the coronary arteries. Green then published his 3-year experience with 165 patients who underwent internal mammary grafting with direct anastomosis to the coronary arteries with a 7.1% overall hospital mortality (Green, 1967). DeBakey and colleagues then published their experience with aortocoronary bypass surgery using saphenous vein grafts through a 7-year follow-up (Garrett et al., 1973), and consequently the Vineberg operation rapidly fell out of favor.

1.2.3. Long-term Angiographic Evaluation After Vineberg Operation

There is a paucity of data on angiographic long-term follow-up after a Vineberg procedure. The most plausible explanation is that prolonged survival in fact is quite rare. Bhayana and co-authors reported an angiographic follow-up with 50% patency of a single graft and 69% patency of a double graft at 1 year. However, 58% of the patients were dead at 10 years (Bhayana et al., 1980). Bigelow and colleagues reported a series of patients with 1- to 13-year follow-up with one patient still alive at 13 years (Bigelow et al., 1966, 1990). Topaz et al. described a patient with patent bilateral mammary arteries 21 years after the Vineberg operation (Topaz et al., 1992). Similarly, Hayward and co-workers reported (Hayward et al., 1991) a 20-year angiographic follow-up of a patient who underwent a double internal mammary implantation. These findings substantiate the view that survival in selected cases depends on the collateral blood flow provided by the mammary implants.

1.2.4. Postmortem Evaluation of Vineberg Operation

Vineberg reported on autopsy studies and fate of 22 internal mammary arteries (IMA) implanted into the left ventricular wall (Vineberg, 1982). In patients who died early, between 6h and 3 weeks after implantation, the IMA was injected with India ink. One of eight grafts was blocked with fresh thrombus whereas the other seven grafts were patent. India ink flowed into the IMA and appeared in the coronary sinuses (Fig. 1-5). This had a strong resemblance to the anatomy described by Wearn et al. (1933) (Fig. 1-1). In the remaining 14 IMA grafts examined at 6 weeks to 4 years postoperatively, only two were blocked. Thus the postmortem data supported angiographic findings indicating patency and communication between the IMA and myocardium.

1.2.5. Surgical Approach After Vineberg Operation

Coronary artery bypass grafting as a second surgery for patients who underwent the Vineberg operation is challenging. Hayward et al. (1991) described a patient for whom such surgical intervention was not possible. However, Topaz et al. (1992) demonstrated the feasibility of coronary artery bypass grafting using saphenous veins in these rare patients but suggested certain precautions such as the use of femoral cannulations for bypass. They also recommended the preservation of the original IMA grafts and avoiding any attempts to use them, either as direct grafts or as free grafts, even if selective angiography demonstrated their patency. In contradiction, Glock and colleagues (1992) reported a successful reoperation on a patient 20 years after Vineberg operation, whereby they ligated the right IMA at the level of the right ventricular wall and created an end-to-side anastomosis to the left anterior descending artery. Interestingly, a histopathologic study of transverse sections of the distal segment of that right IMA showed adequate preservation of the internal and external

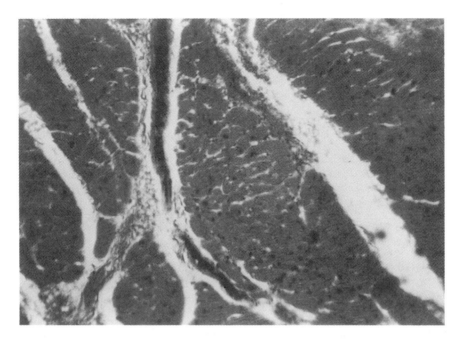

FIGURE 1-5. Photomicrograph of patient who died 82 hours after surgery. Spaces filling with India ink suggestive of sinusoids are seen between myocardial muscle bundles. (Reprinted with permission of the publisher from Vineberg AM, *Myocardial Revascularization by Arterial/Ventricular Implants*, p. 333. Boston, Massachusetts, John Wright/PSG, 1982).

elastic lamina. The intima exhibited moderate thickening, but there were no features of atherosclerosis present in the artery. The postoperative patency of the "converted" right IMA was confirmed by arteriography 10 days after surgery.

1.3. SUMMARY

Modern coronary artery bypass surgery is a standard operative approach for direct revascularization in patients with severe coronary artery disease. The current state-of-the-art operation is the culmination of extensive basic research, clinical experience, and innovative methods of revascularization spanning at least 70 years. The road to contemporary operations includes several milestone surgical methods. Among these landmarks were the Beck operation and the Vineberg operation. In retrospect, it is often easy to criticize certain medical innovations and to dismiss them as unscientific, immature. or noncom-

prehensive. Nevertheless, because there are no short cuts in science, we could not have performed current state-of-the-art coronary revascularization, surgical and percutaneous alike, without the lessons learned from the scientific gains and failures of the pioneers in cardiovascular medicine.

ACKNOWLEDGMENT

The author gratefully acknowledges the editorial assistance of Laurie Topaz and Michelle Gilbert in the preparation of this chapter.

References

Beck CS, Stanton E, Batiuchok W et al. Revascularization of heart by graft of systemic artery into coronary sinus. *JAMA* 1948; 137: 436–442.

Bhayana JN, Gage AA, Takaro T. Long-term results of internal mammary artery implantation for coronary artery disease: a controlled trial. *Ann Thor Surg* 1980; 29: 234–242.

Bigelow WG, Aldridge HE, MacGregor DC. Internal mammary implantation (Vineberg operation) for coronary artery disease. *Ann Surg* 1966; 164: 457–464.

Boyd DP. The Vineberg operation: some pros and cons. *Surg Clin N Am* 1970; 50: 579–584.

Dobell ARC. Arthur Vineberg and the internal mammary artery implantation procedure. *Ann Thorac Surg* 1992; 53: 167–169.

Effler DB, Sones FM Jr, Groves LK et al. Myocardial revascularization by Vineberg's internal mammary artery implant. *J Thorac Cardiovasc Surg* 1965; 50: 527–531.

Favaloro RG, Effler DB, Groves LK et al. Myocardial revascularization by internal mammary artery implant procedures. *J Thorac Cardiovasc Surg* 1967; 54: 359–370.

Garrett HE, Dennis EW, DeBakey ME. Aortocoronary bypass with saphenous vein graft: seven year follow-up. *JAMA* 1973; 223: 792–794.

Glock Y, Girbet G, Delisle MB et al. From Vineberg to bypass: a "second-hand" internal mammary artery. *J Cardiovasc Surg* 1992; 33: 502–504.

Glover RP, Davila JC, Kyle RH et al. Ligation of the internal mammary arteries as a means of increasing blood supply to the myocardium. *J Thorac Surg* 1957; 34: 661–678.

Gorlin R, Taylor WJ. Myocardial revascularization with internal mammary artery implantation: current status. *JAMA* 1969; 207: 907–913.

Green GE. Internal mammary artery-to-coronary anastomoses: three year experience with 165 patients. *Ann Thorac Surg* 1972; 14: 260–271.

Hayward RH, Korompai FL, Knight WL. Long-term follow-up of the Vineberg internal mammary artery implant procedure. *Ann Thorac Surg* 1991; 51: 1002–1003.

Hudson CL, Moritz AR, Wearn JT. The extracardiac anastomoses of the coronary arteries. *Soc Exp Med* 1932; 56: 91–939.

Kolessov VI. Mammary artery—coronary artery anastomosis as method of treatment for angina pectoris. *J Thorac Cardiovasc Surg* 1967; 54: 535–544.

Mundth ED, Austen WG. Surgical measures for coronary heart disease. *N Engl J Med* 1975; 293: 13–19.

Salerno TA, Keith FM, Charrette EJP. Cardioplegic arrest in patients with previous Vineberg implants. *J Thorac Cardiovasc Surg* 1979; 78: 760–771.

Sewell WH. The current status of surgery for coronary artery disease. *Vasc Surg* 1976; 10: 285.

Sones FM Jr, Shirey EK. Cinecoronary arteriography. *Mod Concepts Cardiovasc Dis* 1962; 31: 735–741.

Stanton EJ, Schildt P, Beck CS. The effect of abrasion of the surface of the heart upon intercoronary communications. *Am Heart J* 1941; 22: 529–538.

Takaro T. The enigma of the Vineberg-Sewell implant operation. *Chest* 1973; 64: 150–151.

Topaz O, Pavlos S, Mackall J et al. The Vineberg procedure revisited: Angiographic evaluation and coronary artery bypass surgery in a patient 21 years following bilateral internal mammary artery implantation. *Cath Cardiovasc Diagn* 1992; 25: 218–222.

Vineberg AM. The development of an anastomosis between the coronary vessels and a transplanted internal mammary artery. *Can Med Assoc* 1946; 55: 117–119.

Vineberg AM. Development of anastomosis between the coronary vessels and a transplanted internal mammary artery. *J Thorac Surg* 1949; 18: 839–850.

Vineberg AM. Clinical results. In *Myocardial Revascularization by Arterial/Ventricular Implants*, ed. A. M. Vineberg. Boston, Massachusetts, John Wright/PSG, 1982, p 330–331.

Vineberg AM, Niloff PH. The value of surgical treatment of coronary artery occlusion by implantation of the internal mammary artery into the ventricular myocardium. An experimental study. *Surg Gynecol Obstet* 1950; 91: 551–561.

Vineberg AM, Walker J. The surgical treatment of coronary artery disease by internal mammary artery implantation: report of 140 cases followed up to thirteen years. *Dis Chest* 1964; 45: 190–206.

Wearn JT, Mettier SR, Klump TG et al. The nature of the vascular communications between the coronary arteries and the chambers of the heart. *Am Heart J* 1933; 9: 143–164.

2

Historical Perspectives and Development of Transmyocardial Revascularization

Mary Cayton, R.N., B.S.N., P.A.

St. Luke's Medical Center Heart and
Lung Institute of Wisconsin
Laser Research Laboratory
Clement Zablocki Department of Veterans Affairs Medical Center
Milwaukee, Wisconsin

and

Mahmood Mirhoseini, M.D.

Department of Cardio-Thoracic Surgery
Medical College of Wisconsin
Department of Cardiovascular and Thoracic Surgery
St. Luke's Medical Center, Heart and
Lung Institute of Wisconsin
Laser Research Laboratory
Clement Zablocki Department of Veterans Affairs Medical Center
Milwaukee, Wisconsin

SUMMARY

Results of early clinical and experimental studies have provided the basis for work in transmyocardial laser revascularization (TMR).

It was hypothesized that channels created by a CO_2 laser would remain patent, perfuse ischemic myocardium (via myocardial sinusoids and collateral circulation), and improve myocardial function.

For patients who do not respond to traditional treatment modalities for coronary artery disease (bypass, PTCA, thrombolytic therapy), TMR may be an alternative treatment or may serve a role in combination with or as an adjunct to other treatments.

The first clinical studies of TMR combined with CABG were done in 1984 in Wisconsin, and improved left ventricular function was noted in patients at follow-up,

Myocardial Revascularization: Novel Percutaneous Approaches, Edited by George S. Abela.
ISBN 0-471-36166-6   Copyright © 2002 Wiley-Liss, Inc.

although actual contribution to perfusion and relief of ischemia cannot be determined with accuracy or certainty.

Methods used to evaluate the actual effects of TMR on myocardial perfusion and function have been difficult to quantify and subject to observer bias.

It was hypothesized that cine magnetic resonance (CMR) imaging would provide quantitative, objective, and state-of-the-art measurements for more precise monitoring of TMR effects.

When assessing laser results, wavelength, power density, thermal injury, laser tissue interactions, optimal spot size, and laser physics must be considered.

2.1. INTRODUCTION

Interest in the heart, its diseases, and how to treat them has fascinated physicians for centuries. Avicenna (1906 ed.) was one of the first to make a diagram of the circulatory system (Fig. 2-1). The *Canon of Medicine* is credited with the preservation of medical knowledge and the dissemination of that knowledge between East and West. Our current knowledge of the heart and its function is based on the foundations of western medicine as outlined by Vieussens (1706), Laennec (1824), Osler (1906), Harvey (1931), and many others. Despite this very early curiosity and fascination, methods to diagnose and treat diseases of the circulatory system have only evolved at a sophisticated level in the last 50 years.

In the twentieth century the incidence of coronary artery disease and its sequelae appears to have increased. Part of this observation is due to advances in diagnostic medicine in the twentieth century, increased life expectancy, and. in an aging population. an increase in the number of those with chronic illness. Negative lifestyle changes, increased stress, and other factors contribute to the significant increase in the number of patients with debilitating ischemic heart disease. To meet the challenge of relieving myocardial ischemia, investigators demonstrated vision and foresight in designing surgical techniques

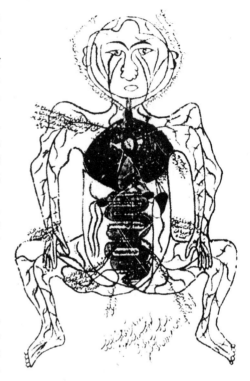

FIGURE 2-1. Illustration of the circulatory system from the *Canon of Medicine* by Avicenna, c930–1037. It is thought to be one of the earliest diagrams of the circulation and perhaps the earliest recognition of its complexity. Both eastern and western physicians relied on these early insights until the mid-seventeenth century.

to provide increased blood flow to compromised coronary artery circulation.

2.2. EARLY EXPERIMENTAL SURGICAL ATTEMPTS TO TREAT CORONARY ARTERY DISEASE

Experimental methods to treat myocardial ischemia have included boring channels by myocardial punch biopsy (Walter et al., 1971, 1973) insertion of T tubes that connected the left ventricular cavity to the myocardium (Massimo and Boffi, 1957), insertion of polyethylene tubes into the heart muscle (Goldman et al., 1956), and needle acupuncture (Sen et al., 1965; Venugopal et al., 1967). Although the methods differed in technique, the concept was the same. The hypothesis was that oxygen-rich blood from the left ventricular cavity could perfuse and nourish ischemic myocardium via the system of myocardial sinusoids and capillary circulation. The results of these various early studies were similar; the blood supply of the left ventricle could perfuse and nourish the myocardium through the alternative circulatory pathways. Initially, left ventricular function and contractility appeared to improve. However, in chronic studies, the initial encouraging results did not last. It is thought that that the injury caused by mechanical trauma, with the sequence of cell infiltration, fibrosis, and scarring, caused closure of the conduits or channels. The results of all of these early experimental studies were similar. The blood supply of the left ventricle would perfuse and nourish the myocardium through the alternative circulatory pathways in the acute setting, but this could not be sustained.

2.3. EARLY CLINICAL ATTEMPTS TO RELIEVE MYOCARDIAL ISCHEMIA BY SURGICAL METHODS

The first clinical attempts to relieve myocardial ischemia by surgical methods included sympathectomy and thyroidectomy (Coffey and Brown, 1922; Blumgart et al, 1933). These modalities were quickly abandoned because of significant systemic complications, side effects, and the realization that coronary ischemia was not relieved by the interventions. Other novel methods demonstrated the emerging understanding of the physiology of the heart. Beck (1933) attempted, with limited success, to introduce angiogenesis by performing myocardial poudrage and omentopexy to stimulate the formation of new myocardial blood vessels. Vineberg (1946) implanted the internal mammary artery directly into the left ventricle to take advantage of the blood-carrying capacity of the myocardial sinusoids. Implanting the mammary artery, and its branches, was successful in early experiments to relieve ischemia in approximately 44% of procedures and was later reported to be effective in 70–80%. Early positive results were sustainable. The results obtained by Vineberg were difficult to reproduce by others because technical considerations and experience were crucial to a good outcome.

2.4. RATIONALE FOR LASER REVASCULARIZATION

Results of these early experimental and clinical studies were the basis for our work in transmyocardial laser revascularization (TMR). We postulated that a major technical development, a new source of energy, the laser, could be used to revascularize the heart. The laser would be used to penetrate the myocardium from the epicardial surface through the endocardium by vaporization of tissue. The mechanical trauma of methods described by earlier investigators could be avoided. The laser would create conduits, or channels. Oxygenated blood of the left ventricle would flow to the ischemic muscle via myocardial sinusoids and alternative circulatory pathways. Maimon (1960) introduced the first operational laser, the ruby laser, in 1960. (Fig. 2-2) Introduction of the carbon dioxide (CO_2) laser (Patel, 1964) followed a few years later, in 1964.

Initial experimentation and studies to ascertain laser-tissue interactions with this exciting new tool took place at our institution as well as at a few other institutions around the world. We concluded that the CO_2 laser, at a wavelength of 10.6 μm, had the desirable properties for TMR. These very important properties included the ability to achieve high energy densities, penetration of tissue with little lateral damage, little thermal damage to adjacent tissue, vaporization of tissue, and a wavelength absorbed by water. The development of the articulated arm to deliver CO_2 laser energy, is a seldom-remarked, but exceedingly important, benchmark in developing medical laser therapies (Fig. 2-3).

Delivery of high-power laser energy with a high power density permitted penetration of the myocardial thickness within milliseconds. Power density [PD = watts × 100/(spot size)^2] determines the rate of tissue vaporization. At low power densities tissue penetration is

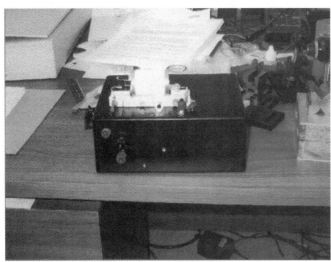

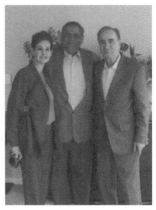

(B)

(A)

FIGURE 2-2. (A) Photograph of the first working laser. A ruby crystal is the active medium. The power supply and excitation mechanism are all contained in this small package. Photo taken in the laboratory of Dr. T. H. Maimon, Vancouver, BC., Canada. (B) T. H. Maimon, Ph.D., far right; Mahmood Mirhoseini, M.D.; center, and Kathleen Maimon, left. On May 15–16, 2000, scientists, physicians, family, and friends gathered, in Vancouver, BC, to honor Dr. Maimon on the 40th "ruby" anniversary of the invention of the laser.

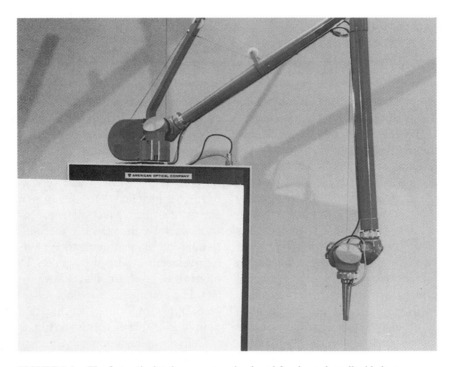

FIGURE 2-3. The first articulated arm system developed for the carbon dioxide laser by Herbert Bredermeir, Ph.D., and associates at American Optical Corporation. The articulated arm was fundamental in allowing the laser to be used for medical applications. Later, more streamlined, articulated arm delivery systems still employ the fundamental concepts used in this delivery system.

slow and damage to marginal or surrounding tissue can be substantial. Although this effect is desired at times, it is contraindicated for TMR. At high power densities the rate of tissue penetration is rapid and the effect on cells surrounding the area of penetration is minimal. Optimal values for surgically useful power densities depend on the nature of the tissue to be vaporized and the spot size of the laser beam. The volume of tissue to be removed will depend on the total beam power and the time of exposure to laser energy. In TMR rapid vaporization of tissues is desired. The CO_2 wavelength is absorbed by water; thus the blood in the left ventricular cavity stops the laser beam, minimizing the chances for damage to structures within the heart.

Our original hypothesis was that channels created by the CO_2 laser would remain patent, perfuse the ischemic myocardium via myocardial sinusoids and collateral circulation, and improve myocardial function. This original hypothesis was the basis for our original work and has been the foundation for our further scientific investigations.

2.5. RATIONALE FOR ALTERNATIVE CIRCULATORY PATHWAYS

Providing an alternative pathway to the coronary circulation was considered a physiological possibility because of the known structure of the heart muscle. Although this hypothesis has been disputed (Pifarrè et al., 1969) there is enough evidence to validate it. As well as being supported by scientific investigation, this thesis is supported by examples from nature. Naturally occurring connections between the heart muscle and ventricular chamber are present in the human heart. During periods of stress or vigorous exercise, as much as 20% of perfusion can occur through the intraventricular coronary connections. Pina et al. (1974, 1983) demonstrated arterio-luminal, veno-luminal, and arterio-thebesian connections with the left ventricle. Flow through these interconnecting vessels increased when a coronary artery was occluded. Early embryonic circulation to the

heart is through alternative pathways. Coronary arteries are not developed in early gestation. The developing heart is perfused through the blood supply of the left ventricle through arterio-luminal and arterio-thebesian connections. Perfusion of the heart in infants with congenital hypoplastic left ventricle is from the blood supply in the left ventricular cavity. In these infants the system of naturally occurring channels and myocardial sinusoids protects the thickened muscle. In the reptilian heart, the coronary artery system is vestigial; perfusion to the heart is from the left ventricular cavity through an intercommunicating system of sinusoids and collateral circulation (Fig. 2-4).

2.6. CENTURIES OF DEVELOPMENT LEADING TO FORTY YEARS OF EXPLOSIVE DEVELOPMENT

Those suffering from angina pectoris refractory to medical management, had few options before the late 1960s and early 1970s, when coronary artery surgery developed (Effler et al., 1965). Controversy, to an extreme degree, regarding coronary bypass existed well into the mid-1970s (Spencer, 1974). By the late and mid-1970s the technique was generally accepted, and by the 1980s it was widely available.

2.7. CURRENT STATUS OF THE TREATMENT OF CORONARY ARTERY DISEASE

There has been a significant increase in the number of options available to treat patients with coronary artery disease. These include improved techniques for coronary artery bypass surgery, minimally invasive surgical techniques, percutaneous balloon angioplasty, the ability to insert stents in a coronary artery, thrombolytic therapy, introduction of agents to promote angiogenesis, and an array of new medications to treat angina (see Chapters 14 and 15). Despite the number of increased options, there are patients who are not candidates for, or who do not respond

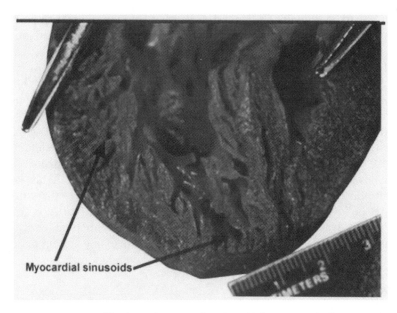

Myocardial sinusoids

FIGURE 2-4.   Reptilian heart demonstrating sinusoidal pattern typically seen in these species. (Courtesy of Dr. Daniel Burkhoff).

to, these treatment modalities. These include those with end-stage coronary artery disease, those who have undergone previous intervention with poor results, and those with diffuse small vessel disease. In carefully selected patients TMR may be an alternative treatment. TMR may also serve a role in combination with, or an as an adjunct to, coronary artery bypass. Although all of the patients who underwent combination procedures did well during the postoperative period, there is controversy regarding the results. Because bypass grafts were inserted at the time of the procedure, quantitative analysis of the results has been difficult.

2.8. BACKGROUND OF EXPERIMENTAL STUDIES

Investigational studies were conducted to determine the feasibility of TMR beginning in 1969. Our colleagues, Dr. Thomas Polyani et al. (personal communication 1996) of the American Optical Corporation (Framingham, MA) loaned us a prototype 450-W CO_2 laser to be used for experimental studies (Fig. 2-5). Early work indicated that focused laser

energy could produce ventricular fibrillation and other cardiac arrhythmia if the impact of laser energy occurred during the vulnerable period of the cardiac cycle. Therefore, we synchronized delivery of laser energy with the electrocardiogram, an easy task today, but sophisticated for that time. To overcome the difficulty of maintaining a constant focal distance, and to provide stability, on the beating heart we developed a focusing tip to attach to the articulated arm (Fig. 2-6). The tip could rest lightly on the surface of the heart. We found that we encountered fewer cardiac arrhythmias when using this tip as opposed to the rather small focusing tip that was standard with the articulated arm.

Several studies were conducted, and reported that showed that channels remained patent in the chronic setting with a canine model (Mirhoseini et al., 1977, 1982, 1996). Myocardial function was improved or preserved. Patent channels were demonstrated at intervals of sacrifice from 4 weeks to 2 years. At reoperation, patent channels could be observed macroscopically. Histopathologic studies confirmed this finding (Fig. 2-7). In one anecdotal case, 3 years after TMR, we

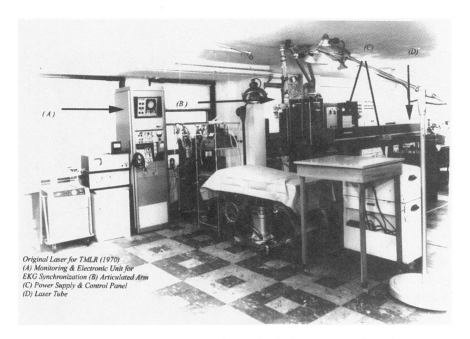

Original Laser for TMLR (1970)
(A) Monitoring & Electronic Unit for
EKG Synchronization (B) Articulated Arm
(C) Power Supply & Control Panel
(D) Laser Tube

FIGURE 2-5. The prototype CO_2 laser system used for the first TMR experimental studies beginning in late 1969 and early 1970. This system was the precursor to later clinical CO_2 laser systems. Photograph taken in our research laboratory in 1970.

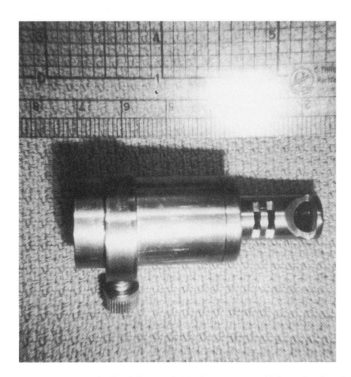

FIGURE 2-6. Focusing tip for delivery of CO_2 laser energy, which we developed to stabilize and provide a consistent focal length for delivery of laser energy to the beating heart. The focal length was 125 mm. It was vented to allow the products of vaporization to escape and to allow for visualization of the target area. The flat ring at the tip provided a platform for the tip to rest on the surface of the heart. The components could be disassembled for cleaning and sterilization.

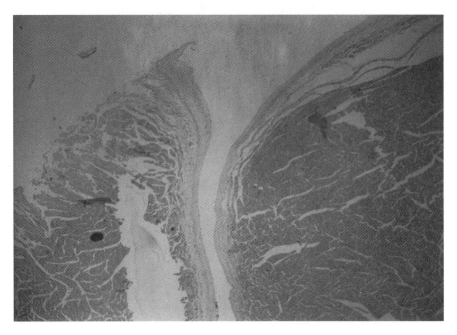

FIGURE 2-7. Photomicrograph of longitudinal section of myocardium 3 months after TMR in experimental canine studies. Channel is patent and endothelialized. (Hematoxylin and eosin stain, magnification ×100).

could induce profuse bleeding of the channels at reoperation. When the heart was exposed after removal of the pericardium, the surface of the heart, in the area that had been revascularized by laser, was dotted with little dark red, raised spots, reminiscent of a pattern of measles. When the surface of the raised spots was removed, we found that they acted like a thrombus "plug" occluding the laser channels. On removal of the plug, there was brisk bleeding from the previously created channels.

Results of the early experimental protocol suggested that clinical application of TMR was a feasible possibility. The drawback was that a high-power CO_2 laser system for clinical use was not available to the surgeon. Our laboratory experiments confirmed that the readily available clinical systems did not have sufficient power to penetrate the beating heart. In 1973, a protocol was developed to assess the possibility of performing TMR on the cooled and arrested heart in conjunction with coronary artery bypass (CABG). Penetration of the ventricular myocardium could be achieved on the still heart by using the lower-power clinical laser systems available at that time.

An experimental protocol designed to modify the high-energy technique was designed. With cardiopulmonary bypass, arresting and cooling the heart, and use of a low-power laser, channels could be made that were similar in size and configuration to those made with the high-power laser (Fig. 2-8). Myocardial wall tension was reduced during cardiac arrest, permitting easier penetration of laser energy. Cooling the tissue allowed heat to dissipate, protecting the muscle from thermal energy. Histologic studies confirmed that the channel configuration was similar to channels made by the high-power laser and patency rates in the experimental setting, were comparable. Until a clinical high-power laser system could be developed, further investigation of the procedure in conjunction with aortocoronary bypass seemed a reasonable alternative.

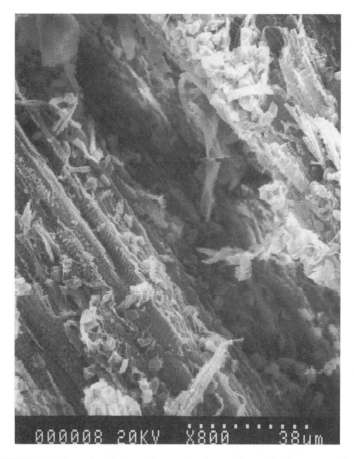

000008 20KV   X800   38μm

FIGURE 2-8.   Scanning electron micrograph of laser channel in the acute setting. Erythrocytes, leukocytes and platelets within the tract. No leukocytic infiltration or necrosis was detected around laser tract.

2.9. THE COMBINED PROCEDURE— FIRST CLINICAL STUDIES (1984)

A clinical protocol designed to assess the safety and possible beneficial outcome of TMR in conjunction with CABG was submitted to the Institutional Review Board (IRB) of St. Luke's Hospital (Milwaukee, WI). The initial submission of the protocol specified that the procedure could be performed on 12 carefully selected patients. The laser had not been used on the human heart before this experimental protocol. Therefore, several presentations of our research results, discussion of the physiologic possibility of alternate circulation pathways, and presentation of what was then known about laser tissue interactions were required. In December 1983, the protocol was approved. At that time the CO_2 laser, as a device, was approved by the U,S, Food and Drug Administration (FDA). There was no requirement for approval of specific operative procedures or techniques. After the series of 12 patients was performed without incident, a review of results from the initial series allowed us to continue to enroll patients in the protocol (Mirhoseini et al., 1988, 1990). An additional 23 patients were treated under the first clinical protocol. During the ensuing years, and as coronary artery surgery developed and presented ever more challenging procedures, it became apparent that there was an increase in the number of patients presenting who were refractory to current treatment methods.

2.10. METHODS AND MATERIALS— THE COMBINED PROCEDURE

Candidates for elective coronary artery bypass, who had an area of ischemia not suitable for graft insertion because of the severity of disease, were selected. Viable muscle in the area intended to be revascularized by laser was a requirement. Baseline and postoperative evaluation included thallium stress test, and echocardiogram. Follow-up studies included thallium stress test, EKG, echocardiogram and clinical evaluation at 3-month intervals for 12 months and then annually. Cardiac catheterization was done at baseline and at 1 year after the procedure, unless otherwise indicated.

The Sharplan 80–100 W CO_2 laser, model 743 (Tel Aviv, Israel) (Fig. 2-9) was used to create the channels. Using conventional coronary bypass techniques all distal coronary anastomoses were completed. During this time the body temperature was brought to 28°C. Before the last proximal anastomosis the heart was chilled to 4°C and the left ventricle was filled with cold cardioplegia solution. Channels ($n = 12–40$) were made in the selected areas. The final anastomosis was completed during the rewarming process. Bleeding from the channels stopped as the patient was weaned from cardiopulmonary bypass and heparinization was reversed.

2.11. RESULTS—THE COMBINED PROCEDURE

In the original series of patients the follow-up is 9–15 years. The results, in summary, showed an increased uptake of isotope during

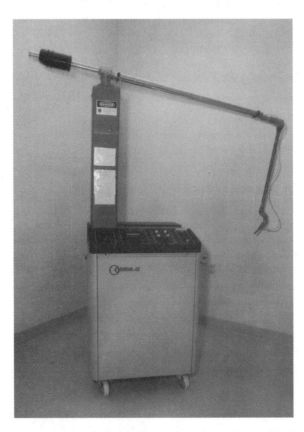

FIGURE 2-9.   Conventional CO_2 laser system used for medical applications in the 1970s. This unit was manufactured by Sharplan Laser Industries, Tel Aviv, Israel and was rated as being capable of delivering up to 80 W at the tissue.

thallium stress testing in the area revascularized by laser in 10 of 12 of the original patients (Fig. 2-10). The increased uptake, noted on initial postoperative evaluations, continued throughout the long-term follow-up. Improved left ventricular function, assessed by regional wall motion, left ventricular ejection fraction, and left ventricular end-diastolic pressure, was noted in all patients in the original series.

With the use of special imaging techniques, the laser channels could be visualized during left ventriculography. Cineangiography equipment (G.E. Medical Systems, Milwaukee, WI) with superior resolution filming on 1-in. film was used. Channels made in the inferior and lateral walls were more likely to be identified than those in the apex or anterior wall (Figs. 2-11 and 2-12). Coincidentally, we observed naturally occurring channels in a patient with coronary artery disease (Fig. 2-13). There were no operative deaths. One patient died of carcinoma of the colon at 1½ years after the combined procedure. A second patient died of carcinoma of the lung

at 4.5 years. An autopsy of this patient was obtained. On microscopic examination, there were numerous laser channels in both cross section and longitudinal section. Channels could be viewed grossly at autopsy. Microscopically, the channels were patent and endothelialized. Immunoperoxidase stain, *Ulex europaeus*, and factor VIII revealed neo-revascularization and angiogenesis surrounding the channels. The lining represented true endothelium (see Chapter 6 and Fig. 6-2).

2.12. CONTINUED STUDIES— THE COMBINED PROCEDURE

The second series of patients in the combined protocol (*n* = 54) have a follow-up ranging from 18 months to 6 years. Patient population included 35 men and 19 women with a mean age of 61 years. Screening for eligibility included myocardial perfusion studies, assessment of left ventricular function and wall motion, clinical evaluation, and assessment of angina class. Parsonnet scores as a predictor of operative risk, ranged from 8 to 25, with a

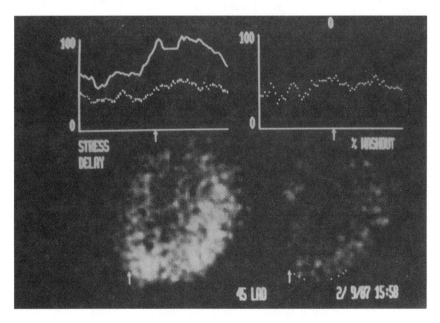

FIGURE 2-10. Thallium stress test 3 years after laser revascularization of the myocardium, combined with coronary artery bypass. Perfusion to the area where the laser was used is demonstrated by an increased pixel count. A bypass graft was not placed in this area (Mirhoseini and Cayton, 1990. Published with permission of Kluwer Academic Publishers.)

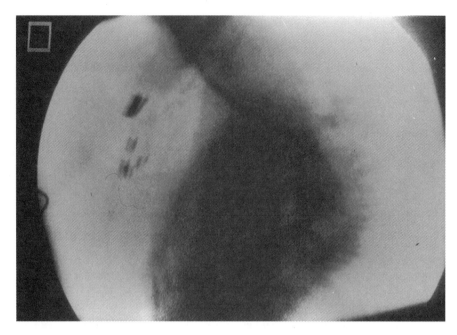

FIGURE 2-11.   Postoperative left ventriculogram, in systole, shows posterior wall laser channels beginning to fill. The image was acquired immediately after the injection of contrast agent.

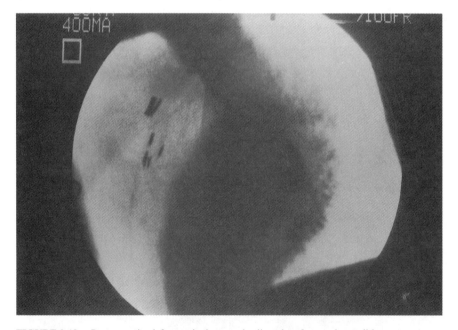

FIGURE 2-12.   Postoperative left ventriculogram, in diastole, of posterior wall laser channels. As the contrast agent empties from the ventricular cavity, the channels can be seen penetrating the thickness of the myocardial wall. Filled channels appear as "rays" projecting from the ventricular cavity (Mirhoseini and Cayton, 1990. Published with permission of Kluwer Academic Publishers.)

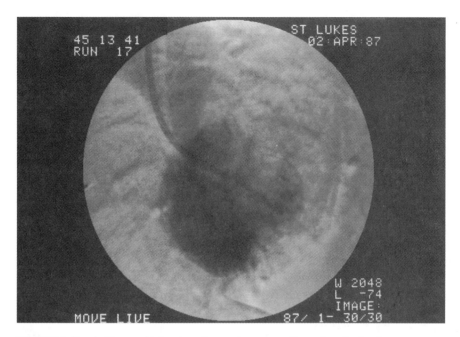

FIGURE 2-13. A 40-year-old female patient underwent cardiac catheterization for angina and suspected coronary artery disease. An incidental finding on left ventriculogram was the presence of naturally occurring channels emanating from the left ventricle.

mean score of 11.4. A score of 10–19 indicates operative risk of 6–19%. A mean of 2.6 grafts were inserted in addition to making the laser channels.

Angina class, classified by the Canadian Cardiovascular Society (CSS), was a mean of 3.11 preoperatively, 0.14 at 12 months, and 0.1 at 24 months. Perfusion and wall motion, assessed by a scoring system with higher numbers indicating increasing dysfunction and zero being normal, improved. Perfusion scores were a mean of 28.6 at baseline and a mean of 3 at 24 months. Wall motion scores were a mean of 15.3 at baseline and a mean of 4 at 24 months. Morbidity was 6% and included renal failure, postcardiotomy syndrome, and respiratory failure. Mortality was 2%.

2.13. DISCUSSION—THE COMBINED PROCEDURE

Although the actual contribution to perfusion and relief of ischemia by the laser channels in the combined procedure cannot be determined with accuracy or certainty, this investigation was important for many reasons. It demonstrated that the laser could safely be used on the human heart. It is important to remember that, at the time we sought approval for the initial clinical study from the IRB, the laser was used only intermittently for some gynecologic procedures, in ophthalmology, and occasionally in neurosurgery. Another infrequent surgical application was for bronchial carcinoma or treatment of vocal cord lesions.

The original study also demonstrated that the channels were patent and endothelialized and that the channels could be visualized by special left ventriculography techniques. An adjunctive treatment option for patients with diffuse disease or no target vessel was now a possibility, and the study suggested that development of a high-power laser system for use on the beating heart or for treatment by laser alone was a viable option.

2.14. TRANSMYOCARDIAL LASER REVASCULARIZATION ON THE BEATING HEART: TREATMENT OF END-STAGE CORONARY ARTERY DISEASE

More than 3,000 patients, world wide, with ischemic coronary artery disease have been treated by TMR to date. In the United States clinical trials to evaluate the safety and efficacy of transmyocardial laser revascularization, under the auspices of the FDA, were required. As a stand-alone procedure, clinical trials began in 1991. The first protocol approved by the FDA, initiated in 1991, was a nonrandomized study. From July of 1996 to August of 1998 a 1:1 randomized trial was conducted. In the randomized trials, one-half of the patients were randomized to continue on medical management and one-half of the patients underwent laser revascularization. Both studies were multicenter trials.

In our own series, 44 patients were enrolled in the nonrandomized trial and 54 in the randomized trial. An additional 20 patients were treated under other parts of the studies or under other protocols.

2.15. METHODS AND MATERIALS: TRANSMYOCARDIAL LASER REVASCULARIZATION ON THE BEATING HEART—NONRANDOMIZED AND RANDOMIZED PROTOCOLS

The patient population for the randomized and nonrandomized trials was essentially the same. Patients with ischemia and viable muscle refractory to medical management and not candidates for coronary artery bypass or percutaneous transluminal angioplasty were selected. Criteria for enrollment included patients with viable myocardium, reversible ischemia of the left ventricular free wall, a left ventricular ejection fraction of 20% or more, and CCS angina class III or IV. Only candidates for elective procedures were enrolled. Criteria for excluding a patient as a candidate for coronary bypass included lack of a target vessel, diffuse disease, and lack of a suitable conduit.

The patient clinical history and mean age for the two protocols were within a decimal point for each study, so they are reported together. Results are given by protocol. All patients were CSS angina class III or IV. Past history included a mean of 1.37 previous coronary artery bypass procedures and a mean of 1.69 previous percutaneous coronary angioplasties. Eighty-six percent had a history of myocardial infarction, thirty-six percent were diabetic, and thirty-two had a history of congestive heart failure. Men outnumbered women by 3:1. The age range was 39–85 years, with a mean age of 60 years for men and 63 years for women.

The procedure was performed through a left anterolateral thoracotomy. A high-power, 850-W peak power, CO_2 laser (PLC Medical Systems, Franklin, MA) was used, in continuous wave, to create channels from the epicardial surface of the left ventricle through the endocardium. Channel size was 0.9 mm. A range of energy from 32 J at 40 ms to 60 J at 75 ms was used. Power requirements were based on the thickness of the myocardium at the point of entry and the overall size of the heart. Energy was delivered in the refractory period of the cardiac cycle and was synchronized with the electrocardiogram. Penetration into the left ventricular cavity was confirmed by transesophageal echocardiogram (Fig. 2-14).

2.16. PATIENT EVALUATION— NONRANDOMIZED STUDY

Patient evaluation for the nonrandomized study, before entry in the protocol, included baseline clinical evaluation, cardiac catheterization, nuclear perfusion studies, and assessment of left ventricular function and wall motion. With the exception of cardiac catheterization, which was performed at 1 year after the procedure, follow-up studies including clinical evaluation, assessment of angina class, nuclear perfusion studies, and assessment of left ventricular function and wall motion were conducted at 3, 6, 9, and 12 months and then annually.

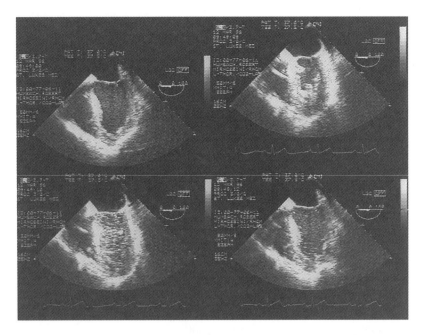

FIGURE 2-14. Transesophageal echocardiogram confirming laser penetration into the ventricular cavity when a laser channel is made. Photograph in the upper left shows the ventricle before laser penetration. The upper right illustrates the moment of penetration by laser energy. The photograph at the lower left shows the products of vaporization being dissipated, and the lower right indicates that the "bubbles" or products of vaporization have cleared the ventricular cavity. The process takes less than 1 s.

2.17. RESULTS—NONRANDOMIZED STUDY

Follow-up in the nonrandomized trial ranges from 4 to 7 years. CSS angina class ( ) was a mean of 3.7 at baseline and a mean of 1.0 at 12 months. Perfusion and wall motion were evaluated by using a scoring system with 0 as the normal score. Perfusion scores were a mean of 29 at baseline, a mean of 8 at 12 months, a mean of 3 at 24 months, and a mean of 1.3 at 36 months. It is interesting to note that regional perfusion improved in the septum, although no channels were made in this area. The mean score for the septum was 4 at baseline, 2 at 12 months, and 1 at 24 months. Wall motion scores were a mean of 18 at baseline, a mean of 3 at 12 months, and a mean of 1 at 24 months. Perioperative mortality was 8%; causes of death included cardiac arrhythmia and, in one instance, hypovolemia, which initiated a spiraling sequence of events that became impossible to reverse in the patient with a borderline ejection fraction of 20% before surgery and a long history of cardiac events. There were no intraoperative deaths. Late mortality was 13%. Causes of death were "silent death," probably resulting from arrhythmia, and noncardiac causes including carcinoma, kidney disease, and complications of Alzheimer disease.

2.18. PATIENT EVALUATION—RANDOMIZED STUDY

In the randomized study, assessment of each patient was performed at baseline. Follow-up studies were performed at 3, 6, 9, and 12 months after treatment by TMR or randomization to medical management. Those who were enrolled in the protocol continue to be evaluated and followed on an annual basis.

Clinical evaluation included history of cardiovascular disease, risk factors, review of cardiac medications, evaluation of comorbidity, and evaluation of angina class according to CSS guidelines. Angina class was evaluated in the clinic and by an independent observer. A quality of life questionnaire (SF-36) and a Seattle Angina Questionnaire (SAQ) were administered to each patient.

Tests included thallium-201 single-photon emission computed tomography (SPECT) at rest and with exercise using dipyridamole at 0.56 mg/kg body weight with 4-h redistribution studies. All tests were performed and images processed in a standardized fashion. Results were evaluated by the nuclear cardiology team at our institution and independently by a core laboratory nuclear cardiologist, who was unaware of patient identity, treatment assignment, and scan date. Multigated acquisition studies (MUGA) were used to evaluate regional wall motion, cardiac function, and ejection fraction. Other tests included echocardiogram, pulmonary function studies, and evaluation for coagulopathy. Those with marginal pulmonary function studies and probability of respirator dependence were determined not eligible, as were those with bleeding disorders.

Those who met the enrollment criteria were randomized, by computer selection, to either medical management or TMR. At our institution, 38 patients were randomized to TMR and 6 to medical management. We participated in the multicenter trial. In the entire multicenter trial there were 192 patients enrolled, with 91 assigned to TMR and 101 assigned to continued medical management.

Assessment of surgical risk in the group randomized to TMR in our study was performed using the Parsonnet scoring system. The mean score was 12.27 (range 3–27), indicating a moderate operative risk between 6% and 17%.

2.19. RESULTS— RANDOMIZED STUDY

Angina class before treatment was a mean of 3.6. At 3 months the mean angina class in our series was 0.5, and at 1 year the mean angina class was 1.0 in the treatment group. Of the patients randomized to medical management, angina class remained the same or was worse in five of six patients at all follow-up intervals. One patient noted moderate improvement after a change in cardiac medications. The mean ejection fraction for those treated by TMR was 55% at baseline, with a range of 22–69%. The mean remained relatively unchanged during the follow-up period; however the range was 30–65% at 6 months; and 40–65% at 12 months. Results of the perfusion scan (SPECT) in the multicenter results have been tabulated. The mean number of segments with reversible ischemia in the TMR group was 7.1 ± 3.7 at baseline. There was an average decrease of 1.5 segments at 3 months, 0.8 segments at 6 months, and 1.4 segments at 12 months in the TMR group. In the medical management group, the mean number of segments with reversible ischemia at baseline was 6.8 ± 3.3. The average number of segments with reversible ischemia increased by 0.8 at 3 months, 0.8 at 6 months, and 1.3 at 12 months. There was not a statistically significant difference in the number of fixed defects in either group at the evaluation intervals. Responses to the SF-36 questionnaire indicated an increase in the quality of life. Perioperative mortality for the TMR group in our series was 3%. There were no operative deaths. Late mortality was 8%. There was no mortality in the medical management group in our series.

2.20. ANALYSIS OF MYOCARDIAL FUNCTION AND PERFUSION OF ISCHEMIC MYOCARDIUM BY CINE RESONANCE IMAGING

Methods to accurately evaluate the effect of TMR on myocardial perfusion and function have been elusive, hard to quantify, and subject to observer bias. The results and mechanisms of action have also been controversial. Although there are a number of sophisticated tests available to globally identify regional wall motion and perfusion, the resolution of most standard testing is about

1 cm. This renders it impossible to identify small or subtle changes in myocardial function and perfusion; nor does it allow evaluation of changes in the microcirculation. There is much controversy as to whether the improvement in angina class and relief of symptoms after TMR correlates with changes in myocardial hemodynamics or if it is caused by an interruption in neurotransmitters. Controversy also exists over the role that channel patency plays in relation to the outcome of TMR. Intuitively, and in our experience, channel patency is important. The effect of TMR on adjacent and remote nonischemic myocardium has not been addressed before our study using magnetic resonance imaging techniques.

Over the last several years, magnetic resonance imaging has become an important clinical tool to assess cardiac morphology and function. Cine magnetic resonance imagining (CMR) is noninvasive and has high temporal and spatial resolution. We hypothesized that CMR would provide quantitative, objective, state-of-the-art measurements for precisely monitoring the effects of TMR. In collaboration with our colleagues, Dr. Norbert Wilke

and Dr. Michael Jerosch-Herold et al. at the University of Minnesota, we performed an acute study to test the hypothesis. From this study we concluded that TMR improved left ventricular function and myocardial blood flow and appeared to protect the myocardium from the effects of acute ischemia (Tables 2-1 and 2-2). We also concluded that quantitative CMR is extremely useful to monitor left ventricular function and perfusion before and after TMR. On the basis of our acute findings we concluded that a chronic study was warranted and could provide valuable information regarding the mechanisms involved in TMR (Mills et al., 1994; Quillen et al., 1992; Wilke et al., 1994, 1995). For the chronic study we attempted to replicate chronic ischemia as seen in our human subjects. It is known that the effects of intervention can be quite different in the acute versus the chronic setting.

2.21. MATERIALS AND METHODS

The study was performed in compliance with all standards of research in animal use and was approved by the hospital committee. A

TABLE 2-1. Acute Myocardial Blood Flow Studies in Swine After TMR

Parameter	Group I Control (n = 5)	Group II LCx Ligation (n = 6)	Group III LCx Ligation & TMR (n = 10)
MBF	1.5 ± 0.8	0.1 ± 0.1*	0.4 ± 0.3*
EN	1.6 ± 0.8	0.2 ± 0.3	1.0 ± 0.5
EN/EP	1.1 ± 0.2	0.2 ± 0**	2.1 ± 1.3**

MBF = myocardial blood flow; EN = endocardial blood flow; EP = epicardial blood flow.
*$P < 0.02$; **$P < 0.05$.

TABLE 2-2. Left Ventricular Function by CMR

Parameter	Group I Control	Group II LCx Ligation	Group III LCx Ligation & TMR
EF%	58 ± 8	35 ± 8	46 ± 1
ESV (ml)	16 ± 6	37 ± 11	28 ± 9
EDV (ml)	39 ± 12	56 ± 13	49 ± 1
PFR (l/mn)	5 ± 2	3 ± 1	4 ± 2

EF = ejection fraction; ESV = end-systolic volume; EDV = end-diastolic volume; PFR = peak filling pressure.

total of 12 swine underwent baseline magnetic resonance imaging studies to measure myocardial function and perfusion. The animals were then subjected to a technique to induce chronic ischemia. Hollow bead embolization, using a custom-made hollow Teflon bead that was introduced fluoroscopically into the lumen of the left circumflex (LCx) coronary artery, was performed. The bead was introduced through a right carotid artery access using an 8-Fr catheter (Bard-USCI, Bellerica, MA). This resulted in gradual occlusion of the LCx. After embolization the animals were then randomized to a control group ($n = 6$) or a TMR treatment group (n = 6). Follow-up cineangiography was done to confirm coronary artery stenosis (Fig. 2-15). The treatment group underwent CMR 1 week after embolization. At 8 weeks after embolization, both groups underwent CMR. Microspheres were injected to determine myocardial blood flow. Image acquisition was obtained, in the lateral decubitus position, under a phased-array body coil in a 1.5-T scanner (Siemens Vision, Germany). Scout images determined the position of the heart. Perfusion images were obtained at rest and during hyperemia. Hyperemia was induced using adenosine (Adenoscan, Fujisawa, IL) titrated to a

maximum dose of 140 µg/kg/min. Perfusion was determined by three short-axis slices through the LV using a single-shot saturation-recovery FLASH sequence with linear k-spacing. A slice thickness of 10-mm spatial resolution and a temporal resolution of 1/image/beat/slice was used. Forty images/slice were acquired with a spatial resolution of 2–3 mm. Gadolinium-DTPA (Mangevist, Schering AG, Germany) at 0.03 mmol/kg was injected for cine imaging. Images were acquired at rest and during dobutamine-induced stress titrated to the target heart rate. Image analysis was blinded. Sets of data (3D) were obtained for stroke volume (SV, ml), cardiac output (CO, ml/min), and ejection fraction (EF, %). Regional wall thickening (RWT, mm) was determined in the septal or remote myocardium and in the lateral or target region. The ischemic area was defined as the area with a wall thickening two standard deviations (SD) below the thickening in the lateral wall of a healthy control group (Fig. 2-16, A and B) (Wilke et al., 1997; Jerosch-Herold et al., 1998).

Perfusion studies were analyzed by applying endocardial and epicardial contours on the image with brightest contrast enhancement in the left ventricle. An automated segmentation algorithm matched the

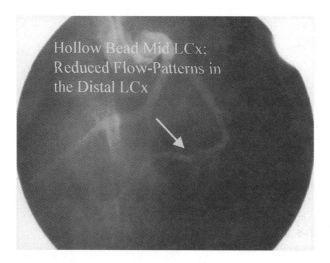

FIGURE 2-15. Angiogram 1 week after hollow bead embolization of the LCx in a swine model. There is reduced distal flow. All animals showed delayed antegrade flow. No collateral circulation could be detected by angiography.

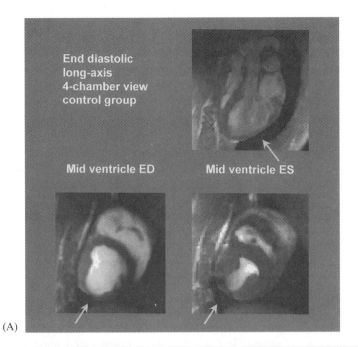

End diastolic
long-axis
4-chamber view
control group

Mid ventricle ED   Mid ventricle ES

(A)

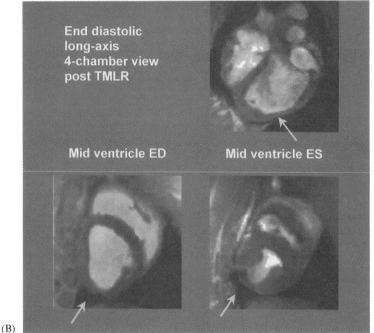

End diastolic
long-axis
4-chamber view
post TMLR

Mid ventricle ED   Mid ventricle ES

(B)

Control (9 wks)   **TMLR - Treated (9 wks)**

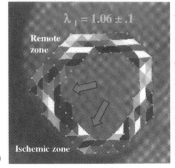

$\lambda_1 = 1.06 \pm .1$

Remote zone

Ischemic zone

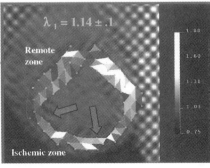

$\lambda_1 = 1.14 \pm .1$

Remote zone

Ischemic zone

(C)

FIGURE 2-16. (A) Example of cine magnetic resonance (CMR) in control swine group demonstrating a nonthickening apical and anterolateral wall. (B) Example of CMR in TMR = treated group showing preserved apical and anterolateral wall thickening. (C) Magnetic resonance tagging technique produced markers or grids. Improvement in the TMR-treated group is displayed by an overall brighter appearance. The TMR-treated group shows a vivid improvement pattern exhibited by the disappearance of black triangles and an increase in the number of gray and light gray triangles.

contours to the remaining images of the slice (Fig. 2-16C).

Myocardial blood flow (MBF, ml/min/g) was determined with radiolabeled microspheres, which were injected at rest and during stress (Fig. 2-17). The amount of necrotic tissue was determined by triphenyltetrazolium chloride (TTC) staining. Necrosis was evaluated by planimetry of the unstained myocardium. Slices were oriented and matched to the MRI.

2.22. RESULTS

At 8 weeks CO and SV were significantly reduced in the control group compared with

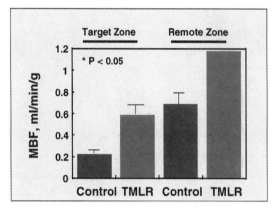

FIGURE 2-17. Myocardial blood flow (MBF in ml/min/g) was determined using radiolabeled microspheres injected at rest and during stress. Target zone was more perfused with TMR vs. control ($P < 0.05$).

the treated group (Table 2-3). There was little difference in RWT in the immediate postoperative period. Thickening in the lateral wall of the treated group improved significantly over 8 weeks. Also, the remote area showed a significantly higher thickening (Table 2-4) compared with the control group.

The baseline values of regional myocardial perfusion, after hollow bead embolization, were markedly reduced in the lateral wall in both groups. The resting and stress perfusion in the lateral wall decreased significantly over 8 weeks in the nontreated group compared with the treated group.

Blood flow data determined by radiolabeled microspheres were in correlation with the imaging data. MBF was significantly higher in the lateral wall in the treated versus. the nontreated group. Stress did not increase MBF in the untreated region (Table 2-5).

TTC staining revealed subendocardial necrosis within the target area in both groups. The percentage of LV necrosis was significantly higher in the nontreated group (6.6 ± 1.6% vs. 3.7 ± 1.5%; $P < 0.01$).

The conclusion reached was that TMR is beneficial in preserving myocardial function and perfusion, at rest and during stress, in chronic ischemia. Myocardial perfusion at rest and during hyperemia was preserved in the TMR-treated group in the distribution of the LCx and remote myocardium. There was improved regional global left ventricular function after TMR. No treatment resulted in deterioration of perfusion and lack of

TABLE 2-3.   Hemodynamic Parameters After LCx Embolization

Parameter	Control		TMR	
	Baseline	8 Weeks	Baseline	8 Weeks
AoP (mmHg)	90 ± 6	92 ± 6	83 ± 8	97 ± 20
EDP (mmHg)	15 ± 7	13 ± 5	12 ± 7	13 ± 2
EDV (ml/kg)	2.5 ± 0.5	1.8 ± 0.3	2.6 ± 0.4	2.3 ± 0.4
ESV (ml/kg)	1.1 ± 0.4	0.8 ± 0.2†	1.1 ± 0.4	1.1 ± 0.4
SV (ml/kg)	1.4 ± 0.3	0.9 ± 0.2§	1.4 ± 0.2	1.3 ± 0.2
CO (ml/kg/min)	158 ± 20§	73 ± 18§	116 ± 23	118 ± 12
EF	56 ± 10	55 ± 6	56 ± 9	55 ± 9

AoP = mean aortic pressure; EDP = end-diastolic pressure; EDV = end-diastolic volume; SV = stroke volume; CO = cardiac output; EF = ejection fraction. §$P < 0.01$ between groups; †$P < 0.05$ between groups.

TABLE 2-4. **Regional Myocardial Thickening by CMR**

Group	LCx Distribution	Baseline		8 Weeks	
		Rest	Stress	Rest	Stress
TMR		0.7 ± 0.3	2.4 ± 0.8*	3.7 ± 1.9‡	4.3 ± 1.7
Control		0.5 ± 0.6	2.4 ± 1.5*	0.5 ± 2.2‡	2.5 ± 1.4
	Remote Myocardium				
TMR		4.9 ± 0.9†	5.1 ± 7†	5.7 ± 1.0	5.2 ± 1.5
Control		4.07 ± 0.7†	5.1 ± 3†	3.7 ± 1.2‡†	4.7 ± 2.5

*$P < 0.02$ compared with rest; †$P < 0.03$ between remote and target region; ‡$P < 0.05$ between groups during follow-up.

TABLE 2-5. **CMR Derived Myocardial Perfusion at Rest and Hyperemia**

LCx Distribution: Group	Baseline			8 Weeks		
	Rest	Hyperemia	PR	Rest	Hyperemia	PR
TMLR	0.7 ± 0.3	11 ± 0.5	1.5 ± 0.4	1.0 ± 0.3	1.3 ± 0.3*	1.4 ± 0.4
Control	0.9 ± 0.3	1.3 ± 0.3	1.6 ± 0.5	0.3 ± 0.1‡	0.5 ± 0.2‡	1.9 ± 0.6
Remote Myocardium:						
TMLR	1.4 ± 0.4†	1.8 ± 0.3*†	1.3 ± 0.2	1.3 ± 0.2	1.9 ± 0.5*	1.5 ± 0.3
Control	1.6 ± 0.2†	1.8 ± 0.2†	1.2 ± 0.1	0.9 ± 0.2†‡	1.5 ± 0.3*†	1.8 ± 0.8

PR = perfusion reserve. *$P < 0.05$ compared with rest; †$P < 0.05$ between regions; ‡$P < 0.02$ between groups during follow-up.

improvement in function. There was more necrotic tissue on TTC staining in the non-treated group. We concluded that CMR is an effective, noninvasive, quantitative method to evaluate patients before and after TMR. One of the great advantages of the method is that it is independent of observer bias.

2.23. DISCUSSION

The clinical data, which are accumulating, as well as the results from experimental studies, may provide answers to some of the fundamental questions that still must be addressed. In-depth explanations of the physiologic mechanisms and technical parameters are still needed. There are many questions to be answered regarding optimal channel size, optimal channel number, channel geometry, and channel patency.

Present systems approved for clinical use need modification. The prototype laser we used in our original experiments was supe-

rior to systems currently available, although the currently approved systems are the only lasers approved for performing the procedure in the United States. Consideration of power density, thermal injury, laser-tissue interactions, optimal spot size, and laser physics must be factored in when assessing results.

There are several parameters we consider extremely important to the long-term success of this procedure. The first is that channel patency should not be ignored as a basic premise. Our goal has always been to create a channel that would remain patent. It has been postulated that the injury caused by creating channels with the Ho: YAG, in which the channels close very early, causes neorevascularization, although the channels are closed. It seems intuitive to believe that channels that remain patent and contribute to angiogenesis would be superior to channels that close. The very early studies to create alternative pathways, which evaluated myocardial revascularization by mechanical methods, failed to provide protection in the chronic phase because of channel closure. The results of our early experimental studies and of the first clinical investigation in the combined procedure support striving for channel patency.

It has been postulated that early closure of the channels is not important and that the laser wavelength is not a significant consideration. It remains our view that the laser wavelength, and its role in tissue interaction, is an extremely important consideration. As in any discipline, a thorough understanding of the equipment, the advantages and disadvantages, and the available alternatives are important to the outcome of the procedure. The current systems available for TMR are the CO_2, Ho:YAG, and excimer. The properties of each system and their advantages and disadvantages are outlined in Tables 2-6 and 2-7. There is a definite need for synchronization of laser energy with the ECG in all laser systems. Arrhythmias caused by the CO_2 laser compared with the Ho:YAG laser are provocative.

An attractive feature, and a reason for the recent enthusiasm, for both the Ho:YAG and

TABLE 2-6.   Major Characteristics of Commonly Used Clinical Laser Systems

Laser	Advantages	Disadvantages	To Be Determined
CO_2 "Heart Laser" 850 W	Penetration of Beating Heart TMLR alone or Combined Procedures Patency Approved System (PMA)	Costly System Costly Disposable Materials Huge, Noisy System	Thermal Injury Long Term TMLR vs. other treatments
CO_2 Low Power	Minimal Thermal Injury Comparative Low Cost Small, Quiet Systems Minimal Disposables (Drape)	w/CABG Only Articulated Arm Not Approved by FDA	Histology? Early Studies Comparable
HO:YAG	Fiberoptic Delivery System Reasonable Cost Percutaneous Or Intraoperative Delivery Approved System	Thermal and Acoustic Injury Expensive Disposables	Early Channel Closure Long Term Effectiveness Is percutaneous advantageous?
Excimer	Fiberoptic Delivery Beating Heart Or w/CABG Approved System	Expensive Systems Expensive Disposables	Thermal Injury? Channel Patency Long Term Effectiveness

TABLE 2-7.   TMR Experiences With Various Commercial Laser Systems*

Laser	Wavelength	Watts	Spot size/mm	Patency	Setting
AO, Inc., CO_2	10.6 μm	450	1.2	5 years Confirmed	Experimental
Sharplan, Inc., CO_2	10.6 μm	80	1.0	4.5 years Confirmed	Clinical & Experimental
PLC, Inc., CO_2	10.6 μm	800	0.9	2 months Confirmed	Clinical & Experimental
Surgilase, Inc.	10.6 μm	100	0.32	Unknown	Clinical
Ho:YAG	2.1 μm	30	1.2	2 months	Experimental
Er:YAG	1.6 μm			N/A—Acute	Experimental
Excimer				2 days	Experimental

* Experience of Dr. M. Mirhoseini and M. Cayton.

excimer laser systems for TMR is the fiberoptic delivery system that allows percutaneous
delivery of laser energy. Current technology
does not support fiberoptic delivery of the
CO_2 wavelength. There are, however limiting
factors. Navigating the catheter to the endocardial site of ischemia can be difficult; this
has been partially solved by electromechanical imaging. There is also difficulty in gauging
the depth of penetration. The risk of perforation of the epicardium in the closed chest
is high. It is known that the channels made
by the Ho:YAG and excimer wavelengths
close because of thermal injury. Percutaneous TMR remains a work in progress.

At 5-year follow-up 73% of patients treated
by TMR are alive and relatively free of debilitating symptoms. Twenty-five percent of
patients are completely free of angina. One
has to take into consideration that the
patients in these studies suffered from
end-stage coronary artery disease and that,
because they were not candidates for other
intervention, the rate of angina would have
been higher if the patient survived, because of
progression of disease. There are no studies
on which to base a comparison; in the randomized studies the numbers are too small,
and follow-up is too short, to suggest a
outcome for nontreated patients.

Our experience has shown that deaths from
cardiac causes occur within the first year after
the procedure; deaths that occur in subsequent years are likely be from causes other
than cardiac and often cannot be discerned at
the time of evaluation.

In the first year after TMR sudden death
syndrome, or silent cardiac death, is of
concern. This is a sudden and unexpected
death in asymptomatic patients. A question
that presents is, if pain as a protective mechanism is eliminated, is the myocardium
stressed beyond its limits because the patient
experiences no pain? The probable cause of
sudden death syndrome is arrhythmia,
although it could also be attributed to
myocardial infarction. It may be prudent to
have electrophysiology studies conducted on
all patients undergoing TMR before discharge form the hospital or at least within the

first 3 months after surgery. A cardiac defib-
rillator can be implanted if warranted. This
may prevent a significant number of silent
deaths.

The outcomes of TMR versus. medical
management must be considered when rec-
ommending surgical treatment to patients
with end-stage ischemic heart disease refractory to medical management. The goals of
treatment are improvement in perfusion to
the ischemic areas, creation of patent channels, preservation (improvement) of function,
and improvement in cardiac performance. The
principle of the four Ps of TMR, perfusion, patency, preservation (of function), and
performance is central.

An advantage of TMR is that it offers
a treatment modality to patients with end-
stage coronary artery disease that is another
alternative to medical management. From
a surgical standpoint, the advantages and
disadvantages are outlined in Table 2-6. The
potential complications of TMR are rupture
of chordae tendineae, which has been unoffi-
cially reported, perforation of other structures, complications of surgery, and laser
hazards.

A subset of patients who can be treated are
those who have undergone orthoptic heart
transplantation and subsequently developed
progressive coronary artery disease. In one of
four patients we treated angina was described
as a component of their disease, although it
is unusual for patients to experience angina
after transplantation. To date we have treated
four patients after heart transplantation with
good results in three of four patients.

2.24. CONCLUSIONS

There are significant numbers of patients with
end-stage coronary artery disease who may
benefit from TMR. Methods of diagnosis and
precise evaluation of results, in addition
to conventional methods, should consider
CMR. Current clinical studies and experience
support this hypothesis. In patients with
end-stage coronary artery disease refractory
to medical management and other treatment
options, TMR may be a viable option.

References

Avicenna A. *Canon de Medicina* (936–1037). 1906; 53.

Beck CS. The development of a new blood supply to the heart by operation. *Ann Surg* 1933; 102: 801–813.

Blungart HL, Risemean JEF, Davis D et al. Congestive heart failure and angina pectoris. The therapeutic effect of thyroidectomy on patients without clinical and pathologic evidence of thyroid toxicity. *Arch Int Med* 1933; 51: 866–877.

Coffey WB, Brown PK. Surgical treatment of angina pectoris. *Arch Int Med* 1923; 31: 200–220.

Effler DB, Sones FM, Favaloro R et al. Coronary endarterotomy with patch-graft reconstruction: clinical experience with 34 cases. *Ann Surg* 1965; 162: 590–601.

Goldman A, Greenstone SM, Preuss FS et al. Experimental methods for producing a collateral circulation to the heart directly from the left ventricle. *J Thorac Surg* 1956; 31: 364–373.

Harvey W. *Excercitatio Anatomica de Motu Cordis et Sanguinis in Animalibus* (1628). Leake CD. Springfield, IL, Charles C. Thomas, 1931.

Jerosch-Herold M, Wilke N, Stillman AE. Magnetic resonance quantification of the myocardial perfusion reserve with a Fermi function model for constraint deconvolution. *Med phys* 1998; 25: 73–84.

Laennec RTH. *On Mediate Auscultation* (1819). Freed, Michael. London, T and G Underwood, 1824.

Maimon TH. Stimulated optical radiation in ruby. *Nature* 1960; 187: 493–494.

Massimo C, Boffi L. Myocardial revascularization by a new method of carrying blood directly from the left ventricular cavity into the coronary circulation. *J Thorac-Cardiovasc Surg* 1957; 34: 257–264.

Mills I, Fallon JT, Wrenn D. Adaptive responses of coronary circulation and myocardium to chronic reduction in perfusion pressure and flow. *Am J Physiol* 1994; 266: H447–H457.

Mirhoseini M. In *Second Henry Ford Hospital International Symposium on Cardiac Surgery*, edited by Davila, JC. New York: Appleton Century Crofts, 1997.

Mirhoseini M, Muckerheide M, Cayton MM. Transventricular revascularization by laser. *Lasers Surg Med* 1982; 2: 187–198.

Mirhoseini M, Shelgikar S, Cayton MM. Clinical and histological evaluation of laser myocardial revascularization. *J Clin Med Surg* 1990; 8: 73–78.

Mirhoseini M, Cayton MM. Revascularization of the heart by laser. *J Microsurg* 1996; 2: 253–260.

Mirhoseini M, Shelgikar S, Cayton MM. New concepts in revascularization of the myocardium. *Ann Thorac Surg* 1988; 45: 415–420.

Osler SW. *The Growth of Truth as Illustrated in the Discovery of the Circulation of the Blood*. London, 1906.

Patel CKN. Continuous wave laser action on vibrational-rotational-transitions of CO_2 *Phys Rev* 1964; 136: A1187–A1193.

Pifarrè R, Jasuja ML, Lynch RD et al. Myocardial revascularization by transmyocardial acupuncture. A physiologic impossibility. *J Thorac Cardiovasc Surg* 1969; 58: 424–431.

Pina JA. Injection-corrosion-fluorescence in the study of human coronary arterial anastomoses. *Acta Anat (Basel)* 1974; 90: 481–488.

Pina JA. General and current morphological aspects of microvascularization. *Acta Med Port* 1983; 4: 433–436.

Polyani TG, Bredemeirer HC, David TW. A CO_2 laser for surgical research. *Med Biol Eng Comp* 1996; 8: 541–548.

Quillen JE, Harrison DG. Vasomotor properties of porcine endocardial and epicardial microvessels. *Am J Physiol* 1992; 262: H1143–H1148.

Sen PK, Udwadia TE, Kinare SG et al. Transmyocardial acupuncture. A new approach to myocardial revascularization. *J Thorac Cardiovasc Surg* 1965; 50: 181–189.

Spencer FC. Acquired heart disease. In *Principles of Surgery*, second edition, edited by Schwartz, Seymour I, Lillehei RC, Thomas SG, Spencer FC, Storer EH., New York: McGraw-Hill, 1974.

Venugopal P, Dutta S, Chitamber I. Evaluation of effectiveness of transmyocardial acupuncture after ligation of anterior descending artery in mongrel dogs, 1967.

Vieussens R. *Nouvelles descourverts sur le coeur*. 1706.

Vineberg AM. Development of an anastomosis in the coronary vessels and a transplanted internal mammary artery. *Can Med Assoc J* 1946; 55: 117–119.

Walter P, Hundeshagen H, Borst HG. Treatment of acute myocardial infarction by transmural blood supply from the ventricular cavity. *Eur Surg Res* 1971; 3: 130–138.

Walter P, Zazvorka F, Hundeshagen H et al. Experimental evaluation of transmural puncture as a treatment of acute myocardial infarction. *Bull Soc Int Chir* 1973; 32: 3–11.

Wilke N, Jerosch-Herold M, Stillman AE et al. Concepts of myocardial perfusion imaging in magnetic resonance imaging. *Magn Reson Q* 1994; 10: 249–286.

Wilke N, Jerosch-Herold M, Wang Y. Myocardial perfusion reserve: assessment with multisection, quantitative, first-pass MR imaging. *Radiology* 1997; 204: 373–384.

Wilke N, Kroll K, Merkle H et al. Regional myocardial blood volume and flow: first-pass MR imaging with polylysine-Gd-DTPA. *J Magn Reson Imaging* 1995; 5: 227–237.

3

Clinical Efficacy and Experience with Transmyocardial Laser Revascularization (TMR)

Keith A. Horvath, M.D.

Northwestern University Medical School
Chicago, Illinois

SUMMARY

Four randomized studies have recently shown TMR to provide significant symptomatic improvement compared with maximal medical therapy.

All the studies reported low perioperative mortality rates, as well as significant symptomatic improvement with patients treated by laser. However, postoperative perfusion scans demonstrated differing results.

To evaluate the results of the four studies, it is important to determine whether patients selected are the same among all studies. For example, in one study there were fewer patients with angina class IV, resulting in a less dramatic success rate.

An advantage to PMR trials over TMR trials is the ability to perform a double-blind randomized placebo-controlled trial because the catheter may be placed against the subendocardium and the laser not fired.

Trials have shown conflicting results with PMR. These may be related to differences in the catheter systems and laser wavelengths used. In both the CO_2 randomized trials there was demonstrable perfusion benefit, whereas PMR has yet to be demonstrated.

Because of the improvement in PMR placebo groups, it may be that the placebo effect is a mechanism in surgical TMR as well; however, long-term benefits with CO_2 lasers argue against this. A better understanding of how TMR does achieve its effects should be elucidated.

3.1. INTRODUCTION

Before the advent of coronary artery bypass grafting (CABG) or percutaneous transluminal coronary angioplasty (PTCA), attempts were made to revascularize the heart by direct perfusion. These were first described by Beck in 1935, who through a number of means achieved at least superficial angiogenesis, primarily as a response to epicardial and pericardial inflammation (Beck, 1935). Later, Vineberg demonstrated that direct perfusion was possible by implanting the internal mammary artery into the myocardium (Vineberg, 1954). Results of this procedure

Myocardial Revascularization: Novel Percutaneous Approaches, Edited by George S. Abela.
ISBN 0-471-36166-6 Copyright © 2002 Wiley-Liss, Inc.

led to neovascularization and collateral formation in some cases. In an effort to recreate the anatomy of the reptilian heart, Sen et al. (1968) and others (Goldman et al., 1956; Massimo and Boffi, 1957) performed direct perfusion by transmyocardial acupuncture. Although these results yielded some success, they were not long lasting, were difficult to reproduce, and, more importantly, were eventually overshadowed by the ability to perform CABG. Although most patients can be treated with conventional methods, such as CABG or PTCA with stenting, there are a significant and growing number of patients who have exhausted the ability to undergo these procedures repeatedly, primarily because of the diffuse nature of their coronary artery disease. As a result of this severe coronary artery disease, they have chronic disabling angina that is refractory to medical therapy. Transmyocardial laser revascularization (TMR) was developed to treat these patients. Although Mirhoseini et al. (1981, 1988) and Okada et al. (1986) used a laser to perform this type of revascularization in conjunction with coronary artery bypass grafting in the early 1980s, the use of a laser as sole therapy required advancements in the technology. After improvements in the laser that allowed TMR to be performed on a beating heart, results from individual institutions (Frazier et al., 1995; Horvath et al., 1996) and from multicenter trials (Dowling et al., 1998; Horvath et al., 1997; Vincent et al., 1997) were reported in 1995 through 1997. Although the outcomes of these trials were encouraging, they lacked an appropriate control group. Recently, four prospective randomized control trials have been published comparing medical management versus TMR in patients with severe angina. Eight hundred and thirty-seven patients were enrolled in these trials, and, by virtue of the one-to-one randomization; one-half of them were treated with the laser and the others continued on maximal medical therapy. All patients were followed for 12 months. One important similarity of these trials was that TMR provided significant symptomatic improvement compared with maximal medical therapy. Although there are other similarities between these studies, there are also significant differences. This review examines the results from these trials in an attempt to provide the reader with an understanding of the clinical efficacy and current experience with TMR.

3.2. METHODS

3.2.1. Patients

The baseline characteristics of patients who underwent TMR are listed in Table 3-1. Although the numbers listed pertain to the TMR patients, because the patients were equally randomized to the medical management group, there were no demographic differences between the groups for any of these trials. The trials employ two different wavelengths of light as their laser source. Burkhoff et al. (1999) and Allen et al. (1999) employed a Ho:YAG laser. Schofield et al. (1999), and Frazier et al. (1999), used a carbon dioxide (CO_2) laser. Schofield's data was obtained

TABLE 3-1.   Baseline Characteristics of TMR Patients

STUDY	Laser	n	Average Age (years)	Female %	CCS Angina Class III	CCS Angina Class IV	Unstable Angina	EF% (mean ± SD)	Previous MI	Previous CABG	Previous PTCA	IDDM	CHF
Schofield et al.	CO_2	188	60	10%	73%	27%	0%	48 ± 9	73%	95%	29%	19%	9%
Burkhoff et al.	Ho:YAG	182	63	11%	37%	63%	0%	50 ± 8	70%	91%	54%	33%	NA
Frazier et al.	CO_2	192	61	19%	31%	69%	8%	50 ± 11	82%	92%	47%	40%	34%
Allen et al.	Ho:YAG	275	60	26%	0%	100%	0%	47 ± 11	64%	86%	63%	46%	17%

CCS = Canadian Cardiovascular System; EF = left ventricular ejection fraction; MI = myocardial infarction; CABG = coronary artery bypass grafting; PTCA = percutaneous transluminal coronary angioplasty; IDDM = insulin-dependent diabetes mellitus; CHF = congestive heart failure; NA = not available.

from a single institution, whereas the others were multi-institutional trials. Approximately 200 patients were enrolled for each study. The average patient age was similar at 61 years, and the majority were male. There were significant differences in the baseline distribution of patients according to Canadian Cardiovascular Society (CCS) angina class. The majority of the patients in Schofield's trial (73%) were in angina class III, with 27% in class IV. These numbers were reversed for the Burkhoff and Frazier trials. One hundred percent of the patients in Allen's trial were in angina class IV. Only Frazier's trial had patients with unstable angina. The ejection fractions for all of the patients were relatively well preserved at 50%. The majority of the patients in all of the trials had a previous myocardial infarction and had some type of previous attempt at revascularization, CABG and/or PTCA. Diabetes was prevalent in three of the trials (40%), whereas only 19% of the patients in Schofield's trial were diabetic. The incidence of preoperative congestive heart failure had a wide range, as the Schofield trial had a 9% incidence and the Frazier trial had a 34% incidence.

The entry criteria were similar. The patients had refractory angina that was not amenable to standard methods of revascularization. They had reversible ischemia based on myocardial perfusion scanning and their ejection fractions were $\geq 25\%$.

Two of the trials, Frazier et al. (1999) and Allen et al. (1999), permitted a crossover from the medical management group to laser treatment for the presence of unstable angina that necessitated intravenous antianginal therapy from which they were unweanable over a period of at least 48 h. By definition, these crossover patients were therefore less stable and significantly different from those who had been initially randomized to TMR or medical management alone.

3.2.2. Operative Technique

All patients underwent a small anterior lateral thoracotomy under general anesthesia. The CO_2 laser (Frazier et al., 1999; Schofield et al., 1999) was used to create a 1-mm channel with a single 25- to 30-J pulse. Transesophageal echocardiography was employed on all of these CO_2-treated patients to confirm transmural penetration of the laser. The Ho:YAG laser (Allen et al., 1999; Burkhoff et al., 1999) achieved a similar 1-mm channel by manually advancing a fiber through the myocardium while the laser was fired. Typical pulse energies were 2 J for this laser with 20–30 pulses required to traverse the myocardium. Confirmation of transmural penetration was primarily by tactile and auditory feedback.

3.2.3. Endpoints

The principal subjective endpoint for all the trials was a change in angina symptoms. This was assessed by the investigator and/or a blinded independent observer. In addition to assigning an angina class, standardized questionnaires such as the Seattle Angina Questionnaire, the Short Form 36 Questionnaire (SF-36), and the Duke activity status index were employed. These tests were used to detect changes in quality of life. Objective measurements consisted of repeated exercise tolerance testing as well as repeat myocardial perfusion scans. Patients were reassessed at 3, 6, and 12 months after randomization.

3.3. RESULTS

3.3.1. Mortality

All the studies reported low perioperative mortality rates, ranging from 1% to 5% (Table 3-2). Predictably, the studies with more patients in class IV or unstable patients had higher mortality rates (Allen et al., 1999; Frazier et al., 1999). Meta-analysis of the 1-year survival demonstrated no statistically significant difference between the patients treated with the laser and those that continued their medical therapy. The odds ratio for 1-year survival in the laser-treated group was 0.988 that of the 1-year survival in the medically treated group, with 95% confidence interval of 0.637, 1.534.

TABLE 3-2.   12-Month Morbidity and Mortality

Studies	Perioperative Mortality TMR	1 Yr. Survival		CHF		MI		Arrhythmias	
		MM	TMR	MM	TMR	MM	TMR	MM	TMR
Schofield et al.	5%	96%	89%	NA	12%	NA	NA	NA	15%
Burkhoff et al.	1%	90%	95%	14%	32%	11%	18%	14%	14%
Frazier et al.	3%	79%	85%	NA	11%	NA	7%	13%	8%
Allen et al.	5%	84%	89%	NA	NA	11%	14%	NA	22%

MM = medical management; TMR = transmyocardial laser revascularization; CHF = congestive heart failure; Arrhythmias = ventricular and atrial arrhythmias; NA = not available.

TABLE 3-3.   1 Year Success Rate

Studies	MM	TMR
Schofield et al.	4%	25%
Burkhoff et al.	11%	61%
Frazier et al.	13%	72%
Allen et al.	32%	76%

Success Rate = proportion of patients who experienced a decrease of 2 or more angina classes.

3.3.2. Morbidity

A comparative assessment for morbidity is difficult because the baseline demographics were not identical between the studies. Additionally, unlike mortality, the exact definition of the various complications varies from one study protocol to the next. However, review of the available rates of postoperative congestive heart failure, myocardial infarction, and arrhythmias demonstrated a higher rate of all of these complications for patients treated with the Ho:YAG laser (Table 3-2).

3.3.3. Angina Class

A blinded independent observer in all studies performed angina class assessment. This was done as either the only angina assessment or in comparison with the investigator's assessment. Significant symptomatic improvement was seen in all studies for patients treated with a laser. Using a definition of success of a decrease of two or more angina classes, all of the studies demonstrated a significant success rate for treatment with the laser, with success rate range from 25% to 76% (Table 3-3). A smaller portion of patients in the medical

management group also experienced symptomatic improvement, and the success rate for these patients ranged from 4% to 32% (Table 3-3). Schofield's study, which started with most of its patients in class III, not surprisingly, showed the lowest success rate. In contrast, Allen showed the largest success rate with all of the patients in class IV at enrollment. Of note, the medical management patient group in Allen's study also showed the largest success rate at 32%.

3.3.4. Quality of Life and Myocardial Function

Quality of life as assessed by the Seattle Angina Questionnaire, the SF-36, and the Duke activity status index, demonstrated significant improvement in the quality of life by all of these indices in the TMR group versus the medical management group for each study. Global assessment of myocardial function by ejection fraction using echocardiography or radionuclide multigated acquisition scans showed no significant change in the ejection fraction of any of the patients, regardless of group assignment or study.

3.3.5. Hospital Admissions

Another indicator of the efficacy of the two treatments was demonstrated in the hospital admissions for unstable angina or cardiac-related events for all the patients. Meta-analysis of the data provided indicates that the 1-year hospitalization rate for patients in the laser-treated group was statistically significantly less than that for those treated medically. The odds ratio for 1-year hospitalization in the laser-treated group was 0.28 that of the 1-year hospitalization for the medically treated group, with an associated 95% confidence interval of 0.192, 0.408.

3.3.6. Myocardial Perfusion

As mentioned, myocardial perfusion scans were obtained preoperatively to verify the extent and severity of reversible ischemia. Postoperative scans demonstrated differing results between the studies. Schofield et al. (1999) divided the left ventricular into five segments and tallied the number of reversible (ischemic) and fixed (scar) defects for both groups. The data was then analyzed and presented as a pooling of all of the defects for all of the patients. Their results demonstrated a decrease in the number of reversible defects for both the TMR and medical management patients. There were 144 reversible defects in the TMR group at baseline and 160 in the medical management group. At 12 months, the TMR group had 78 reversible defects and the medical management group had 86. These numbers result in an overall improvement for both groups. The fixed defects showed little change in the TMR group, 65 at baseline and 69 at 12 months. However, there was a near doubling of the fixed defects in the medical management group from 38 at baseline to 68 at 12 months. These totals yield a 5% change for the TMR group and a doubling of the percentage for the medical management group (8–17%) over 1-year follow-up. Burkhoff et al. (1999), using polar plot analysis of the perfusion data, reported their results in percentage of ischemic (reversible) myocardium, which on average was 14% for TMR patients and 13% for the medical management patients at baseline. The percentage of infarcted myocardium (fixed defects) was 9% for TMR patients and 13% for the medical management patients at baseline. At 12 months, the reversible myocardium was 11% in the TMR group and 12% in the medical management group. The percentage of infarcted myocardium was 11% in both groups at 12 months. These values for both

types of defects did not differ significantly from each other or from the baseline measurement. Frazier, using a 24-segment model, also determined the number of reversible and fixed defects at baseline, which was the same for both groups. There was a 20% improvement in the perfusion of previously ischemic areas in the TMR group, whereas there was a 27% worsening of the perfusion of ischemic areas in the medical management group at 12 months. There was no difference in the number of fixed defects (scar) between the groups at 12 months, nor was there a significant change in the number of fixed defects for each patient compared with their baseline scans. The perfusion results from all of these studies are represented in Figure 3-1 and are expressed as changes in infarcted or ischemic myocardium at 1 year. The perfusion analysis employed by Allen et al. is not delineated in their text. However, they reported no significant differences between the TMR group and the medical management group with respect to reversible or fixed defects at baseline. There was no significant change from the baseline at 12 months in either the fixed or reversible defects in either group as well.

3.3.7. Exercise Tolerance

The aforementioned are results that are common to all of the studies. Additional functional assessment by exercise tolerance testing was also performed. Treadmill testing employed the modified Bruce protocol, in which exercise intensity was increased every 3 min. TMR patients of Schofield et al. (1999) had a 40-s increase in their exercise time compared with the medical management group at 12 months. This difference between the groups was not statistically significant. However, there was a 70-s improvement over the baseline for the TMR group and only a 5-s improvement for the medical management group. Burkhoff et al. (1999) reported an average of a 65-s increase in the TMR group at 12 months compared with their baseline with an average of a 46-s decrease in the medical management group over the same interval. This created a median difference

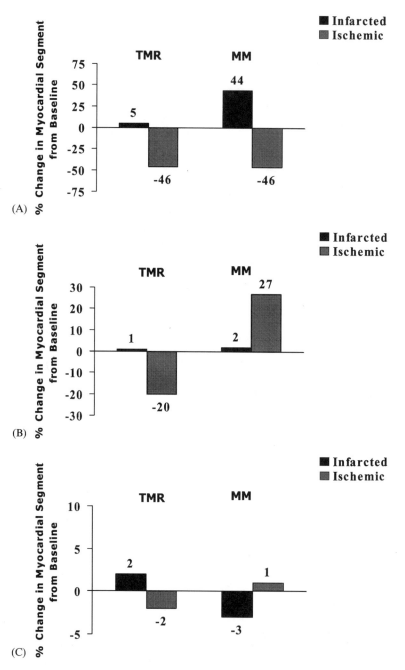

FIGURE 3-1.   Change in myocardial perfusion 1 year after medical management (MM) or transmyocardial laser revascularization (TMR). (A) Significant decrease in ischemic myocardium treated with CO_2 TMR ($P < 0.05$) without a significant change in infarcted areas. Decrease in ischemic myocardium for MM patients because of a concomitant increase in infarcted myocardium (Schofield et al., 1999). (B) Significant decrease in ischemic myocardium treated with CO_2 TMR, coupled with a significant increase in ischemic myocardium for MM patients ($P < 0.05$). No significant change in infarcted areas for either group (Frazier et al., 1999). (C) Perfusion was not changed after Ho:YAG TMR (Burkhoff et al., 1999).

between the groups of 111s. Allen et al. (1999) instituted exercise treadmill testing in substitution for thallium scanning midway through their study. Treadmill tests were performed at baseline. Using the Naughton protocol for a subset of patients, they showed a statistically significant improvement in exercise tolerance in the TMR versus the medical management group as measured by metabolic equivalents at 12 months. Exercise treadmill testing was not part of Frazier's study.

3.3.8. Medications

The protocols were established such that the TMR patients would continue on their maximum medical therapy and be weaned as tolerated. For each study, the frequencies of antianginal and cardiovascular drugs were similar between the two groups at baseline. Schofield reported a decrease in TMR patients' nitrate use at 12 months from 86% to 69%, compared with the use of the medical management patients, which increased slightly from 79% to 82%. Burkhoff (1999) reported "little change in overall pattern of medications during the study" for both groups. Frazier et al. (1999) reported 60% decrease in nitrate usage among the TMR patients, whereas the medical management patients had a 22% increase in their use of nitrates. They also noted that the overall medications decreased or remained unchanged in 83% of the TMR patients and, conversely, the use of medications increased or remained unchanged in 86% of the medical management patients.

3.3.9. Crossover

As previously mentioned, Allen and Frazier had crossover groups for patients who failed medical therapy. These crossover rates were 32% and 60%, respectively. Once treated with TMR, the crossover patients had a higher perioperative mortality rate, 9%. After the initial perioperative period, their survival was the same as that of the other group and their angina relief was the same as that of those originally assigned to the TMR group.

3.4. DISCUSSION

Almost 10 years have passed since the first patients were treated with a laser as sole therapy for their end-stage coronary artery disease. Since then, over 6,000 patients have undergone the procedure around the world. In addition to these patients who have undergone the procedure as sole therapy, an increasing number of patients are being treated with TMR in combination with coronary artery bypass grafting (Trehan et al., 1998). The procedure has also been performed as percutaneous myocardial revascularization (PMR) via a peripheral artery access in a smaller number of patients (Kim et al., 1997; Lauer et al., 1999a, 1999b; Leon et al., 2000; Oesterle et al., 1998, 2000; Shawl et al., 1999; Stone et al., 2000).

The purpose of this review is to examine the clinical efficacy of TMR on basis of the most recent publications of prospective randomized controlled trials using the procedure as sole therapy for severe angina. There is a growing body of literature, both experimental and clinical, on this topic. The four studies reviewed here highlight important issues in understanding and applying TMR.

In evaluating the results, particularly in making comparisons, it is critical to determine whether the patients selected for the procedure are the same between the studies under comparison. In this series, the study by Schofield had significantly fewer patients in angina class IV. The result is that a less dramatic success rate was seen. Additionally, fewer patients were at risk of becoming unstable or needing to crossover. This is an important distinction. One of the lessons learned from Frazier's study was that patients who underwent TMR less than 2 weeks after an episode of unstable angina requiring intravenous medications had a significantly higher perioperative mortality rate (22% for the unstable patients and 1% for the stable patients). For all of the patients in all of the studies, there was a similar symptomatic response. This success rate in the relief of angina as a result of TMR was accompanied by improvements in the quality of life for these patients. Interestingly, the perfusion results did not mirror these clinical outcomes. One would not expect an anatomic study (perfusion scan) to correlate perfectly with symptoms. For example, the size of a patient's reversible defect was not always reflected by the severity of his/her symptoms. Be that as it may, a significant perfusion benefit was noted in Frazier's study. Schofield's results indicated a similar decrease in the number of reversible defects for TMR and medical management patients. A careful review of Schofield's data indicates that the decrease in the number of reversible defects for the medical management patients is likely due to a doubling of the number of fixed defects for the same patients. The TMR patients did not exhibit this increase in fixed defects. As a result, for both of these studies, an argument could be made that perfusion is improved for patients treated with TMR. A similar perfusion benefit was not seen by Burkhoff or Allen, the principal difference being that a Ho:YAG laser was used in the latter studies and a CO_2 laser in the former. The argument is made that the present methods of perfusion imaging may not be sensitive enough; however, they appear sensitive enough to detect improvement in patients treated with the CO_2 laser. This may also indicate that the mechanism of action for Ho:YAG TMR is not an increase in myocardial perfusion.

The lack of improvement in myocardial perfusion after Ho:YAG TMR may be one reason that a recent report documented a loss of the long-term symptom relief in patients treated with a Ho:YAG laser (De Carlo et al., 2000). Significant short-term angina relief was demonstrated at 1 year, as the average angina class fell from 3.5 ± 0.5 at baseline to 1.8 ± 0.8 at 1 year ($P < 0.01$). However, the average angina class at 3 years after Ho:YAG TMR had significantly increased to 2.2 ± 0.7 ($P = 0.003$ vs. 1 year). Additionally, at 3 years only 30% of the patients had a two-class angina improvement compared to their baseline and 70% had a one-class improvement. Long-term results with a CO_2 laser were markedly different. Recently reported, these results demonstrated a decrease in angina

class from 3.7 ± 0.4 at baseline to 1.5 ± 1.0 at 1 year ($p = 0.0001$). This was unchanged from the 1.5 ± 1.0 average angina classes at 1 year of follow-up ($P =$ not significant vs. 5 years). Additionally, 68% of the patients at 5 years had two or more angina class improvement and 23% had a one-class improvement. This loss of clinical effectiveness seen with a Ho:YAG laser was also noted in a direct clinical comparison (Lansing et al., 1998, 2000). In a review of 460 patients treated by a single investigator using both devices, the angina improvements seen with CO_2 were greater than with Ho:YAG (Lansing et al., 2000). At 12 months the majority of CO_2 patients were in class I or angina free, whereas the majority of the Ho:YAG patients were in class II.

This distinction in wavelengths of light between Ho:YAG and CO_2 may have increasing importance because PMR (which also employs a Ho:YAG laser) has failed to demonstrate a perfusion benefit and perhaps even a significant clinical benefit. PMR employs a Ho:YAG laser and a catheter-based delivery system in which the laser fiber is placed against the endocardium and fired, creating a nontransmural 3- to 4-mm depression in the subendocardial layer (Kim et al., 1997; Lauer et al., 1999a, 1999b; Leon et al., 2000; Oesterle et al., 1998, 2000; Shawl et al., 1999; Stone et al., 2000). In a randomized controlled trial comparing PMR and maximal medical therapy, the results at 12 months indicated a significant increase in exercise tolerance and a decrease in symptoms for PMR-treated patients (Oesterle et al., 2000). However, the symptomatic improvement with PMR was not as great as had been seen with TMR, with only 34% of the patients in angina class II or lower. Additionally, the improvement in exercise tolerance was less than that in PMR-treated patients, with an average increase of 90s for the PMR patients and 150 s for the TMR patients (Oesterle et al., 2000). This comparison of PMR and TMR indicates that the revascularization is more effective with TMR.

One advantage that PMR trials have over the surgical TMR trials is the ability to perform a double-blind randomized placebo-controlled trial. The catheter may be placed against the subendocardium and the laser not fired. Recent reports of the 6-month data of such a trial (Leon et al., 2000) have indicated that the placebo group had the same results as the PMR-treated group. There was no difference in the exercise tolerance at 6 months between the groups, despite a significant increase in exercise tolerance for each group versus their baseline. Forty-two percent of the placebo group achieved a greater than two angina class reduction in symptoms at 6 months. However, another randomized placebo study, the BELIEF Trial using a different laser catheter system that penetrates the muscle, demonstrated a significant improvement in symptoms and exercise performance (Nordrehaug et al., 2001). As a result of the improvement in the PMR placebo group, it has been suggested that the placebo effect may be an important mechanism of surgical TMR as well. Unfortunately, it is impossible to run a double-blind surgical trial. Patient expectations for the surgical procedure certainly may generate a placebo effect. However, the long-term benefits seen with the CO_2 laser argue against the placebo effect, and more salient and objective data have also been obtained. In addition to the symptomatic improvement, CO_2 TMR has been demonstrated via numerous studies to improve myocardial perfusion by nuclear SPECT scans (Frazier et al., 1999; Horvath et al., 1997; Schofield et al., 1999) as well as PET scans (Cooley et al., 1996; Frazier et al., 1995; Kadipasaoglu and Frazier, 1999). A significant decrease in number of reversible or ischemic myocardial defects without an increase in the number of fixed or infarcted areas has been demonstrated with CO_2 in comparison of TMR patients both against their baseline and versus patients randomized to medical management (Frazier et al., 1999; Schofield et al., 1999). Further evaluation using other objective measures such as dobutamine stress echocardiography (Donovan et al., 1997) CINE and contrast-enhanced MRI (Horvath et al., 2000) demonstrated improvement in myocardial function and decrease in myocardial ischemia without an increase in

myocardial infarction in patients treated with CO_2 TMR. This evidence is not subject to the placebo effect and has been analyzed by readers blinded to the treatments that the patients received. A better understanding of the mechanisms whereby TMR achieves its effect is needed and is the impetus for ongoing studies. Additionally, the enhancement of these results by combining laser revascularization with conventional revascularization (i.e., CABG) as well as with other types of unconventional revascularization (i.e., gene therapy) will undoubtedly be the focus of investigations of the future. CO_2 TMR has demonstrated a perfusion benefit in both of the CO_2 randomized trials. Ho:YAG TMR or Ho:YAG PMR has yet to demonstrate a perfusion benefit.

ACKNOWLEDGMENTS

I acknowledge the statistical assistance of Michele Parker in review of the statistical analyses performed in these studies and subsequent meta-analysis of the results. I also thank Carleen Guzman for her assistance in the preparation of this manuscript.

References

Allen KB, Dowling RD, Fudge TL et al. Comparison of transmyocardial revascularization with medical therapy in patients with refractory angina. *N Engl J Med* 1999; 341: 1029–1036.

Beck CS. The development of a new blood supply to the heart by operation. *Ann Surg* 1935; 102: 801–813.

Burkhoff D, Schmidt S, Schulman SP et al. Transmyocardial laser revascularization compared with continued medical therapy for treatment of refractory angina pectoris: a prospective randomized trial. *Lancet* 1999; 354: 885–890.

Cooley DA, Frazier OH, Kadipasaoglu KA et al. Transmyocardial laser revascularization: clinical experience with 12-month follow-up. *J Thorac Cardiovasc Surg* 1996; 111: 791–799.

De Carlo M, Milano AD, Pratali S et al. Symptomatic improvement after transmyocardial laser revascularization: how long does it last? *Ann Thorac Surg* 2000; 70: 1130–1133.

Donovan CL, Landolfo KP, Lowe JE et al. Improvement in inducible ischemia during dobutamine stress echocardiography after transmyocardial laser revascularization in patients with refractory angina pectoris. *J Am Coll Cardiol* 1997; 30: 607–612.

Dowling RD, Petracek MR, Selinger SL et al. Transmyocardial revascularization in patients with refractory, unstable angina. *Circulation* 1998; 98 (*Suppl* II): II-73–II-76.

Frazier OH, Cooley DA, Kadipasaoglu KA et al. Myocardial revascularization with laser: preliminary findings. *Circulation* 1995; 92 (*Suppl* II): II-58–II-65.

Frazier OH, March RJ, Horvath KA. Transmyocardial revascularization with a carbon dioxide laser in patients with end-stage coronary artery disease. *N Engl J Med* 1999; 341: 1021–1028.

Goldman A, Greenstone SM, Preuss FS et al. Experimental methods for producing a collateral circulation to the heart directly from the left ventricle. *J Thorac Surg* 1956; 31: 364–374.

Horvath KA, Mannting F, Cummings N et al. Transmyocardial laser revascularization: operative techniques and clinical results at two years. *J Thorac Cardiovasc Surg* 1996; 111: 1047–1053.

Horvath KA, Cohn LH, Cooley DA et al. Transmyocardial laser revascularization: results of a multicenter trial with transmyocardial laser revascularization used as sole therapy for end-stage coronary artery disease. *J Thorac Cardiovasc Surg* 1997; 113: 645–654.

Horvath KA, Kim RJ, Judd RM et al. Contrast enhanced MRI assessment of microinfarction after transmyocardial laser revascularization (abstract). *Circulation* 2000; 102: II-765.

Kadipasaoglu KA, Frazier OH. Transmyocardial laser revascularization: effective laser parameters on tissue oblation and cardiac perfusion. *Semin Thorac Cardiovasc Surg* 1999; 11: 4–11.

Kim CB, Kesten R, Javier M et al. Percutaneous method of laser transmyocardial revascularization. *Cathet Cardiovasc Diagn* 1997; 40: 223–228.

Lansing AM. Transmyocardial revascularization: mechanism of action with CO_2 and Ho:YAG lasers. *J Thorac Cardiovasc Surg* 1998; 115: 1392.

Lansing AM. Transmyocardial revascularization: late results and mechanisms of action. *J Ky Med Assoc* 2000; 98: 406–412.

Lauer B, Junghans U, Stahl F et al. Catheter-based percutaneous myocardial laser revascularization in patients with end-stage coronary artery disease. *J Am Coll Cardiol* 1999a; 34: 1663–1670.

Lauer B, Junghans U, Stahl F et al. Catheter-based percutaneous myocardial laser revascularization in patients with end-stage coronary artery disease (abstract). *J Am Coll Cardiol* 1999b; 33: 381A.

Leon MB, Baim DS, Moses JW et al. A randomized blinded clinical trial comparing percutaneous laser myocardial revascularization (using Biosense LV mapping) vs. placebo in patients with refractory coronary ischemia (abstract). *Circulation* 2000; 102: II-565.

Massimo C, Boffi L. Myocardial revascularization by a new method of carrying blood directly from the left ventricular cavity into the coronary circulation. *J Thorac Surg* 1957; 34: 257–264.

Mirhoseini M, Cayton M. Revascularization of the heart by laser. *J Microsurg* 1981; 2: 253–260.

Mirhoseini M, Shelgikar S, Cayton MM. New concepts in revascularization of the myocardium. *Ann Thorac Surg* 1988; 45: 415–420.

Oesterle SN, Reifart NJ, Meier B et al. Initial results of laser-based percutaneous myocardial revascularization for angina pectoris. *Am J Cardiol* 1998; 82: 659–662.

Oesterle SN, Sanborn TA, Ali N et al. Percutaneous transmyocardial laser revascularization for severe angina: the PACIFIC randomized trial. *Lancet* 2000; 356: 1705–1710.

Okada M, Ikuta H, Shimizu K et al. Alternative method of myocardial revascularization by laser: experimental and clinical study. *Kobe J Med Sci* 1986; 32: 151–161.

Schofield PM, Sharples LD, Caine N et al. Transmyocardial laser revascularization in patients with refractory angina: a randomized controlled trial. *Lancet* 1999; 353: 519–524.

Sen PK, Daulatram J, Kinare SG et al. Further studies in multiple transmyocardial acupuncture as a method of myocardial revascularization. *Surgery* 1968; 64: 861–870.

Shawl FA, Domanski MJ, Kaul U et al. Procedural results and early clinical outcome of percutaneous transluminal myocardial revascularization. *Am J Cardiol* 1999; 83: 498–501.

Stone GW, Rubinstein P, Schmidt D et al. A prospective, randomized, multicenter trial of percutaneous transmyocardial laser revascularization in patients with non-recanalizable chronic total occlusions (abstract). *Circulation* 2000; 102: II-689.

Trehan N, Mishra Y, Mehta Y et al. Transmyocardial laser as an adjunct to minimally invasive coronary artery bypass grafting for complete myocardial revascularization. *Ann Thorac Surg* 1998; 66: 1113–1118.

Vinberg A. Clinical and experimental studies in the treatment of coronary artery insufficiency by internal mammary artery implant. *J Int Coll Surg* 1954; 22: 503–518.

Vincent JG, Bardos P, Kruse J et al. End stage coronary artery disease treated with the transmyocardial CO_2 laser revascularization: a chance for the 'inoperable' patient. *Eur J Cardiothorac Surg* 1997; 121: 888–894.

II

Biological Responses and Mechanisms of Action of Myocardial Revascularization

4

Angiogenesis Versus Arteriogenesis: Can Different Transmyocardial Revascularization Approaches Be Distinguished?

Renu Virmani, M.D., Frank D. Kolodgie, Ph.D., Andrew Farb, M.D., and Allen P. Burke, M.D.

Department of Cardiovascular Pathology
Armed Forces Institute of Pathology
Washington, DC

SUMMARY

Intramyocardial channel formation has been proposed as the mechanism of improved myocardial oxygenation and cardiac benefit. The three forms of channel formation discussed herein are angiogenesis, arteriogenesis, and vasculogenesis.

Angiogenesis is defined as "the sprouting of capillaries in avascular regions from pre-existing cells." Vessels formed by this process may act as conduits for inflammatory cells during healing rather than supporting actual blood flow.

"The development of muscular collateral blood vessels in-situ from pre-existing arteriolar anastomoses supplying ischemic beds" defines arteriogenesis. This process has two phases of development: remodeling and proliferation.

Vasculogenesis is constituted by "the synthesis of arteries de novo."

The hypothesis that oxygenated blood from the left ventricular cavity could perfuse myocardium by attempting to partially recreate embryonic or cold-blooded vertebrate circulation led to the creation of TMR.

To achieve the primary goal of myocardial revascularization, angiogenesis would need to support the distribution of the blood within the myocardium, whereas arteriogenesis would need to initially provide blood flow. TMR currently appears to promote primarily angiogenesis within the area of the channels and must be used judiciously when attempting to help the failing heart.

4.1. INTRODUCTION

In the early 1980s, Rahimtoola found a significant improvement in left ventricular

Myocardial Revascularization: Novel Percutaneous Approaches, Edited by George S. Abela.
ISBN 0-471-36166-6 Copyright © 2002 Wiley-Liss, Inc.

function after coronary revascularization in selected patients with depressed ventricular performance (Rahimtoola et al., 1981). He postulated that the mechanism of poor myocardial contractility was chronic ischemia, which could be improved by revascularization. Presumably, viable, potentially functional myocardium was present but was in a depressed, "hibernating" state (Rahimtoola, 1989, 1999). In many patients, diffuse coronary artery atherosclerosis precludes surgical or intravascular treatment to alleviate chronic ischemia. As an alternative therapy, transmyocardial laser revascularization (TMR), a procedure performed at the time of open-heart surgery, was introduced to create myocardial channels to support the flow of oxygenated blood directly from the ventricular cavity to the ischemic myocardium (Mirhoseini et al., 1981). The benefits of TMR have been shown in experimental models of hibernating myocardium, in which gradual coronary occlusion leads to depressed myocardial contractility. These studies have demonstrated the feasibility of intramyocardial channel creation without causing additional ventricular dysfunction. The method used to create channels does not appear to be specific, because similar results have been produced by needle-induced trauma, or so-called transmyocardial revascularization angiogenesis (Chu et al., 1999).

Rather than serving as a permanent conduit, over time, newly created channels heal and become filled with areas of collagen and neoangiogenesis. Neoangiogenesis has been proposed as the mechanism of improved myocardial oxygenation and cardiac benefit. Although the clinical effectiveness of such revascularization techniques remains controversial for the improvement of cardiac function and exercise capacity, most studies have shown relief of angina symptoms.

Whether angiogenesis secondary to intramyocardial channel formation can enhance blood flow to the failing heart is debatable. The best argument against this hypothesis involves tumor formation, in which regions demonstrating a rich neovasculature often accompany large areas of necrosis. Therefore, neovascularity does not necessarily confer viability; certain types of vessels formed in response to injury may directly influence myocardial perfusion, resulting in improved functional recovery. In this review, we discuss the different types of new vessel formation, namely, angiogenesis, arteriogenesis, and vasculogenesis. We then focus on the various mechanisms of vessel development. Finally, our report on the pathologic changes in animals and humans after transmyocardial revascularization is presented to further clarify the goals of intramyocardial revascularization.

4.2. CURRENT DEFINITIONS OF ANGIOGENESIS, ARTERIOGENESIS, AND VASCULOGENESIS

4.2.1. Angiogenesis

The sprouting of capillaries (endothelium-derived vascular spaces) in avascular regions from pre-existing vessels is referred to as angiogenesis. Angiogenesis in nature is seen during wound healing and inflammation, in areas of ischemia, in the female reproductive organs, and in tumor growth beyond a critical size (Cines et al., 1998; Pepper, 1997). The process of endothelial cell sprouting gradually leads to the development of a lumen proximal to the proliferating end of the nascent vessel. Capillary maturation is accompanied by the generation of the basement membrane associated with smooth muscle cells to stabilize the endothelium. The ability of these vessels to conduct the blood flow to ischemic tissue is uncertain; often, capillaries end abruptly or travel in haphazard directions. Rather than supporting blood flow, vessels formed by angiogenesis may be conduits for inflammatory cells involved in the healing process. Probably the best example of functional angiogenesis is complete recanalization of an occlusive thrombus to the point where blood flow to a previously ischemic bed is at least partially restored.

4.2.2. Arteriogenesis

The remodeling or expansion of pre-existing vessels defines arteriogenesis (Fig. 4-1).

Collateral Vessel Enlargement
(Arteriogenesis)

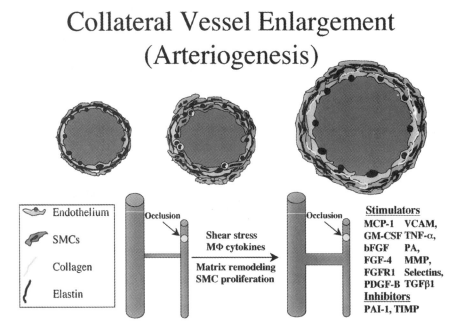

FIGURE 4-1. Cartoon diagram illustrating arteriogenesis through collateral vessel enlargement. Normal collateral on the left undergoes positive remodeling after coronary artery occlusion. Early remodeling shows invasion of inflammatory cells and partial dissolution of the internal elastic lamina with invasion of periendothelial cells (SMCs/pericytes). These cells help change the endothelial phenotype to a more quiescent state and provide structural integrity. As remodeling advances, there is continued thickening of the arterial wall by migration and proliferation of smooth muscle cells and matrix synthesis (modified from Carmeliet, *Nat Med* 2000; 6: 389–395).

Arteriogenesis is the development of muscular collateral blood vessels in situ from pre-existing arteriolar anastomoses supplying ischemic beds. Collateral arteriogenesis has two phases of development, proliferation and remodeling. Proliferation occurs in the vessel wall and involves endothelial and smooth muscle cells. The smooth muscle cells first change their phenotype to a synthetic state and then proliferate and migrate into the intima. There they actively synthesize extracellular matrix, proteoglycans, collagen, and elastin (Schaper et al., 1996). This phase is followed by eutropic remodeling, a process in which vessel diameters increase up to 20-fold. Remodeling requires dissolution or weakening of smooth muscle cell-to-cell or cell-to-matrix adhesion that allows the vessel to dilate and remodel. The precise stimuli for arteriogenesis are not well defined; apoptosis of smooth muscle cells via tumor necrosis factor-α (TNF-α) produced by macrophages may be involved. In addition, matrix lysis by urokinase-type plasminogen activator and its inhibitor plasminogen activator inhibitor-1 (PAI-1), which are upregulated by both basic fibroblast growth factor (bFGF) and vascular endothelial cell growth factor (VEGF) may also play a role (Pepper et al., 1987, 1990a, 1990b). Unlike angiogenesis, the development of collateral vessels by arteriogenesis is not dependent on ischemia but rather on shear stress-induced upregulation of angiogenic factors and inflammatory cells like macrophages.

4.2.3. Vasculogenesis

The synthesis of arteries de novo constitutes vasculogenesis. During embryonic development, early vascular plexus forms from mesoderm by the maturation of angioblasts, which

Coronary Vasculogenesis

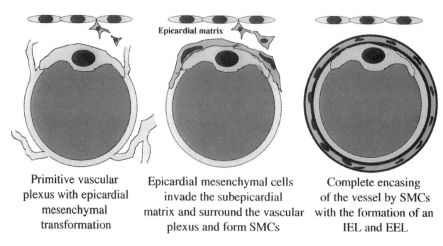

Epicardial matrix

| Primitive vascular plexus with epicardial mesenchymal transformation | Epicardial mesenchymal cells invade the subepicardial matrix and surround the vascular plexus and form SMCs | Complete encasing of the vessel by SMCs with the formation of an IEL and EEL |

FIGURE 4-2.   Cartoon diagram illustrating the mechanisms of coronary vasculogenesis in the developing heart (adapted from Dettman et al., *Dev Biol* 1998; 193: 169–181).

subsequently differentiate into blood vessels. Because vasculogenesis can also occur from circulating endothelial cell progenitors or angioblasts from human peripheral blood, it has been proposed that endothelial progenitors may be useful for augmenting collateral vessel growth in ischemic myocardial tissue (Asahara et al., 1997). Development of coronary arteries begins with angioblasts, which are derived from the proepicardial organ (protrusions of mesothelial cells on the right side of the sinus venosus) that invade the epicardium and differentiate into endothelium-lined capillary plexus (Carmeliet, 2000).

Initially, the primitive myocardium derives its oxygen via diffusion from the ventricular cavity, which is facilitated by the presence of prominent trabeculae on the endocardial surface. On the 11th embryonic day, the myocardium is infiltrated by primitive vascular plexus, which eventually becomes mature epicardial coronary arteries by acquiring a smooth muscle cell covering (Dettman et al., 1998). The coronary smooth muscle cells are derived from the epicardium, from which the epithelial cells transform into mesenchymal tissue that traverses the subepicardial matrix

to the point where the coronary arteries are developing (Fig. 4-2). The smooth muscle cells cover the endothelium-lined plexus when they penetrate the aorta. A higher blood pressure may be the reason why these plexuses become invested with smooth muscle cells, however, the signals that control this phenomenon remain unclear.

4.2.4. Mechanisms of Angiogenesis/Arteriogenesis

A balance of positive and negative regulators determines angiogenic endothelial responses. The list of these factors is rapidly expanding and beyond the scope of this review (Carmeliet, 1996, 2000). Both stimulator and inhibitory factors coexist in normal endothelium and, quiescence is maintained by the dominance of negative regulators. The most studied positive regulators of angiogenesis are mitogens such as VEGF, acidic fibroblast growth factor (aFGF), and bFGF. Of these, VEGF is the most potent during the phase of endothelial activation. Although transforming growth factor β (TGF-β) and TNF-α are negative regulators in vitro, they are angiogenic in vivo and stimulate direct-acting positive regulators produced by inflammatory cells.

Some of the nonchemokine factors implicated as positive regulators of angiogenesis include nitric oxide, angiopoietin (Ang-1 and -2), proteases of the plasminogen activator, matrix metalloproteinases, chymase, and heparinase. Other negative promoters of angiogenesis include inhibitors of matrix degrading proteolytic enzymes (TIMPs), thrombospondin, angiostatin, retinoids, interferon-β, interleukin-12, and hyaluronan.

Alterations in endothelium-cell matrix interactions promote the effects of angiogenic stimuli through multiple integrins that provide the link between the extracellular matrix and cytoskeletal elements (Cines et al., 1998). Integrin-ligand interactions trigger cytoskeletal organization and facilitate migration, cell replication, and apoptosis (Cines et al., 1998). Integrin-associated signaling pathways are likely to be diverse, and it is possible that the cell receptors required for angiogenesis during embryogenesis differ from those required for collateral vessel formation in adults (Cines et al., 1998).

In the myocardium, both angiogenesis and arteriogenesis are stimulated after tissue injury, although the extent of which may vary depending on the underlying trauma. Although ischemia is believed to be the driving force for angiogenesis, recent studies in chronically ischemic pigs in which the "ischemia" was relieved by beta-blockers showed no effect on the development of arteriogenesis (collateral circulation). Perhaps other stimuli such as local inflammation and/or sheer stress are more important for regulation of vessel growth in the ischemic heart.

Under certain conditions, arterioles can form larger-diameter arteries by undergoing degradation of the internal elastic lamina associated with smooth muscle cell and endothelial cell proliferation. The proliferating cells may secrete other components of the vessel wall such as elastic and collagen fibers and proteoglycans. These collateral vessels then remodel to form larger-caliber muscular

arteries that can begin to carry blood at high volumes. Thoma's "law of histomechanics," published in 1893, first described the positive relationship between blood flow velocity and artery size. This dependence plays a central role in coronary atherosclerosis. In early coronary atherosclerosis with up to 40–50% luminal narrowing, vessel size increases because of positive remodeling and normal blood flow is maintained (Glagov et al., 1987). However, severely stenotic vessels tend to show a reduction in size as blood flow is reduced.

Fluid shear stresses can act as remodeling forces, and increases in hemodynamic shear forces have been shown to upregulate adhesion molecules expressed on the endothelium. These adhesion molecules can attract circulating monocytes and stimulate the production of bFGF and platelet-derived growth factor (PDGF), which can lead to proliferation of endothelial and smooth muscle cells (Sampath et al., 1995). Mechanical strain on endothelial cells after induction of coronary artery stenosis can increase monocyte chemotactic protein-1 (MCP-1), facilitating monocyte adherence and migration into the wall of collateral arteries (Ito et al., 1997b; Wang et al., 1995).

Angiogenesis in vivo has been shown to be dependent on specific isoforms of VEGF. In transgenic mice with exclusive expression of the $VEGF_{120}$ isoform ($VEGF_{120/120}$), which lack the isoforms of 164 and 188 amino acids, Carmeliet et al. have shown impaired myocardial angiogenesis, fewer coronary vessels, and fewer smooth muscle α-actin-positive cells (Carmeliet et al., 1996). Myocyte size was 40% larger than in normal mice, and the myocyte-to-capillary ratio was increased because myocyte hypertrophy is a response to reduced perfusion. Abnormal capillaries were observed, characterized by irregular, tortuous, and dilated vessels, an indication of incomplete remodeling. The functional consequences of these vascular effects were reduced contractility, impaired relaxation, dilated ischemic cardiomyopathy, pump failure, and death. The hearts of $VEGF_{120/120}$ mice expressed reduced levels of PDGF-B, whereas the levels of Ang-1 were normal. These data support the importance of isoforms $VEGF_{164}$ and $VEGF_{188}$ for the development of both angiogenesis and arteriogenesis, the impairment of which results in ischemic cardiomyopathy. Although these studies suggest that events during embryogenesis have consequences after birth, they may not be applicable in the adult. Therefore, it seems most likely that different VEGF isoforms have varied biologic effects and specific VEGF isoforms may be important for optimal angiogenesis.

Chronic inflammation has been shown to affect cell proliferation, vessel formation, and enlargement, and Thurston et al. have shown that the type of inflammation influences the angiogenic response (Thurston et al., 1998). These authors used a model of chronic airway inflammation, produced by *Mycoplasma pulmonis*, in mice that were either resistant or susceptible to the development of trachitis. Tracheal vascularity (angiogenesis) was assessed in whole mounts after the tracheas were removed, opened flat, and stained. Mild inflammation resulted in the doubling of vessels in the trachea, and there was a parallel increase among capillaries and venules. In contrast, severe inflammation was associated with no change in the vessel number or length; instead, vessel diameter and endothelial cell number doubled, and the proportion of venules also doubled with a corresponding decrease in capillaries (Thurston et al., 1998). It is conceivable that needle or laser trauma to heart may promote an inflammatory response, which may not be uniform, especially in humans with other underlying diseases. Therefore, differences in the inflammatory infiltrate after injury may influence the types of vessels generated and the clinical success of the treatment.

4.3. TRANSMYOCARDIAL REVASCULARIZATION IN ANIMALS AND HUMANS

Transmyocardial revascularization evolved from the hypothesis that oxygenated blood from the left ventricular cavity could perfuse the myocardium in an attempt to partially recreate embryonic or cold-blooded vertebrate circulation. Typically, Ho:YAG or CO_2 lasers are used for TMR. In animals, regardless of the laser source, it has been conclusively shown that channel closure develops 6–24 h after their creation by occlusive thrombi consisting of platelets, fibrin, and trapped red blood cells. The myocardium bordering the channel shows a band of myocyte coagulation necrosis and contraction band necrosis, which is five to seven cell layers thick. The thrombus organizes by the formation of granulation tissue, which consists of neoangiogenesis and chronic inflammatory cells with interspersed myofibroblasts, which are visible between 1 and 2 weeks after laser injury. The granulation tissue is finally replaced by collagenous scar tissue interspersed with a paucity of capillaries; these capillaries have never been conclusively shown to increase blood flow into the myocardium surrounding the region of the laser channels (Fisher et al., 1997; Horvath et al., 1995; Mirhoseini and Cayton, 1981; Whittaker et al., 1993).

At early time points, the thermal injury produced by CO_2 laser is less pronounced compared with that produced by Ho:YAG laser; however, by 6 weeks the histologic appearance and degree of neovascularization are indistinguishable between these laser energy sources (Fisher et al., 1997). Channel formation is not associated with left ventricular dysfunction (Hughes et al., 1998). Myocardial infarct size in the rat, an animal with poor collaterals, has been reported to decrease after the creation of myocardial channels, and this effect is independent of whether lasers or needles were used to create the channels (Whittaker et al., 1996).

Early clinical follow-up studies after TMR have mostly been encouraging (Cooley et al., 1996; March, 1999; Mirhoseini et al., 1988). A multicenter study in the United States showed improvement in anginal symptoms and myocardial perfusion (Horvath et al., 1997). A randomized study from the United Kingdom also demonstrated a reduction in anginal symptoms; however, no clinical improvements were noted in mean treadmill exercise time or 12-min walking distance. Furthermore, no differences in survival time between TMR and medical treatment were observed (Schofield et al., 1999).

Of the few published studies on the histologic changes of TMR in humans, all have shown very similar morphology to that reported in animals (Burkhoff et al., 1996; Gassler et al., 1997; Sigel et al., 1998). The pathology of eight cases of TMR has been reported, and we have examined another three hearts in our laboratory. Soon after the laser channels are formed, platelets, fibrin, red blood cells, and acute inflammatory cells occlude channels. The myocardium surrounding the channel shows a clear zone of myocyte coagulation necrosis with infiltration of neutrophils (Fig. 4-3). Between the viable myocardium and the region of coagulation necrosis, there is a zone of contraction band necrosis. The surrounding vessels are congested, and occasionally the laser may disrupt muscular arteries, resulting in extravasation of red blood cells and thrombosis, if they happen to be in the laser energy field (Gassler et al., 1997; Sigel et al., 1998). On the epicardial surface, the channels are funnel shaped and are occluded by fibrinous material. The endocardial channels are also sealed by fibrinous material, which either is on the same level with the surrounding endocardium or may protrude into the ventricular cavity (Gassler et al., 1997).

At 1–3 weeks after TMR, there is a pronounced healing response at the mouth of the channel created by the laser tract relative to the inner myocardium. This accelerated phase of healing is characterized by fibrin and collagen deposition in association with macrophages, lymphocytes, scattered red blood cells, and rare neutrophils. In contrast, intramyocardial channels show a greater accumulation of fibrin, red blood cells, macrophages, and inflammatory cells compared with the mouth of the channel. At this phase, a few cells within the laser tract react positively with antibodies to CD31 and von Willebrand factor (vWf), providing evidence for the presence of new endothelium-lined structures. The surrounding myocyte necrosis associated with channel formation is no longer evident. Some cases have microscopic areas of necrotic debris with focal surrounding granulomas and a foreign body giant cell reaction.

Late histologic changes (>2 months) after clinical TMR consist of fibrous tissue scar-

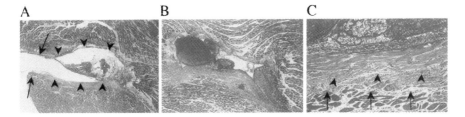

FIGURE 4-3. A 66-year-old woman underwent transmyocardial laser revascularization (TMR) 3 days before death. At autopsy, myocardial channels could be easily discerned grossly with focal areas of hemorrhage within the myocardium and fibrinous pericarditis. Microscopic sections (A) show the mouth of the channel (arrows) on the endocardial surface with focal presence of fibrin clot and platelets. A border zone of surrounding myocardial necrosis (arrowheads) is present. A high-power view of a channel in the midmyocardium is shown in B. The channel is filled with thrombus, and the surrounding myocardium has a zone of coagulation necrosis. In C, a high-power view of the channel wall shows luminal fibrin thrombus with surrounding coagulation necrosis (arrowheads). The normal myocardium is separated from the zone of coagulation necrosis by a layer of contraction band necrosis (arrows). At the border zone between viable and necrotic myocardium, neutrophils are present (arrowheads).

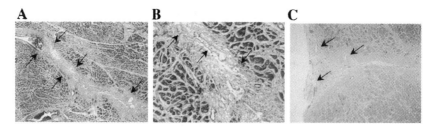

FIGURE 4-4. A 61-year-old man died 70 days after TMR. The channels at this stage could not be identified by gross examination. Histologically (A), in the area of TMR treatment, loosely filled fibrocollagenous tracts could be identified (arrows). Within the channel, multiple capillaries (arrows) were identified with only rare arterioles (B). In C, coronary section from a 66-year old man who underwent TMR 2 years before death is shown. Note that TMR channels are difficult to identify histologically. The channel is fully healed with collagenous dense scarring and a few interspersed small capillaries (arrows).

ring, sparse macrophage infiltration with an interspersed capillary network, scattered small veins, and rare arterioles. With time, the fibrous tissue is transformed into a dense collagenous scar with fewer endothelium-lined capillaries (Fig. 4-4). The capillary lining of endothelial cells are both CD31 and vWf positive. The mouth of the channel becomes completely filled with fibrous tissue, and there is no direct communication between the ventricular cavity and the capillary network within the fibrous channel. Similarly, epicardial openings are completely filled with fibrous scars and may appear as depressions microscopically. No evidence of cellular proliferation has been found at early, intermediate, or late phases of healing.

4.4. TRANSMYOCARDIAL "NONLASER" REVASCULARIZATION IN ANIMALS

We have recently examined porcine hearts from animals that had transmyocardial revascularization by mechanical needle puncture, cryotherapy, or radio frequency at varying intervals after treatment (see Chapters 10, 11). The healing response was similar in the three treatments and was complete by 1 month, with scar areas showing muscular arteries, arterioles, and neocapillaries. A detailed morphometric analysis of the number of different types of vessels was performed in hearts exposed to cryotherapy. The regions of interest included the treatment site, areas bordering 1 mm and 2 mm around the treatment site, and a remote "control" area greater than 2 mm away from the treatment site. The number of muscular arteries was greatest within the treatment site compared with bordering regions and was least in the control area. Arterioles were maximal in the border regions compared with the control or treatment sites; there were no differences in the number of arterioles between the control and treatment sites. In contrast, neocapillaries were maximal in the control area and minimal in the treatment site. Measurement of left ventricular ejection fraction failed to show and any untoward effects of cryotherapy.

Similar results were found in another preliminary study of mechanical myocardial channeling using a needle (Fig. 4-5). Transmyocardial revascularization performed 2 months earlier markedly reduced ST segment elevation, lowered the frequency of premature ventricular contractions (PVCs) and episodes of ventricular fibrillation after left anterior decending coronary artery (LAD) occlusion (Slepian et al., 2000). Despite these encouraging results, it is not clear whether the benefit is derived from the creation of conductance vessels or from some nonspecific effect of healed myocardial injury.

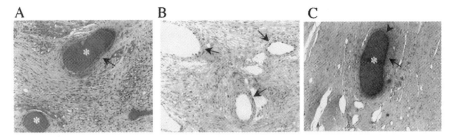

FIGURE 4-5. Sections of pig myocardium at 1 week (A and B) and 30 days (C) after transmyocardial revascularization. A, arteriogenesis showing early vessel formation in a channel created by blunt trauma (Movat pentachrome). A developing muscular artery within an area of granulation tissue and proteoglycan matrix is shown (arrow); note that the vessel is filled with barium gelatin (asterisk), suggestive of flow. B, immunostaining of the same area as in A using an antibody directed against bromodeoxyuridine to identify extensive proliferation within endothelial cells and smooth muscle cells of the developing vessels. The arrows in panel B represent vessels showing a positive reaction for bromodeoxyuridine. C, mature dilated muscular artery within a scar showing a well-developed medial layer (arrow) and external elastica (arrowhead); asterisk shows barium gelatin.

4.5. CAN ARTERIOGENESIS BE DEMONSTRATED IN ANIMALS?

The most comprehensive experimental work on in vivo arteriogenesis comes from the laboratory of Wolfgang Schaper et al. in their studies in rabbits and dogs (Schaper and Ito, 1996). In a model of bilateral femoral artery occlusion in the rabbit, corkscrew collateral arteries in the thigh are apparent by 1 week and are associated with active proliferation of endothelial and smooth muscle cells. There was a sixfold increase in the maximum collateral conductance in the first week in the rabbit thigh. In regions without a perfusion deficit, collateral vessels were observed. In areas with a perfusion deficit, there were no visible collateral vessels, but there was evidence of capillary proliferation, or angiogenesis. These data show that angiogenesis occurs in regions of ischemia, whereas collateral growth occurs in the absence of ischemia and may be the result of the presence of a pressure gradient rather than ischemia (Fig. 4-6) (Ito et al., 1997a).

Other studies by the same group demonstrated increased numbers of monocyte/macrophages in the area of the enhanced vascular growth. MCP-1 gene expression and protein secretion are upregulated by shear stress and cyclic strain on endothelial cells (Wang et al., 1995). MCP-1 infusion, in the model of bilateral femoral artery occlusion, increased both collateral and peripheral conductance (Ito et al., 1997b). Histologic and angiographic findings suggested that the increase in conductance is caused by enhanced vessel growth, either through greater accumulation of macrophages or by an unknown direct proliferative effects of MCP-1 on smooth muscle cells and endothelial cells. Other growth factors such as VEGF, aFGF, bFGF, insulin-like growth factor-1 (IGF-1), and PDGF are also potentially involved in the process of collateralization.

4.6. HOW TO ACHIEVE INCREASE BLOOD FLOW INTO THE ISCHEMIC MYOCARDIUM

The development of collateral circulation may offer the possibility to alter the natural history of coronary atherosclerotic disease (Wolf et al., 1998). Collateral vessels, on demand, have the capability to expand their diameter by a factor of 20 and increase their flow capacity by 10 (Schaper, 1979; Schaper

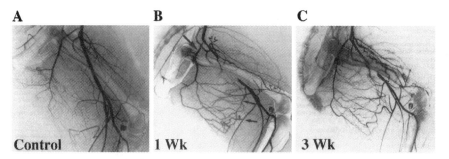

FIGURE 4-6. Development of collateral arteries after femoral artery occlusion in the rabbit. Postmortem angiogram from a control animal without femoral artery occlusion (A); no visible collaterals are present. One week after femoral artery occlusion (B), collaterals are visible in the quadriceps muscle (large open arrows) and entering the sapena parava and magna artery (small solid arrows). The large solid arrow indicates the arteriae genuales in the adductor muscle originating from the arteria femoralis profunda. Three weeks after femoral artery occlusion, the collateral arteries are substantially increased (Reproduced with permission from Ito WD et al. Angiogenesis but not collateral growth is associated with ischemia after femoral artery occlusion. *Am J Physiol* 1997; 273: H1255–H1265).

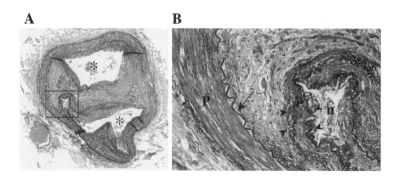

FIGURE 4-7. An epicardial coronary artery from a young patient whose heart showed a healed myocardial infarction. Although the artery at the time of infarction was totally occluded by a thrombus (A), the thrombus is focally replaced by recanalized arteries (asterisk), which have well-formed vessel walls inside the epicardial muscular artery. A high-power view of the area outlined by the black box in A is shown in B. Note the parent artery (P) with its internal elastic lamina (arrow); within the lumen of this artery is another new muscular artery (n) with its own internal and external elastic laminae and media (between arrowheads). This morphology confirms the possibility of creating new arteries with normal histologic characteristics.

and Ito, 1996). Clinically, it is common to see total occlusion of a vessel in the absence of a myocardial infarction, because of collateral development. However, there is marked individual variability and interspecies variability among animal models. Some humans have the intrinsic ability to form muscular arteries "de novo" that contains a well-formed media and internal elastic lamina (Fig. 4-7). Large

epicardial collaterals may exist in dogs and humans, but in the pig and in some humans, only small collaterals are found. The small vessel collaterals are the result of small capillary growth or angiogenesis (Risau, 1993). The large epicardial collaterals develop from enlargement of pre-existing interarteriolar connections (arteriogenesis) (Wolf et al., 1998). Because of the complexities of vessel

A. Normal
myocardium

B. Myocardial infarction
with angiogenesis

C. Arteriogenesis and
angiogenesis in an area
of infarction

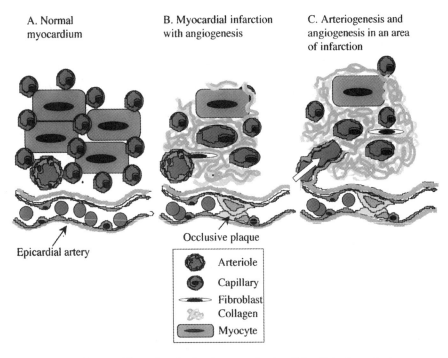

Epicardial artery

Occlusive plaque

	Arteriole
	Capillary
	Fibroblast
	Collagen
	Myocyte

FIGURE 4-8. Cartoon illustrating the development of epicardial collateral arteries in
response to coronary artery occlusion. Normal myocardium shows numerous
capillaries and arterioles and a patent epicardial coronary artery (A). A myocardial
infarction resulting from an occlusive atherosclerotic plaque; the distal myocardial
vascular bed shows a healed myocardial infarction, because no collateral arteries were
formed (B). Nevertheless, the infarcted area contains a large number of capillaries
(angiogenesis), but the blood flow to this bed is inadequate for maintaining normal
contractility. When there is both arteriogenesis (large white arrow) and angiogenesis
from epicardial collateral formation, the myocardium around the area of previous
infarct will no longer be ischemic (C). Thus, for effective treatment of myocardial
ischemia, the development of epicardial collateral arteries is required rather than small
capillaries.

development and our naive understanding of
the underlying mechanisms, the formation of
new vessels by physical injury or the overexpression of angiogenic genes alone may not
afford much patient benefit. This may result
from the wrong type of vessel being formed
and anatomic limitations to adequate supply
of the distal ischemic bed.

The primary goal of myocardial revascularization should involve the creation of large
epicardial or intramyocardial collateral arteries proximal to the site of coronary occlusion that branch and anastamose to the
arterial circulation within the zone of ischemia (Fig. 4-8). This would require arteriogenesis to provide blood flow initially and

angiogenesis to support the distribution of
the blood within the myocardium. Transmyocardial revascularization thus far appears
to promote angiogenesis only within the
area of the channels. Although arteriogenesis
after transmyocardial revascularization has
been observed in the nonischemic pig model,
it remains to be proven whether these newly
developed vessels would relieve chronic
ischemia. The demonstration of true arteriogenesis would involve demonstration of
"corkscrew" epicardial collaterals in a large
animal (e.g., adult pig) within 6 weeks after
the procedure. Postmortem angiography
using bismuth and gelatin at physiologic pressure of 80–100mmHg in arteries predilated

with papaverine would be an appropriate method to demonstrate large collateral vessels. Histologic examination must also be performed to demonstrate endothelial and smooth muscle cell proliferation within the collateral vessel wall and the occurrence of remodeling over time. Although myocardial sections in the region of ischemia may show capillary formation, this does not necessarily constitute true arteriogenesis.

4.7. CONCLUSION

For patients with diffuse coronary artery disease and refractory ischemia, transmyocardial revascularization alone or in combination with gene therapy is increasingly becoming popular for improving myocardial perfusion. Our understanding of the requirement to create functional large muscular arteries in the clinical setting is evolving. The current knowledge of the precise genetic and/or protein factors associated with arterial development is insufficient to precisely regulate vessel development in the adult heart. Thus treatment with transmyocardial revascularization and/or gene therapy as a rationale for promoting angiogenesis in an attempt to rescue the failing heart should be judicious. For patients with intractable angina and no recourse, these treatments may be advocated only when the patient and the community have a clear understanding that these are palliative procedures of which relief of angina has proven to be the only benefit.

References

Asahara T, Murohara T, Sullivan A et al. Isolation of putative progenitor endothelial cells for angiogenesis. *Science* 1997; 275: 964–967.

Burkhoff D, Fisher PE, Apfelbaum M et al. Histologic appearance of transmyocardial laser channels after 4 1/2 weeks. *Ann Thorac Surg* 1996; 61: 1532–1534.

Carmeliet P, Ferreira V, Breier G et al. Abnormal blood vessel development and lethality in embryos lacking a single VEGF allele. *Nature* 1996; 380: 435–439.

Carmeliet P. Mechanisms of angiogenesis and arteriogenesis. *Nat Med* 2000; 6: 389–395.

Chu V, Kuang J, McGinn A et al. Angiogenic response induced by mechanical transmyocardial revascularization. *J Thorac Cardiovasc Surg* 1999; 118: 849–856.

Cines DB, Pollak ES, Buck CA et al. Endothelial cells in physiology and in the pathophysiology of vascular disorders. *Blood* 1998; 91: 3527–3561.

Cooley DA, Frazier OH, Kadipasaoglu KA et al. Transmyocardial laser revascularization: clinical experience with twelve-month follow-up. *J Thorac Cardiovasc Surg* 1996; 111: 791–797.

Dettman RW, Denetclaw W Jr., Ordahl CP et al. Common epicardial origin of coronary vascular smooth muscle, perivascular fibroblasts, and intermyocardial fibroblasts in the avian heart. *Dev Biol* 1998; 193: 169–181.

Fisher PE, Khomoto T, DeRosa CM et al. Histologic analysis of transmyocardial channels: comparison of CO_2 and holmium:YAG lasers. *Ann Thorac Surg* 1997; 64: 466–472.

Gassler N, Wintzer HO, Stubbe HM et al. Transmyocardial laser revascularization. Histological features in human nonresponder myocardium. *Circulation* 1997; 95: 371–375.

Glagov S, Weisenberg E, Zarins CK et al. Compensatory enlargement of human atherosclerotic coronary arteries. *N Engl J Med* 1987; 316: 1371–1375.

Horvath KA, Smith WJ, Laurence RG et al. Recovery and viability of an acute myocardial infarct after transmyocardial laser revascularization. *J Am Coll Cardiol* 1995; 25: 258–263.

Horvath KA, Cohn LH, Cooley DA et al. Transmyocardial laser revascularization: results of a multicenter trial with transmyocardial laser revascularization used as sole therapy for end-stage coronary artery disease. *J Thorac Cardiovasc Surg* 1997; 113: 645–653.

Hughes GC, Lowe JE, Kypson AP et al. Neovascularization after transmyocardial laser revascularization in a model of chronic ischemia. *Ann Thorac Surg* 1998; 66: 2029–2036.

Ito WD, Arras M, Scholz D et al. Angiogenesis but not collateral growth is associated with ischemia after femoral artery occlusion. *Am J Physiol* 1997a; 273: H1255–H1265.

Ito WD, Arras M, Winkler B et al. Monocyte chemotactic protein-1 increases collateral and peripheral conductance after femoral artery occlusion. *Circ Res* 1997b; 80: 829–837.

March RJ. Transmyocardial laser revascularization with the CO_2 laser: one year results of a randomized, controlled trial. *Semin Thorac Cardiovasc Surg* 1999; 11: 12–18.

Mirhoseini M, Cayton MM. Revascularization of the heart by laser. *J Microsurg* 1981; 2: 253–260.

Mirhoseini M, Shelgikar S, Cayton MM. New concepts in revascularization of the myocardium. *Ann Thorac Surg* 1988; 45: 415–420.

Pepper MS, Vassalli JD, Montesano R et al. Urokinase-type plasminogen activator is induced in migrating capillary endothelial cells. *J Cell Biol* 1987; 105: 2535–2541.

Pepper MS. Manipulating angiogenesis. From basic science to the bedside. *Arterioscler Thromb Vasc Biol* 1997; 17: 605–619.

Pepper MS, Belin D, Montesano R et al. Transforming growth factor-beta 1 modulates basic fibroblast growth factor-induced proteolytic and angiogenic properties of endothelial cells *in vitro*. *J Cell Biol* 1990a; 111: 743–755.

Pepper MS, Montesano R. Proteolytic balance and capillary morphogenesis. *Cell Differ Dev* 1990b; 32: 319–327.

Rahimtoola SH. The hibernating myocardium. *Am Heart J* 1989; 117: 211–221.

Rahimtoola SH. Concept and evaluation of hibernating myocardium. *Annu Rev Med* 1999; 50: 75–86.

Rahimtoola SH, Grunkemeier GL, Teply JF et al. Changes in coronary bypass surgery leading to improved survival. *JAMA* 1981; 246: 1912–1916.

Risau W. Development of the vascular system in organs and tissues. *Collateral Circulation—Heart, Brain, Kidney, Limbs*. Boston: Kluwer Academic, 1993.

Sampath R, Kukielka GL, Smith CW et al. Shear stress-mediated changes in the expression of leukocyte adhesion receptors on human umbilical vein endothelial cells in vitro. *Ann Biomed Eng* 1995; 23: 247–256.

Schaper W. Collateral circulation. V. Mechanisms of collateral enlargement. *The Pathophysiology of Myocardial Perfusion*. Amsterdam: Elsevier/North-Holland Biomedical, 1979.

Schaper W, Ito WD. Molecular mechanisms of coronary collateral vessel growth. *Circ Res* 1996; 79: 911–919.

Schofield PM, Sharples LD, Caine N et al. Transmyocardial laser revascularisation in patients with refractory angina: a randomised controlled trial. *Lancet* 1999; 353: 519–524.

Sigel JE, Abramovich CM, Lytle BW et al. Transmyocardial laser revascularization: three sequential autopsy cases. *J Thorac Cardiovasc Surg* 1998; 115: 1381–1385.

Slepian MJ, LePrince P, Toporoff B et al. Myocardial conditioning via mechanical channeling plus healing limits ischemic consequences of acute coronary occlusion (abstract). *J Am Coll Cardiol* 2000; 35 (*Suppl* A): 369A.

Thurston G, Murphy TJ, Baluk P et al. Angiogenesis in mice with chronic airway inflammation: strain-dependent differences. *Am J Pathol* 1998; 153: 1099–1112.

Wang DL, Wung BS, Shyy YJ et al. Mechanical strain induces monocyte chemotactic protein-1 gene expression in endothelial cells. Effects of mechanical strain on monocyte adhesion to endothelial cells. *Circ Res* 1995; 77: 294–302.

White FC, Carroll SM, Magnet A et al. Coronary collateral development in swine after coronary artery occlusion. *Circ Res* 1992; 71: 1490–1500.

Whittaker P, Kloner RA, Przyklenk K. Laser-mediated transmural myocardial channels do not salvage acutely ischemic myocardium. *J Am Coll Cardiol* 1993; 22: 302–309.

Whittaker P, Rakusan K, Kloner RA. Transmural channels can protect ischemic tissue. Assessment of long-term myocardial response to laser- and needle-made channels. *Circulation* 1996; 93: 143–152.

Wolf C, Cai WJ, Vosschulte R et al. Vascular remodeling and altered protein expression during growth of coronary collateral arteries. *J Mol Cell Cardiol* 1998; 30: 2291–2305.

5

Revascularization Versus Denervation: What Are the Mechanisms of Symptom Relief?

G. Chad Hughes, M.D., and James E. Lowe, M.D.

Division of Thoracic and Cardiovascular Surgery
Duke University Medical Center
Durham, North Carolina

SUMMARY

Numerous hypotheses have been offered to explain the decrease in angina after TMR.

One early theory focused on "patent channels," but this has fallen out of favor.

Two mechanisms that are important to clinical benefits of TMR are laser-induced angiogenesis and regional myocardial denervation.

Regional myocardial denervation is a result of TMR; however, it does not appear to account for long-term clinical results and may in fact allow silent ischemia in the early postoperative period.

Angiogenesis is the most likely mechanism of action responsible for clinical improvement after TMR, and research should be done to find ways to increase or augment this process.

Current studies are focused on which process of TMR—laser energy versus mechanical means—yields greater neovascularization.

5.1. INTRODUCTION

In the United States alone, up to 200,000 patients annually may be eligible for transmyocardial laser revascularization (TMR) (Mukherjee et al., 1999), with a range of potential indications including sole therapy for refractory angina pectoris in end-stage coronary artery disease, combined therapy with bypass grafting or angioplasty for nonrevascularizable territories, and treatment of coronary vasculopathy after cardiac transplantation (Hughes et al., 1999c) (see Chapter 19). Despite this potentially wide application, the mechanism of action of TMR remains controversial (Brinker, 1999). Since the original description (Mirhoseini and Cayton, 1981), numerous hypotheses have been put

Myocardial Revascularization: Novel Percutaneous Approaches, Edited by George S. Abela.
ISBN 0-471-36166-6   Copyright © 2002 Wiley-Liss, Inc.

forward to explain the observed reductions in angina class seen after the procedure. These postulated mechanisms have focused mainly on direct myocardial perfusion via patent channels, myocardial denervation, and therapeutic angiogenesis (Roethy et al., 1999).

The original hypothesized mechanism of action of TMR was the so-called "patent channel theory" (Hughes et al., 1999c), whereby the laser channels were thought to connect with the left ventricular cavity and remain patent, thus providing a direct source for oxygenated blood to perfuse the myocardium (Horvath et al., 1995; Mirhoseini et al., 1986; Okada et al., 1991). The rationale behind the procedure was an attempt to surgically mimic the reptilian pattern of myocardial circulation, in which blood flows directly into myocardial tissue from the ventricular cavity (Kohmoto et al., 1997b; Sen et al., 1965). However, this theory of chronically patent channels has generally fallen out of favor. Numerous studies in various animal models (Hardy et al., 1990; Hughes et al., 2000a; Kohmoto et al., 1996; Kohmoto et al., 1997a; Landreneau et al., 1991; Mueller et al., 1998; Whittaker et al., 1993) have demonstrated no physiologically meaningful increase in myocardial blood flow via TMR channels in the acute setting. These studies have been supplemented by histologic findings in both experimental animals (Fisher et al., 1997; Fleischer et al., 1996; Hughes et al., 1999d; Malekan et al., 1998a, 1998b) and autopsy studies (Burkhoff et al., 1996; Burkhoff et al., 1997; Gassler et al., 1997; Krabatsch et al., 1996; Sigel et al., 1998), demonstrating that channels do not maintain patency but rather fill with organized thrombus and become surrounded by granulation tissue. Over the course of several weeks, the thrombus undergoes progressive organization to finally replace the channel region with fibrous tissue (Fisher et al., 1997) (Fig. 5-1).

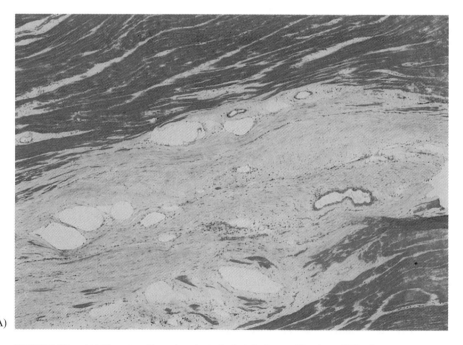

(A)

FIGURE 5-1. (A) Hematoxylin and eosin stain (original magnification ×100) of a TMR channel sectioned longitudinally shows a hypocellular region representing the channel remnant at 6 months after TMR. (B) Masson's trichrome staining (original magnification ×100) shows the TMR channel remnant to be filled with blue staining connective tissue (Reproduced with permission from the Society of Thoracic Surgeons, Hughes et al., 1998).

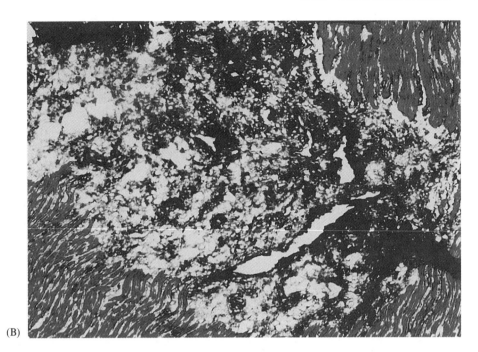

(B)

FIGURE 5-1. *Continued.*

Burkhoff and colleagues have coined the term "channel remnant" (Burkhoff et al., 1997) to describe these regions.

Clinical results support these observations. In our experience, improvement in anginal class after the procedure is typically delayed by weeks to months (Landolfo et al., 1999), a finding inconsistent with an acute increase in myocardial blood flow via patent channels. Likewise, there appears to be a significant incidence of myocardial ischemia in the first 48 h postoperatively (Hughes et al., 1999a), with the majority of perioperative morbidity and mortality secondary to ischemic complications (Hughes et al., 1999b). This again argues against an acute improvement in myocardial perfusion in the early postoperative period.

Because of the overwhelming evidence that the channels do not remain patent, the two mechanisms currently felt to be most likely responsible for the clinical benefits of TMR are laser-induced regional myocardial denervation and laser-induced angiogenesis (see Chapter 6). The theory behind regional denervation is that TMR produces local destruction of nerve fibers in the treated myocardial regions such that patients experience a reduction in angina without any significant increase in myocardial perfusion. The angiogenesis hypothesis, on the other hand, holds that laser injury leads to new blood vessel growth with an improvement in angina symptoms caused by an increase in oxygen delivery. The evidence surrounding each of these mechanisms is presented in this chapter with an emphasis on work from our laboratory. Because in the clinical setting TMR is applied to regions of chronically ischemic, yet viable (hibernating) myocardium, we (St. Louis et al., 2000) have developed an animal model using microswine to reproduce this state, which allows us to study the potential mechanism(s) of action of TMR under conditions similar to those seen clinically (Fig. 5-2).

5.2. MYOCARDIAL DENERVATION

Because of the apparent disparity in the clinical arena between reductions in angina class and improved perfusion after TMR (Sundt and Kwong, 1999), denervation has been suggested as a potential mechanism of action of the procedure. Kwong and colleagues (1997)

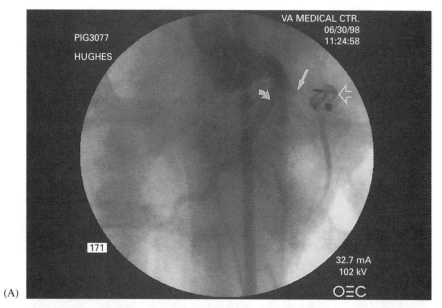

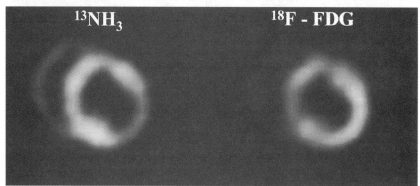

FIGURE 5-2. (A) Coronary angiogram demonstrating the experimental model of hibernating myocardium used in our laboratory. A radiolucent hydraulic occluder (straight arrow) and ultrasonic flow probe (open arrow) are placed around the proximal left circumflex coronary artery (LCx). The flow probe readings are used to guide the production of an approximately 90% stenosis of the proximal LCx. The result is an area of chronic ischemia in the lateral and posteroinferior walls of the left ventricle supplied by the LCx. Note normal caliber left anterior descending coronary artery (curved arrow) (Reproduced with permission from the Society of Thoracic Surgeons, Hughes et al., 1999f). (B) Positron emission tomography ^{13}N-ammonia perfusion scan (left) performed 2 weeks after production of the LCx stenosis demonstrating a flow defect in the lateral and posteroinferior walls of the left ventricle as seen on short-axis view. Corresponding ^{18}F-fluorodeoxyglucose uptake scan is seen on the right, showing a relative increase in glucose utilization in the region of the flow defect consistent with preserved myocardial viability. This flow-metabolism mismatch is characteristic of chronic hibernating myocardium. (Reproduced with permission from the Society of Thoracic Surgeons, Hughes et al., 1998).

were the first to present evidence for regional myocardial denervation after TMR. They used a Ho:YAG laser to perform TMR in nonischemic canine myocardium and demonstrated diminished cardiac afferent nerve function, as assessed by blood pressure response to epicardial application of bradykinin (Fig. 5-3), as well as regional sympathetic

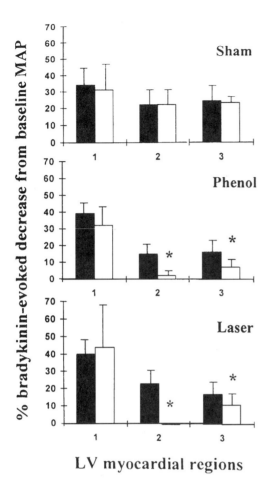

FIGURE 5-3. Hemodynamic response to bradykinin stimulation in base (1), mid (2), and apical (3) regions of the heart preoperatively (black bars) and 2 weeks after (open bars) holmium:YAG TMR (bottom graph). Note significant reduction in hemodynamic response in mid and apical regions of TMR-treated hearts indicating afferent denervation (TMR performed in midregion of heart only and consequently afferent innervation preserved in base). The results seen after TMR are similar to those after topical phenol treatment of the myocardium (middle graph), a well-established technique for producing local denervation. There was no difference in hemodynamic response pre-versus 2 weeks postoperatively in sham animals undergoing thoracotomy but no TMR (top graph) (* indicate $p < 0.05$ for post- versus preoperative values) (Reproduced with permission from the Society of Thoracic Surgeons, Sundt and Kwong, 1999).

denervation, manifest as a loss of the sympathetic neural-specific enzyme tyrosine hydroxylase, in the lased regions 2 weeks after the procedure. They performed a follow-up

study (Kwong et al., 1998) in which partial-thickness laser channels, similar to those produced during percutaneous myocardial laser revascularization, also produced denervation, although not to the degree observed with full-thickness TMR. These findings have been demonstrated by other laboratories as well (Kwong et al., 1997). However, Hirsch et al. (1999), using direct neural stimulation techniques, found that nonischemic canine myocardium was innervated 30 min after Ho:YAG TMR. Whether these discordant results are caused by the short time after TMR at which innervation was assessed or by the alternative experimental methods used is unclear. What is clear is that TMR invokes an intense inflammatory response in the lased regions (Hughes et al., 1999d), a response that likely plays a large role in the local destruction of nerve fibers. This inflammatory response is in its early stage of development 30 min postoperatively. Consequently, one might speculate that were the studies of Hirsch and colleagues to be repeated several days or weeks after TMR, different results might be obtained.

Denervation has been demonstrated clinically as well. Al-Sheikh and colleagues (1999) used C-11 hydroxyephedrine (HED) positron emission tomographic (PET) scanning to assess regional sympathetic innervation in human subjects after TMR. HED is an inactive norepinephrine analog and a highly specific tracer of presynaptic nerve terminals (Al-Sheikh et al., 1999). Using this tracer, they demonstrated sympathetic denervation in the lased regions of six of eight patients 2 months after Ho:YAG TMR.

If TMR produces regional denervation, one might expect ischemia occurring in the postoperative period to be clinically silent. We have investigated this phenomenon in 21 patients undergoing CO_2 TMR (Hughes et al., 1999a) and found that more than 50% had ischemic electrocardiographic changes in the first 48 h postoperatively. This ischemia was clinically silent in over 60% of the patients. These findings lend further support to the hypothesis that TMR produces regional myocardial denervation.

The aforementioned experimental studies (Hirsch et al., 1999; Kwong et al., 1997; Kwong et al., 1998) were carried out in nonischemic hearts and only examined myocardial innervation after TMR with a Ho:YAG laser. In addition, these studies did not examine whether the observed regional denervation persists long term after the procedure. Prior work after myocardial infarction, another potential cause of regional myocardial denervation, demonstrated that reinnervation to the infarct zone occurs during the 6 months after infarction (Fallen et al., 1999). Consequently, we sought to explore whether a similar phenomenon might occur after TMR. Using the previously described model of hibernating myocardium, we examined regional myocardial sympathetic innervation 6 months after TMR with the three laser systems currently in clinical use, namely, Ho:YAG, CO$_2$, and xenon chloride excimer.

Myocardial sympathetic innervation was assessed using techniques similar to those of Kwong et al. (Kwong et al., 1997, 1998). Specifically, immunohistochemistry for anatomic localization and immunoblotting for protein quantification of tyrosine hydroxylase, a neural-specific enzyme found in sympathetic efferent nerves (Fleming-Jones and McFadden, 1995; Oki et al., 1994) were performed. This enzyme is involved in the biosynthesis of norepinephrine from tyrosine, a reaction unique to nervous tissue (Wooten and Coyle, 1973). The cardiac visceral afferent nerve fibers responsible for the pain of angina pectoris and the sympathetic efferent fibers travel together in a subepicardial location adjacent to the coronary vasculature (Kwong et al., 1997), thus making tyrosine hydroxylase a reasonable surrogate for cardiac afferent nerve damage. Using these techniques, we have found evidence for regional sympathetic denervation in the lased regions 3 days after TMR (Figs. 5.4 and 5.6) (Hughes et al., 1999g), consistent with the results of prior studies. However, when examined 6 months postoperatively, TMR-treated myocardium appears to be innervated, as evidenced by equal concentrations of tyrosine hydroxylase in lased and nonlased regions of the heart (Fig. 5-5). Immunohistochemistry confirmed the presence of tyrosine hydroxylase in myocardium adjacent to the TMR channel remnants 6 months postoperatively (Fig. 5-6).

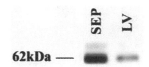

FIGURE 5-4. Representative immunoblot demonstrating tyrosine hydroxylase protein in lased left circumflex and untreated septal myocardium 3 days after holmium:YAG TMR. Note significant reduction in tyrosine hydroxylase protein in lased regions. LV = lased left circumflex region myocardium; SEP = nontreated septal myocardium (Courtesy of Hughes et al.).

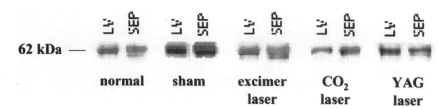

FIGURE 5-5. Representative immunoblot showing tyrosine hydroxylase protein in normal, untreated hibernating (sham), and lased (excimer, CO$_2$, YAG) myocardium. There is no difference in tyrosine hydroxylase protein concentration between any of the regions by quantitative densitometry. LV = lased left circumflex region myocardium; SEP = septal myocardium; excimer = xenon chloride excimer laser; CO$_2$ = carbon dioxide laser; YAG = holmium:YAG laser (Courtesy of Hughes et al.).

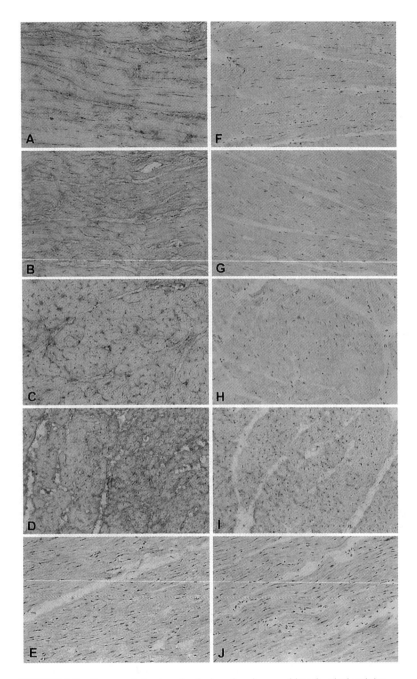

FIGURE 5-6. Representative tyrosine hydroxylase immunohistochemical staining (original magnification ×200) of lased (A–C) and sham-operated (D) left circumflex myocardium 6 months postoperatively as well as lased left circumflex myocardium 3 days postoperatively (E). Panels on the left have been stained with an antibody specific for tyrosine hydroxylase (stains red) and demonstrate myocardium immediately adjacent to holmium:YAG (A), CO_2 (B), and excimer (C) laser channel remnants (channel remnants not in field of view), as well as nonlased sham-operated left circumflex myocardium (D), and left circumflex myocardium adjacent to a holmium:YAG channel remnant 3 days postoperatively (E). Panels on the right (F–J) are the corresponding regions stained with a non-sense murine IgG monoclonal antibody to serve as a negative control. Note intact tyrosine hydroxylase staining in myocardium surrounding the laser channel remnants (A–C) 6 months postoperatively. Staining does not differ from nonlased hibernating left circumflex myocardium (D). By contrast, note marked reduction in tyrosine hydroxylase staining 3 days after TMR (E) (Courtesy of Hughes et al.).

Consequently, the data accrued from our laboratory and others seem to support the hypothesis that TMR produces regional myocardial denervation in the treated regions. However, reinnervation of the TMR-treated regions appears to occur, as evidenced by immunohistochemical staining and Western blot analysis showing normal levels of tyrosine hydroxylase in the lased regions 6 months postoperatively (Hughes et al., 1999g). Consequently, because reductions in angina after TMR persist beyond 6 months (Allen et al., 1999; Burkhoff et al., 1999; Frazier et al., 1999; Schofield et al., 1999), denervation does not appear to account for the long-term clinical results. Nevertheless, denervation remains clinically important, as it may allow silent ischemia in the early postoperative period, as described previously. Because of this potential for creating silent ischemia, patients undergoing TMR should be followed with serial electrocardiograms and cardiac enzymes to monitor for ongoing ischemia in the early postoperative period, as well as continued aggressive anti-ischemic medical management. Finally, sympathetic denervation, as seen after TMR, may promote denervation hypersensitivity, in which there is a heightened adrenoreceptor response to circulating catecholamines in the denervated regions. In theory, this may predispose to ventricular arrhythmias (Fallen et al., 1999), although this does not appear to be clinically relevant in our experience.

5.3. THERAPEUTIC ANGIOGENESIS

Angiogenesis is defined as the formation of new blood vessels from preexisting vessels by the process of cellular outgrowth (see Chapter 4). In mature organisms, endothelial cells do not normally proliferate unless stimulated by wounding, inflammation, or other pathological conditions (Ware and Simons, 1997). New blood vessel formation is a complex process involving several steps, including breakdown of the existing extracellular matrix underlying the endothelium, smooth muscle and endothelial cell migration, adhesion, and proliferation, formation of new vascular structures,

and deposition of a new extracellular matrix. A number of growth factors are capable of promoting angiogenesis, including the vascular endothelial growth factor (VEGF), fibroblast growth factor (FGF), and transforming growth factor (TGF) families, hepatocyte growth factor (HGF), and platelet-derived growth factor (PDGF), among others (Ware and Simons, 1997). Angiogenesis may represent an alternative mechanism for the clinical improvement seen after TMR.

Hardy et al. (1987) in 1987 were among the first investigators to note new blood vessels in the region of TMR channels. They used a low-power CO_2 laser to produce channels in normal canine myocardium and found histologic evidence for new blood vessel formation as early as 5 days postoperatively. Since that early work, numerous investigators (Fisher et al., 1997; Hughes et al., 1998; Hughes et al., 2000b; Kohmoto et al., 1997a; Kohmoto et al., 1998; Mack et al., 1997; Malekan et al., 1998b; Pelletier et al., 1998; Yamamoto et al., 1998) have published experimental studies carried out in nonischemic as well as ischemic myocardium documenting neovascularization in the region of the TMR channels at various time points postoperatively. These data have been confirmed in autopsy studies of patients undergoing TMR as well (Burkhoff et al., 1997; Gassler et al., 1997; Krabatsch et al., 1996).

After TMR, neovascularization appears to be enhanced both within the channel remnant and in the myocardium immediately surrounding the channels (Hughes et al., 1998; Kohmoto et al., 1998; Yamamoto et al., 1998). Kohmoto and colleagues (1998) performed both CO_2 and Ho:YAG TMR in normal canine myocardium and studied the animals for 2–3 weeks. Routine hematoxylin and eosin as well as immunohistochemical staining for the endothelial cell marker factor VIII and proliferating cell nuclear antigen (PCNA), a marker of cellular proliferation, were performed. They found a significant increase in vascular density within the channel remnants as well as in the myocardium surrounding the channels, with vessels within the remnants appearing to extend out into the surrounding myocardium. These vessels stained positive for PCNA, indicating that they were new and actively growing. These PCNA-stained vessels were observed only in the region of the channel remnants, which is consistent with the fact that active cell proliferation is rare in normal myocardium (Kohmoto et al., 1998). This study clearly demonstrates that vascular growth is stimulated within and immediately surrounding TMR channel remnants up to 3 weeks postoperatively.

Most of the studies investigating the effects of TMR on blood vessel growth have been performed in nonischemic animal models over relatively short time periods postoperatively. We have examined the neovascularization response 6 months after TMR in our porcine model of hibernating myocardium (Hughes et al., 1998). Using immunohistochemical staining for the endothelial cell-specific antibodies anti-factor VIII-related antigen and anti-human tie-2, we were able to clearly document a significant increase in vascular density in lased hibernating myocardium 6 months after TMR with both Ho:YAG and CO_2 lasers (Fig. 5-7). The neovessels did not stain for Flt4, a unique marker of lymphatic endothelial cells (Kaipainen et al., 1995), thus indicating that the observed vessels were truly vascular in origin (Hughes et al., 1999e). The vessels were further characterized by staining with HHF-35, an anti-smooth muscle actin antibody, and anti-collagen IV, an antibody to the collagen component of normal basement membrane. Compared with normal penetrating intramyocardial blood vessels, the neovessels demonstrated relatively increased staining with HHF-35 and decreased staining with anti-collagen IV (Fig. 5-8). These findings are typical of collateral vessels formed via arteriogenesis (the growth of arteries from pre-existing arterioles) and involved in improving blood flow to ischemic tissues (Schaper and Ito, 1996; Schaper et al., 2000).

PET and dobutamine stress echocardiography (DSE) before and 6 months after TMR in these same animals demonstrated a significant increase in myocardial blood flow (Fig. 5-9) and contractile reserve (Fig. 5-10) in the lased regions. These improvements were not seen in chronically ischemic animals undergoing sham thoracotomy (Hughes et al., 1999f). Similar results have been reported by other investigators (Horvath et al., 1998; Yamamoto et al., 1998).

The mechanism responsible for the observed neovascularization response after TMR appears to be related, at least in part, to an upregulation in angiogenic growth factor levels in the lased regions. Pelletier and colleagues (Pelletier et al., 1998) demonstrated a significant increase in tissue levels of the angiogenic growth factors TGF-β and basic FGF over ischemic controls up to 8 weeks postoperatively in a rat model of TMR. A follow-up study from the same laboratory (Chu et al., 1999) using a porcine ischemic model found an increase in VEGF protein levels 1 week postoperatively in treated regions. Likewise, using a similar porcine model (Horvath et al., 1999), Horvath et al. showed a twofold increase in VEGF messenger RNA in association with a threefold increase in vascular density in the lased regions 6 weeks after CO_2 TMR compared with untreated controls.

Finally, a major question remaining is whether laser energy is necessary for the angiogenic response and, if so, which of the numerous clinically available laser systems is superior. Several studies have suggested that the angiogenic response to TMR is a nonspecific response to injury, which may be produced using mechanical means. Malekan et al. (Malekan et al., 1998b) found no significant difference in vascular density in normal ovine myocardium 4 weeks after treatment with CO_2 laser or mechanical drill, both of which significantly increased vascular density over untreated control regions. Likewise, Chu et al. (Chu et al., 1999) found a similar increase in VEGF protein levels as well as vascular density 1 week after TMR using either a CO_2 laser or an 18-gauge hypodermic needle in chronically ischemic porcine hearts. Mack and colleagues (Mack et al., 1997), on the other hand, found significantly greater neovascularization 30 days after treatment with

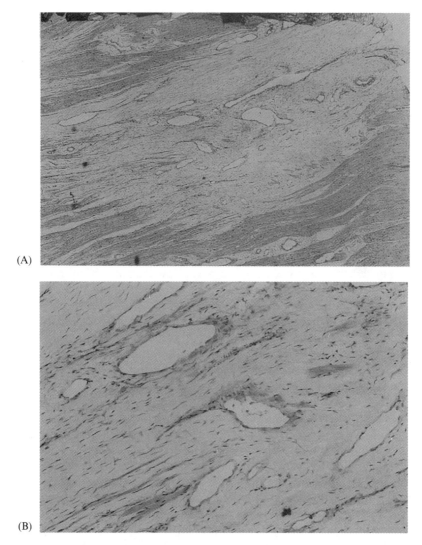

(A)

(B)

FIGURE 5-7. (A) Longitudinal section of a TMR channel stained using anti-human tie-2 (×100), an antibody specific for the soluble extracellular domain of the TEK protein, a receptor tyrosine kinase expressed exclusively in endothelial cells. Note the numerous red staining blood vessels within and adjacent to the channel remnant. (B) Higher magnification (×330) of the center of the channel remnant in (A), again demonstrating immunostaining (antigen appears red) of endothelial cells in the walls of the neovessels (Reproduced with permission from the Society of Thoracic Surgeons, Hughes et al., 1998).

excimer TMR as compared to nonlased channels in nonischemic sheep hearts.

Mechanical means of performing TMR produce tissue effects confined to their path through the myocardium. Lasers, on the other hand, produce a zone of reversible injury distant from the laser channels (Hardy et al., 1987), the degree of which varies with the type of laser used (Hunter and Dixon, 1985). As described previously, inflammation is an important potential contributor to angiogenesis and inflammatory cells such as macrophages and neutrophils infiltrating the region of laser injury may release numerous cyto-

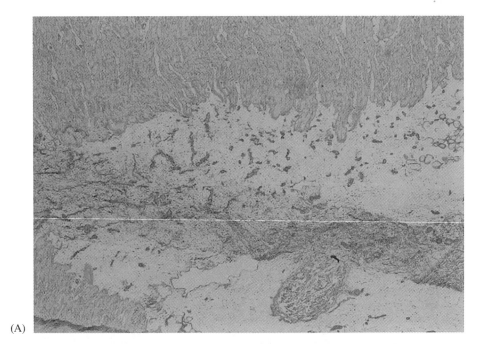

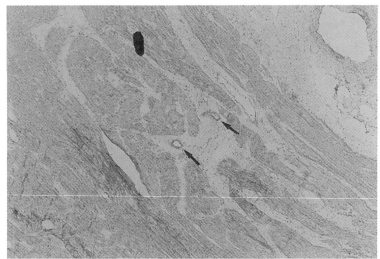

(A)

(B)

FIGURE 5-8. HHF-35 (anti-smooth muscle actin) staining (original magnification ×40) of (A) numerous red-staining neovessels within a TMR channel and (B) normal penetrating intramyocardial vessels (arrows). Note relatively increased HHF-35 staining of neovessels versus normal vessels. Anti-collagen IV staining (×200) of (C) neovessel (arrow) at periphery of TMR channel and (D) normal penetrating vessels (arrows). Note relatively decreased collagen IV staining of neovessel versus normal vessels (Reproduced with permission from the Society of Thoracic Surgeons, Hughes et al., 1998).

kines capable of stimulating the expression of angiogenic growth factors, upregulating their receptors, and downregulating naturally present angiogenesis inhibitors (Schaper and Ito, 1996; Ware and Simons, 1997). Consequently, one might hypothesize that the use of laser energy, with its increased inflammatory response, might yield greater neovasculariza-

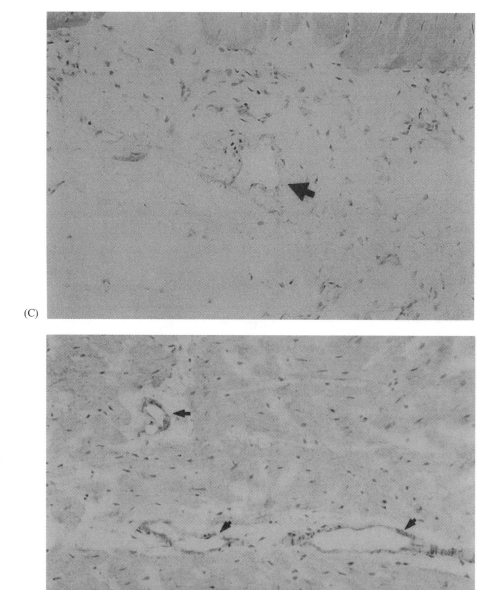

(C)

(D)

FIGURE 5-8.   *Continued.*

tion for a given number of channels compared with mechanical means. However, other energy sources, such as radio frequency ablation, might also be effective in inducing reversible myocardial injury and a secondary angiogenic response at a distance from their site of direct myocardial application and thus might be used for TMR in the future (Roethy et al., 1999).

We have compared the long-term angiogenic response after TMR with Ho:YAG, CO_2, and xenon chloride excimer lasers

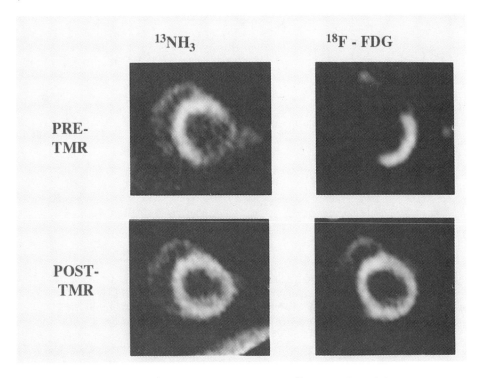

FIGURE 5-9. Baseline positron emission tomography (PET) ^{13}N-ammonia perfusion scan (top left) demonstrating a flow defect in the lateral and posteroinferior walls of the left ventricle as seen on the short-axis view. Corresponding ^{18}F-fluorodeoxyglucose uptake scan is seen on the top right, showing a relative increase in glucose utilization in the region of the flow defect consistent with preserved myocardial viability. (Bottom) Corresponding post-TMR PET scan from the same animal. Note the increase in ^{13}N-ammonia accumulation in the lased left circumflex distribution 6 months postoperatively (bottom left), consistent with increased blood flow. There is more homogeneous ^{18}F-fluorodeoxyglucose uptake (bottom right) associated with this improvement in blood flow (Reproduced with permission from the Society of Thoracic Surgeons, Hughes et al., 1999f).

(Hughes et al., 2000b). Both the Ho:YAG and CO_2 lasers are infrared lasers that use thermal ablation to create transmyocardial channels. Excimer lasers, on the other hand, are "cold" lasers that operate deep within the ultraviolet spectrum and produce tissue ablation via dissociation of molecular bonds (Mack et al., 1997). Consequently, excimer lasers are more purely ablative and produce less damage to surrounding myocardium than the infrared lasers. Of the infrared lasers, Ho:YAG produces greater lateral thermal damage than CO_2 (Deckelbaum, 1994). Using our model of hibernating myocardium, we found a significant increase in myocardial blood flow by PET and contractile reserve by DSE 6 months

after TMR with both the Ho:YAG and CO_2 lasers. No significant change in regional perfusion or function was seen 6 months after excimer TMR or sham thoracotomy. Likewise, significantly greater neovascularization was observed in the Ho:YAG and CO_2 lased regions than with either the sham procedure or excimer TMR (Fig. 5-11). Ho:YAG laser treatment appeared to invoke a greater neovascularization response than CO_2 laser treatment at 6 months postoperatively, although both were associated with an improvement in regional perfusion and function. In this study, TMR was performed according to the clinical protocol with a channel density of approximately 1 per cm^2. These results demonstrate

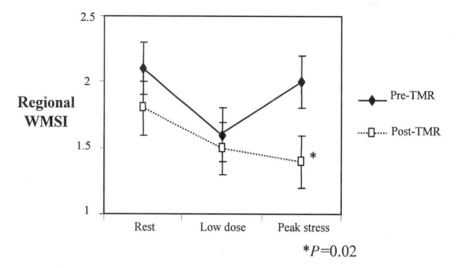

FIGURE 5-10.   Mean regional wall motion score index (WMSI) (1 = normal, 2 = hypokinetic, 3 = akinetic, 4 = dyskinetic) at rest, low stress, and peak stress for the lateral and posteroinferior walls of the left ventricle before and 6 months after their treatment with TMR. Note the trend toward improved resting function and the significant improvement in regional WMSI at peak stress 6 months after TMR (Reproduced with permission from the Society of Thoracic Surgeons, Hughes et al., 1999f).

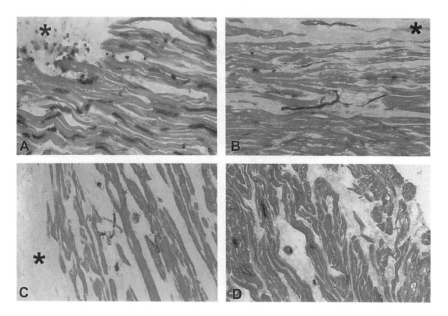

FIGURE 5-11.   Endogenous endothelial alkaline phosphatase staining (original magnification ×100) of representative sections from hibernating myocardium lased with holmium:YAG (A), CO_2 (B), and excimer (C) lasers and from nonlased hibernating myocardium (D) in a sham group animal. Note the progressive decrease in blue staining intensity, characteristic of endothelial cells, from A through D (* indicate location of TMR channel remnant) (Reproduced with permission from the Society of Thoracic Surgeons, Hughes et al., 2000b).

that infrared lasers produce a greater angiogenic response than excimer laser TMR.

This is supported by recent work demonstrating a dose response to the number of channels produced with the excimer laser. Using a porcine ischemic model, Lee and colleagues (Lee et al., 1999) found no increase in perfusion 4 weeks after treatment of a given area of myocardium with 10 excimer-lased channels but a significant increase when the same area was treated with 50 channels. These findings support the hypothesis that angiogenesis is related to inflammation, as a greater number of channels are needed to produce a given level of inflammatory response with the excimer compared with the infrared lasers. Likewise, if one considers that myocardial injury after excimer TMR is rather analogous to that seen after mechanical TMR, that is, essentially confined to the path through the myocardium, then the above data also suggest that infrared laser might be superior to mechanical TMR for inducing angiogenesis as well.

In summary, TMR clearly induces neovascularization in the lased regions, likely via an upregulation of the angiogenesis/arteriogenesis cascade secondary to the associated inflammatory response after laser injury. The new blood vessels have been demonstrated experimentally to be present at least 6 months postoperatively and are associated with improved regional perfusion and function in animal studies. Whether laser energy is necessary for producing this sustained angiogenic response remains unclear, although for a given channel density per area of myocardium, it appears that infrared lasers are superior to excimer laser and, likely, mechanical means of channel production in stimulating new blood vessel growth.

5.4. SUMMARY

Of the various mechanisms postulated to underlie the observed reductions in angina seen in the months to years after TMR, angiogenesis appears most likely to be responsible. Myocardial denervation clearly occurs in the early postoperative period and may persist for several weeks to months. However, reinnervation of the lased myocardial regions has been demonstrated experimentally, and thus denervation likely does not explain the long-term benefits of the procedure. Angiogenesis, on the other hand, has been observed both in humans and experimental animals and appears to be present long term after TMR. This angiogenic response has been associated with improved perfusion and function in chronic animal studies and likely is the predominant mechanism responsible for the long-term reductions in angina seen after the procedure. Why improvements in myocardial blood flow have been less consistent in the clinical arena is unclear, although marked improvements have been noted in individual cases (Hughes et al., 1999c) while in others little change is seen. This lack of consistency may relate to the fact that the perfusion changes are likely relatively small and the clinical population heterogeneous in terms of the degree of their pretreatment coronary disease and perfusion deficits, thus making detection of significant improvement difficult in individual studies containing relatively small numbers of patients. Regardless, the weight of the evidence favors angiogenesis as the mechanism of action, and, consequently, further studies are needed to better understand the mechanisms behind the angiogenic response as well as methods of augmenting or accelerating the process so that the clinical benefits of the procedure might be maximized.

References

Allen KB, Dowling RD, Fudge TL et al. Comparison of transmyocardial revascularization with medical therapy in patients with refractory angina. *N Engl J Med* 1999; 341: 1029–1036.

Al-Sheikh T, Allen KB, Straka SP et al. Cardiac sympathetic denervation after transmyocardial laser revascularization. *Circulation* 1999; 100: 135–140.

Brinker JA. A tunnel at the end of the light? *J Am Coll Cardiol* 1999; 34: 1671–1674.

Burkhoff D, Fisher PE, Apfelbaum M et al. Histologic appearance of transmyocardial laser channels after $4^{1}/_{2}$ weeks. *Ann Thorac Surg* 1996; 61: 1532–1534.

Burkhoff D, Fulton R, Wharton K et al. Myocardial perfusion through naturally occurring subendocardial channels. *J Thorac Cardiovasc Surg* 1997; 114: 497–499.

Burkhoff D, Schmidt S, Schulman SP et al. Transmyocardial laser revascularisation compared with continued medical therapy for treatment of refractory angina pectoris: a prospective randomized trial. *Lancet* 1999; 354: 885–890.

Chu VF, Giaid A, Kuang JQ et al. Angiogenesis in transmyocardial revascularization: comparison of laser versus mechanical punctures. *Ann Thorac Surg* 1999; 68: 301–308.

Deckelbaum LI. Cardiovascular applications of laser technology. *Lasers Surg Med* 1994; 15: 315–341.

Fallen EL, Coates G, Nahmias C et al. Recovery rates of regional sympathetic reinnervation and myocardial blood flow after acute myocardial infarction. *Am Heart J* 1999; 137: 863–869.

Fisher PE, Khomoto T, DeRosa CM et al. Histologic analysis of transmyocardial channels: comparison of CO_2 and holmium:YAG lasers. *Ann Thorac Surg* 1997; 64: 466–472.

Fleischer KJ, Goldschmidt-Clermont PJ, Fonger JD et al. One-month histologic response of transmyocardial laser channels with molecular intervention. *Ann Thorac Surg* 1996; 62: 1051–1058.

Fleming-Jones RM, McFadden PN. A denaturant-insoluble form of tyrosine hydroxylase in PC12 pheochromocytoma cells. *J Protein Chem* 1995; 14: 275–282.

Frazier OH, March RJ, Horvath KA. Transmyocardial revascularization with a carbon dioxide laser in patients with end-stage coronary artery disease. *N Engl J Med* 1999; 341: 1021–1028.

Gassler N, Wintzer HO, Stubbe HM et al. Transmyocardial laser revascularization. Histological features in human nonresponder myocardium. *Circulation* 1997; 95: 371–375.

Hardy RI, Bove KE, James FW et al. A histologic study of laser-induced transmyocardial channels. *Lasers Surg Med* 1987; 6: 563–573.

Hardy RI, James FW, Millard RW et al. Regional myocardial blood flow and cardiac mechanics in dog hearts with CO_2 laser-induced intramyocardial revascularization. *Basic Res Cardiol* 1990; 85: 179–197.

Hirsch GM, Thompson GW, Arora RC et al. Transmyocardial laser revascularization does not denervate the canine heart. *Ann Thorac Surg* 1999; 68: 460–468.

Horvath KA, Smith WJ, Laurence RG et al. Recovery and viability of an acute myocardial infarct after transmyocardial laser revascularization. *J Am Coll Cardiol* 1995; 25: 258–263.

Horvath KA, Greene R, Belkind N et al. Left ventricular functional improvement after transmyocardial laser revascularization. *Ann Thorac Surg* 1998; 66: 721–725.

Horvath KA, Chiu E, Maun DC et al. Up-regulation of vascular endothelial growth factor mRNA and angiogenesis after transmyocardial laser revascularization. *Ann Thorac Surg* 1999; 68: 825–829.

Hughes GC, Lowe JE, Kypson AP et al. Neovascularization after transmyocardial laser revascularization in a model of chronic ischemia. *Ann Thorac Surg* 1998; 66: 2029–2036.

Hughes GC, Landolfo KP, Lowe JE et al. Diagnosis, incidence, and clinical significance of early postoperative ischemia after transmyocardial laser revascularization. *Am Heart J* 1999a; 137: 1163–1168.

Hughes GC, Landolfo KP, Lowe JE et al. Perioperative morbidity and mortality after transmyocardial laser revascularization: incidence and risk factors for adverse events. *J Am Coll Cardiol* 1999b; 33: 1021–1026.

Hughes GC, Abdel-aleem S, Biswas SS et al. Transmyocardial laser revascularization: experimental and clinical results. *Can J Cardiol* 1999c; 15: 797–806.

Hughes GC, Annex BH, Yin B et al. Transmyocardial laser revascularization limits in vivo adenoviral-mediated gene transfer in porcine myocardium. *Cardiovasc Res* 1999d; 44: 81–90.

Hughes GC, Annex BH, Peters KG et al. Lymphatic angiogenesis induced by transmyocardial laser revascularization. *Ann Thorac Surg* 1999e; 68: 295–296.

Hughes GC, Kypson AP, St.Louis JD et al. Improved perfusion and contractile reserve after transmyocardial laser revascularization in a model of hibernating myocardium. *Ann Thorac Surg* 1999f; 67: 1714–1720.

Hughes GC, Baklanov DV, Annex BH et al. Denervation is not the long-term mechanism of action of transmyocardial laser revascularization (abstract). *Circulation* 1999g; I-249.

Hughes GC, Shah AS, Yin B et al. Early postoperative changes in regional systolic and diastolic left ventricular function after transmyocardial laser revascularization. A comparison of holmium:YAG and CO_2 lasers. *J Am Coll Cardiol* 2000a; 35: 1022–1030.

Hughes GC, Kypson AP, Annex BH et al. Induction of angiogenesis after TMR: a comparison of holmium:YAG, CO_2, and excimer lasers. *Ann Thorac Surg* 2000b; 70: 504–509.

Hunter JG, Dixon JA. Lasers in cardiovascular surgery-current status. *West J Med* 1985; 142: 506–510.

Kaipainen A, Korhonen J, Mustonen T et al. Expression of the fms-like tyrosine kinase 4 gene becomes restricted to lymphatic endothelium during development. *Proc Natl Acad Sci USA* 1995; 92: 3566–3570.

Kohmoto T, Fisher PE, Gu A et al. Does blood flow through holmium:YAG transmyocardial laser channels? *Ann Thorac Surg* 1996; 61: 861–868.

Kohmoto T, Fisher PE, Gu A et al. Physiology, histology, and 2-week morphology of acute transmyocardial channels made with a CO_2 laser. *Ann Thorac Surg* 1997a; 63: 1275–1283.

Kohmoto T, Argenziano M, Yamamoto N et al. Assessment of transmyocardial perfusion in alligator hearts. *Circulation* 1997b; 95: 1585–1591.

Kohmoto T, DeRosa CM, Yamamoto N et al. Evidence of vascular growth associated with laser treatment of normal canine myocardium. *Ann Thorac Surg* 1998; 65: 1360–1367.

Krabatsch T, Schaper F, Leder C et al. Histological findings after transmyocardial laser revascularization. *J Card Surg* 1996; 11: 326–331.

Kwong KF, Kanellopoulos GK, Nickols JC et al. Transmyocardial laser treatment denervates canine myocardium. *J Thorac Cardiovasc Surg* 1997; 114: 883–890.

Kwong KF, Schuessler RB, Kanellopoulos GK et al. Nontransmural laser treatment incompletely denervates canine myocardium. *Circulation* 1998; II-67–II-71.

Landolfo CK, Landolfo KP, Hughes GC et al. Intermediate-term clinical outcome following transmyocardial laser revascularization in patients with refractory angina pectoris. *Circulation* 1999; II-128–II-133.

Landreneau R, Nawarawong W, Laughlin H et al. Direct CO_2 laser "revascularization" of the myocardium. *Lasers Surg Med* 1991; 11: 35–42.

Lee LY, Lee KT, Woo CS et al. TMR dose response: evidence of enhanced perfusion in a porcine ischemic model after 50 vs. 10 channel TMR (abstract). *Circulation* 1999; 100: I-249.

Mack CA, Magovern CJ, Hahn RT et al. Channel patency and neovascularization after transmyocardial revascularization using an excimer laser. Results and comparisons to nonlased channels. *Circulation* 1997; 96: II-65–II-69.

Malekan R, Kelley ST, Suzuki Y et al. Transmyocardial laser revascularization fails to prevent left ventricular functional deterioration and aneurysm formation after acute myocardial infarction in sheep. *J Thorac Cardiovasc Surg* 1998a; 116: 752–762.

Malekan R, Reynolds C, Narula N et al. Angiogenesis in transmyocardial laser revascularization. A nonspecific response to injury. *Circulation* 1998b; 98: II-62–II-65.

Mirhoseini M, Cayton MM. Revascularization of the heart by laser. *J Microsurg* 1981; 2: 253–260.

Mirhoseini M, Cayton MM, Shelgikar S et al. Laser myocardial revascularization. *Lasers Surg Med* 1986; 6: 459–461.

Mueller XM, Tevaearai HH, Genton CY et al. Transmyocardial laser revascularization in acutely ischaemic myocardium. *Eur J Cardio-thorac Surg* 1998; 13: 170–175.

Mukherjee D, Bhatt DL, Roe MT et al. Direct myocardial revascularization and angiogenesis—How many patients might be eligible? *Am J Cardiol* 1999; 84: 598–600.

Okada M, Shimizu K, Ikuta H et al. A new method of myocardial revascularization by laser. *Thorac Cardiovasc Surg* 1991; 39: 1–4.

Oki H, Inoue S, Makishima N et al. Cardiac sympathetic innervation in patients with dilated cardiomyopathy: immunohistochemical study using anti-tyrosine hydroxylase antibody. *Jpn Circ J* 1994; 58: 389–394.

Pelletier MP, Giaid A, Sivaraman S et al. Angiogenesis and growth factor expression in a model of transmyocardial revascularization. *Ann Thorac Surg* 1998; 66: 12–18.

Roethy W, Yamamoto N, Burkhoff D. An examination of potential mechanisms underlying transmyocardial laser revascularization induced increases in myocardial blood flow. *Semin Thorac Cardiovasc Surg* 1999; 11: 24–28.

Schaper W, Ito WD. Molecular mechanisms of coronary collateral vessel growth. *Circ Res* 1996; 79: 911–919.

Schaper W. Quo vadis collateral blood flow? A commentary on a highly cited paper. *Cardiovasc Res* 2000; 45: 220–223.

Schofield PM, Sharples LD, Caine N et al. Transmyocardial laser revascularization in patients with refractory angina: a randomised controlled trial. *Lancet* 1999; 353: 519–524.

Sen PK, Udwadia TE, Kinare SG et al. Transmyocardial acupuncture. A new approach to myocardial revascularization. *J Thorac Cardiovasc Surg* 1965; 50: 181–189.

Sigel JE, Abramovich CM, Lytle BW et al. Transmyocardial laser revascularization: three sequential autopsy cases. *J Thorac Cardiovasc Surg* 1998; 115: 1381–1385.

St. Louis JD, Hughes GC, Kypson AP et al. An experimental model of chronic myocardial hibernation. *Ann Thorac Surg* 2000; 69: 1351–1357.

Sundt TM III, Kwong KF. Clinical experience with the holmium:YAG laser for transmyocardial laser revascularization and myocardial denervation as a mechanism. *Semin Thorac Cardiovasc Surg* 1999; 11: 19–23.

Ware JA, Simons M. Angiogenesis in ischemic heart disease. *Nat Med* 1997; 3: 158–164.

Whittaker P, Kloner RA, Przyklenk K. Laser-mediated transmural myocardial channels do not salvage acutely ischemic myocardium. *J Am Coll Cardiol* 1993; 22: 302–339.

Wooten GF, Coyle JT. Axonal transport of catecholamine synthesizing and metabolizing enzymes. *J Neurochem* 1973; 20: 1361–1371.

Yamamoto N, Kohmoto T, Gu A et al. Angiogenesis is enhanced in ischemic canine myocardium by transmyocardial laser revascularization. *J Am Coll Cardiol* 1998; 31: 1426–1433.

6

Potential Mechanisms of Myocardial Revascularization Techniques: Channels, Functional and Structural Remodeling, Angiogenesis, Denervation, or Placebo

Elie Hage-Korban, M.D., Khaled Ghosheh, M.D.,
Hongbao Ma, Ph.D., Ruiping Huang, Ph.D.,
Oliver G. Abela, and George S. Abela, M.D., M.Sc., M.B.A.

Department of Medicine
Division of Cardiology
Michigan State University
East Lansing, Michigan

and

Rakesh C. Arora, M.D.

Cardiac Surgery, Dalhousie University
Halifax, Nova Scotia, Canada

SUMMARY

Several mechanisms are proposed as possible ways of angina relief after PMR. These include 1) creation of transmyocardial channels, 2) mechanical effects of remodeling, 3) angiogenesis resulting from the thermal and mechanical injury, 4) direct or indirect denervation, 5) remodeling of the intrinsic nervous system, 6) altered myocardial function, and 7) the placebo effect.

PMR/TMR in animals has been found to enhance vascular growth of both large and small arteries in the ischemic myocardium; however, the mechanism responsible for improvement in symptoms and exercise tolerance in humans has yet to be discovered.

Myocardial Revascularization: Novel Percutaneous Approaches, Edited by George S. Abela.
ISBN 0-471-36166-6   Copyright © 2002 Wiley-Liss, Inc.

Concern has been raised in the DIRECT Trial regarding "placebo effect" in patients who undergo PMR procedures, but this was offset by recent results of a double blinded placebo study from Norway, the BELIEF Trial, showing significant improvement in symptoms and exercise tolerance with PMR.

Multiple mechanisms are probably at work after PMR. In the early phase denervation may provide symptom relief, whereas in latter stages angiogenesis may have a greater role.

6.1. INTRODUCTION

The premise of laser revascularization is based on the early work of Wearn et al. (1922, 1933), who described arterioluminal and arteriosinusoidal vessels as direct connections between the blood in the ventricular chamber and the myocardium. Thus it seemed obvious to attempt to perfuse the myocardium by creating direct channels with the left ventricular cavity. Several earlier techniques were investigated to achieve that goal, including the insertion of a T-tube implant between the ventricular chamber and the muscle or mechanical boring by needle acupuncture (Goldman et al., 1956; Sen et al., 1965). None of these techniques was found to be successful in perfusing ischemic myocardium. Almost a half-century later, there was a resurgence of the concept of direct myocardial reperfusion, stimulated by an increasing number of patients with coronary artery disease who were not candidates for standard revascularization techniques. Transmyocardial revascularization (TMR) with laser was proposed as a novel technique using this concept to supply oxygenated blood to the ischemic myocardium (Mirhoseini and Cayton, 1981). Numerous animal and human studies have been performed to test this concept. However, despite the clinical relief of angina and improved functional status in the patients treated with TMR, the mechanism of this and related procedures remains unclear. In this chapter we present data supporting and negating various proposed mechanisms including direct channel perfusion, angio-

genesis, laser-induced myocardial remodeling, altered mechanical function, denervation, and placebo effects.

6.2. DIRECT MYOCARDIAL PERFUSION BY CHANNELS

The creation of channels by laser or other methods is thought to transect the myocardium and connect with the intramyocardial vascular network. Wearn et al. initially described this network as a sinusoidal system, but other investigators challenged this observation and proposed more of a vascular network that may even involve the lymphatics or just distorted coronary veins (Chiu and Scott, 1973). Thus the attempt to mimic the "reptilian heart" physiology by TMR may be too simplistic.

In the 1960s, Pifarré et al. indicated that it was physiologically impossible for blood to flow from the ventricular chamber to the myocardium during either systole or diastole. Using various animal models, they demonstrated that the pressure within the myocardium was always greater than the pressure within the ventricle; hence, no flow would be possible (Pifarré et al., 1962, 1969). However, several investigators recently postulated that an endocardial-epicardial pressure gradient could allow transmyocardial blood flow. Hardy et al. demonstrated that the endocardial-epicardial gradient increased with progressive rise in left ventricular pressure and that ventricular systolic pressure greater than 207 ± 16.1 mmHg permitted the entry of microspheres into the TMR channels (Hardy et al., 1990). This simulates the conditions often seen in the ischemic myocardium (Kohmoto et al., 1996). Others have observed radiographic contrast as well as ultrasonic medium filling the transmyocardial channels during systole (Berwing et al., 1996; Kim et al., 1999).

Another aspect of this controversy revolved around channel patency. Abela et al. demonstrated patent channels in the myocardium of an acute dog model using an argon laser delivered via an optical fiber extended from a hollow electrode-tipped catheter under fluoroscopic guidance (Abela et al., 1983; Curtis et

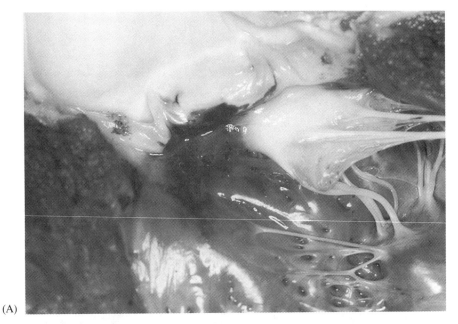

(A)

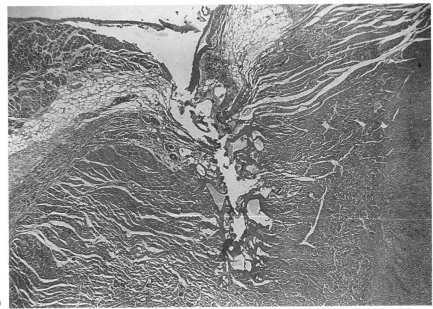

(B)

FIGURE 6-1. (A) Heart of dog after laser exposures from the right ventricle. Left ventricular chamber with an area of thermal necrosis and hemorrhage below the aortic valve. No perforation of the septum is noted. (B) Histologic cross section of crater at the tricuspid valve ring. A channel of vaporized myocardial tissue is seen extending about halfway through the interventricular septum below the fibrous body (Reprinted with permission of Futura Publishing Co.)

al., 1989) (Fig. 6-1). Similarly, Horvath et al. demonstrated patent channels in an ovine (sheep) model that were associated with improved myocardial function (Horvath et al., 1996). Mirhoseini et al. demonstrated patent and endothelialized channels in dog myocardium several years after TMR with a high-power CO_2 laser (Mirhoseini and

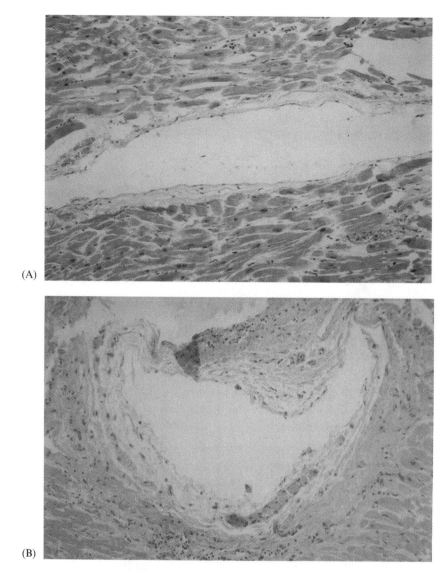

(A)

(B)

FIGURE 6-2.   Photomicrographs of myocardium from patient who received TMR 4.5 years after a combined procedure (TMR and coronary artery bypass surgery). Channels are seen to be patent and lined with endothelium both in longitudinal (A) and cross-sectional views (B) (hematoxylin and eosin) (Courtesy of M. Mirhoseini and M. Cayton, St. Luke's Hospital, Milwaukee, WI.)

Cayton, 1981). Subsequently, Mirhoseini reported similar findings in several patients who died 2–5 years after TMR (Mirhoseini et al., 1986) (Fig. 6-2). He speculated that using high-power CO_2 laser energy that penetrates the full thickness of the myocardium with a single pulse, the channels are less likely to thrombose and become fibrosed. His rationale was that these very high-energy pulses limit collateral thermal tissue injury.

Cooley et al. made similar observations in humans after TMR (Cooley et al., 1994). They corroborated the presence of patent channels in patients who died at 3 months after TMR. Other investigators also showed evidence of long-term channel patency and increased perfusion to the myocardium in the areas treated with TMR (Conger et al., 1995; Hughes et al., 1999).

However, other investigators have demonstrated occluded channels after TMR treatment in animal models and in patients who subsequently died. These channels were occluded by fibrin thrombus and granulation tissue infiltrates by 2–3 weeks after the procedure. Moreover, Landreneau et al. (1991) and Hardy et al. (1990) were not able to find any evidence of myocardial perfusion by microsphere techniques under normal physiologic conditions. In an acute ischemic dog model Whittaker et al. (1993) showed that TMR using a Ho:YAG laser did not improve myocardial perfusion. Also, Eckstein et al. could not demonstrate any benefit on myocardial perfusion in a model of acute ischemia in sheep (Eckstein et al., 1999). No patent channels were detected by histology or by magnetic resonance imaging. In an acute ischemic pig model, Mueller et al. consistently demonstrated that TMR channels were occluded by thrombus on the same day after the procedure and were scarred after 28 days (Mueller et al., 1999a, 1999b). Kohmoto et al. also concluded in a dog model that there was not significant blood flow through the TMR channels in both the acute and subacute setting at 2 weeks (Kohmoto et al., 1996). A similar conclusion was proposed by Glasser et al., who noted that channels were occluded and fibrosed at the time of autopsy in four patients shortly after TMR (Gassler et al., 1997). Additional autopsy studies in humans demonstrated that channels do not remain patent (Burkhoff et al., 1996).

The controversy over channel patency and myocardial viability in ischemic regions has been hotly debated based on conflicting results already mentioned. Some of this discrepancy may be explained by the use of various animal models as well as various laser systems. For example, the ovine and pig models have end coronary arteries whereas the dog model is widely known to have good collateral circulation, making it difficult to compare the TMR effects on ischemic myocardium. Another confounding factor is

the various types of laser wavelengths used. Each laser wavelength and energy delivery has different tissue effects that can alter the outcome significantly. For example, laser channels made with CO_2 laser were found to have longer patency compared with channels created with needle puncture (Whittaker et al., 1999). Also, with regard to the patient studies, it has been argued that those patients who died do not represent a true benefit because those patients did not survive because of procedure failure. Consequently, those who were alive may be benefiting from the TMR effects.

Other studies using positron emission tomography (Frazier et al., 1995) (Fig. 6-3) and sestamibi (Horvath et al., 1996) scanning studies have indicated that myocardial perfusion is improved in treated areas 3–6 months after operation, with a statistical increase in the ratio between endocardial and epicardial myocardial perfusion.

Most clinical trials have demonstrated angina relief and improved cardiac performance after TMR. However, the mechanism of these observations remains to be established. If direct perfusion of the myocardium by channel formation were the primary mechanism, the maximum benefit would be expected almost immediately after the procedure. Although some patients have reported some immediate improvement in symptoms after TMR, the majority of improvement has been several months (i.e., 6 months) after treatment. Subjective improvement scores were also corroborated by objective measures. These included increased time on exercise stress test and less ischemia by myocardial perfusion imaging. Hence, being inconsistently patent, anatomic channels could not be the sole mechanism responsible for the beneficial effects noted after TMR.

6.3. MECHANICAL EFFECTS DUE TO MYOCARDIAL REMODELING

One mechanism that may contribute to symptom relief is the acute and chronic effects of laser on mechanical properties of the myocardium. Acute changes were

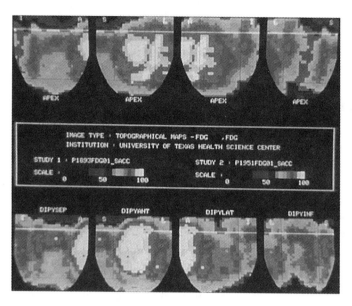

FIGURE 6-3. Computer-processed images of positron emission tomography from patient with inferior wall ischemia before and after TMR. The images after TMR show reduction of ischemia. Areas of ischemia are depicted in green and perfused areas in orange and red (Courtesy of O.H. Frazier, Texas Heart Institute, Texas Heart Institute Journal.) (See color plates.)

described by Lutter et al., who examined the histology of laser channels and interstitial microskeleton (Lutter et al., 1999a). They demonstrated that the CO_2 laser channels were open at 2 h after lasing. The channels were lined by a zone of carbonization surrounded by an outer zone of necrosis with a rim of myofibrillar degeneration and edema. Neutrophils were also seen infiltrating these sites. Some of these channels had direct connections to small vessels and were filled with erythrocytes. However, in a study using Ho:YAG (2.1 μm) in an ischemic pig model, examination of older channels by Mueller et al. (1998) revealed that the majority of these were occluded by fibrous tissue. These channels exhibited an elliptic morphology, and those that were patent had a lumen dimension smaller than the channel size noted immediately after lasing. The degree of vascularization within the scar tissue replacing the channel lumen was highly variable. The elliptic morphology of the channels may be a result of asymmetric distribution of the thermal spread. This is thought to be caused

by the direction of myocardial muscle fibers and the diversion of the laser beam by the local architecture (Mueller et al., 1998, 1999a). In another study (Whittaker et al., 1999), a frequency tripled Nd:YAG laser with γ—355 nm at 5–6; 6–10 mJ/pulse and 10 Hz and 9 ns pulse wide was used. It was found that at 2–5 months after lasing in rat hearts, collagen fibers adjacent to open channels were aligned parallel to the channel. However, adjacent to the closed channels, the fibers were aligned in a perpendicular fashion to the original channel direction (Fig. 6-4). Thus the method of laser application, the amount of laser energy used, and the type of wavelength applied all determine the amount of thermal injury that is a crucial determinant of long-term channel patency.

In another experiment Mueller et al. (1999b) analyzed the morphologic evolution of TMR channels in a pig model. Mueller focused on the reduction of the channel area resulting from the scarring process. He noted marked cicatricial contraction of the channel area by 1 month. Under the Laplace law, the

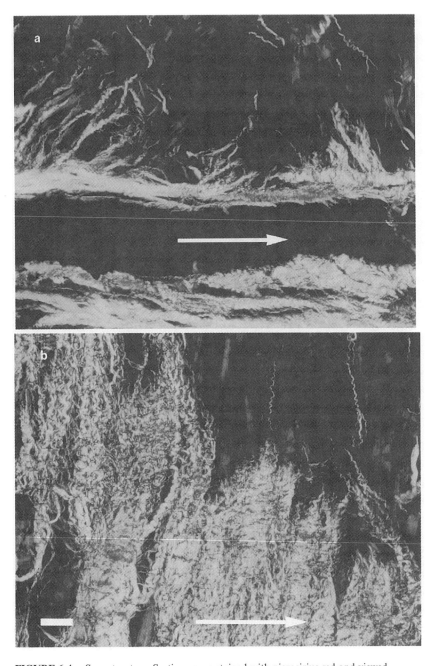

FIGURE 6-4.   Scar structure. Sections were stained with picrosirius red and viewed with polarized light. Collagen fibers appear yellow/orange, and muscle appears green. (A) Open channel. Collagen fibers are aligned parallel to the long axis of the channel (arrow) and perpendicular to adjacent muscle. (B) Closed channel. Collagen fibers are aligned perpendicular to the direction of the original channel (arrow) and parallel to adjacent muscle. Scale bar = 50 μm (Reprinted by permission of Dr. Peter Whittaker, Wiley-Liss, Inc., a subsidiary of John Wiley & Sons., Inc.)

contraction effect reduces the left ventricular cavity diameter and therefore diminishes wall stress and hence oxygen consumption.

This concept has been further investigated by Whittaker et al. (1999), who used the Nd:YAG laser to create channels 4 weeks after myocardial infarction in a rat model. Laser treatment remodeled the rat hearts and restored the three-dimensional shape of the left ventricle as compared to nonlased controls. This remodeling was accompanied by a 25% reduction in cavity volume and corresponding reductions in cross-sectional areas and diameters. By microscopy, Whittaker found that collagen fibers in laser-treated scars were straighter than those in the untreated scars. Collagen scars were always more coherently aligned in the treated rats compared with the nontreated rats. This finding suggests that such fibers were connected to those contracted and straightened directly by the temperature increase. Whittaker concluded that laser treatment of scar tissue successfully reversed ventricular expansion associated with transmural infarction.

6.4. ANGIOGENESIS

Angiogenesis is the sprouting of capillaries in hypovascular regions from preexisting vessels (see Chapters 4 and 5). This is often noted in areas of wound healing, inflammation, ischemia, and tumor growth. Laser energy during channel creation initiates similar local signals for angiogenesis. Although many of these channels closed with time, the effect of this local signal for angiogenesis seemed to persist. This potential mechanism was postulated after the region surrounding the channel remnant was noted to have endothelium-lined areas containing red blood cells. This has been confirmed by histologic studies with special staining using antibodies to factor VIII defining the endothelial surface lining of new blood vessels in lased areas. This was elegantly illustrated by Domkowski et al. (2001) (Fig. 6-5).

Other investigators provided further evidence in support of the angiogenesis mecha-

nism. Kohmoto et al. related the benefit from laser revascularization to increased vessel density that increased blood flow capacity in the vicinity of the laser channels (Kohmoto et al., 1997). They created an average of 12 transmural channels (approximately 1 channel/cm^2) in a region of the heart of mongrel dogs using Ho:YAG laser ($n = 4$) or a CO_2 laser ($n = 4$). The dogs were euthanized 2–3 weeks after the TMR procedure, and transmural tissue cubes of the myocardium containing one or two channels were excised and serially sectioned in a plane perpendicular to the channel at 2-mm intervals. Slides from Ho:YAG-made channels and CO_2-made channels were analyzed, and the area around each channel remnant was divided into two concentric ovals. Samples remote from the area of laser treatment served as controls. Slides stained for factor VIII revealed increased number of vessels in the area surrounding the channel remnants. These demonstrated vascular structures of various sizes originating from the channel and extending to the surrounding normal myocardium. Included were capillaries and vessels of intermediate size lined by one or more layers of smooth muscle. Such vessels are infrequently found in normal myocardium. Thus Kohmoto et al. concluded that vascular growth is stimulated in a region of myocardium measuring a 3-mm diameter from the epicenter of the channel. This process was observed as early as 2 weeks after channel creation and may be explained by the thermoacoustic injury surrounding the channel that may stimulate the inflammatory response liberating cytokines and growth factors.

Fisher and colleagues studied the tissue response to TMR in normal canine myocardium (Fisher et al., 1997). They performed histologic staining on the lased tissue and demonstrated that the channel consisted of small central lumen surrounded by an organizing fibrin thrombus with prominent neovascularization. They speculated that this intrachannel thrombus itself contains growth factors and other mediators that stimulate

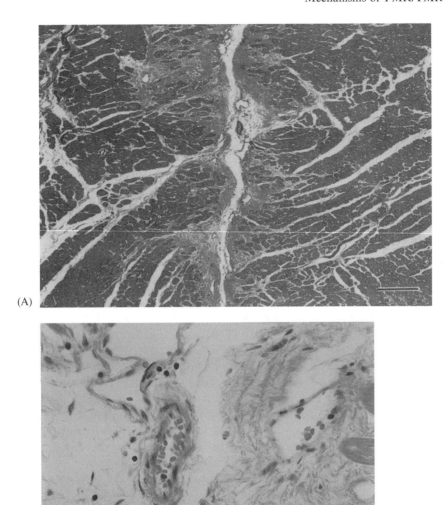

(A)

(B)

FIGURE 6-5. (A) Photomicrograph of myocardium from patient who received TMR 7 months before heart transplantation for progressive ischemia and failure despite early relief from symptoms for 6 months. Lased channel remnants demonstrating minimal scarring in surrounding myocardium with numerous blood vessels branching from the channel. (B) Photomicrograph of high-power magnification showing neoblood vessels containing red blood cells. (C) Factor VII antibody stain demonstrates endothelial lined vessels adjacent to channel remnant (Domkowski PW, Biswas SS, Steenbergen C et al. Histological evidence of angiogenesis 9 months after transmyocardial laser revascularization. *Circulation* 2001; 103: 469–471. Reproduced with permission of Lippincott Williams and Wilkins.) (See color plates.)

angiogenesis in surrounding tissues. Also, they proposed that the original channel might even serve as a scaffold or skeleton for endothelial migration and proliferation, which seems to be an appealing yet unproven con-

cept. Spanier et al. performed a similar experiment in the same model but in the presence of ischemia (Spanier et al., 1997). TMR was performed over the LAD territory in 7 of 14 mongrel dogs after ligating all its visible

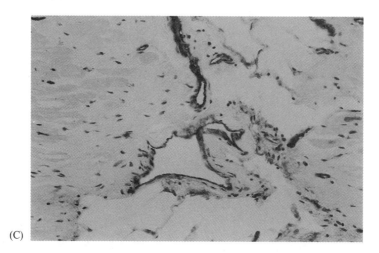

(C)

FIGURE 6-5. *Continued.*

collaterals. An ischemic challenge was then induced by placing ameroid constrictors on the proximal LAD artery. The control group ($n = 7$) had no TMR. Bromodeoxyuridine (BrdU) was administered subcutaneously as a method to assess cellular proliferation in four dogs from each group on postoperative days 7, 14, and 28. The animals were killed 8–9 weeks after surgery, and samples from the LAD region of the hearts were obtained as well as samples from the left circumflex region that served as controls. At 2 weeks, many vessels were seen within the channel remnants, and they were lined with endothelial cells as evidenced by factor VIII staining. BrdU assays also showed evidence of vascular growth that was concentrated in the channel remnants and, to a lesser extent, in the small communicating vessels that extend to the surrounding myocardium. Vessels of different sizes were observed as far as 5 mm from the channel remnant, with evidence of BrdU incorporation as well as immunohisto-chemical staining for smooth muscle and endothelial cells. In the ischemic areas of the control animals, vascular growth was noticed, but to a much lesser degree than in the treatment group. When the vascular density was quantified, it was found to be 50% greater in the TMR group than in the control group. Moreover, the incorporation of BrdU in the vascular cells was about four times greater in

the TMR regions of the treatment group compared with the ischemic regions of the control group. From these observations, Spanier et al. concluded that TMR enhances vascular growth of both small and large arteries in ischemic myocardium. However, the fact remains that the real mechanism responsible for the observed improvement of ischemic symptoms and exercise performance after TMR remains to be elucidated in humans.

6.5. EFFECTS ON MYOCARDIAL FUNCTION

The impact of laser revascularization on myocardial function has been studied by several researchers in animal models as well as in human subjects. Early studies that investigated the effect of laser irradiation on left ventricular function by angiography did not demonstrate any significant myocardial dysfunction. A study was performed by Vincent and colleagues using a catheter-directed fiberoptic system to evaluate the effect of Nd:YAG laser on myocardial function for the purpose of ventricular arrhythmia ablation (Curtis et al., 1990). They detected a reduction in left ventricular ejection fraction from 0.65 to 0.54 immediately after irradiation. However, at 1-week follow-up wall motion had recovered to normal baseline. Mueller et al. found, in a pig model of acute ischemia, that laser treatment depressed myocardial contractility acutely as assessed by echocardiography but recovered in 30 min, suggesting good myocardial tolerance to TMR (Mueller et al., 1998). However, this improvement in recovery did not exceed the baseline function. In that setting, lasing did not seem to improve or worsen myocardial contractility. Lutter et al. found that CO_2 laser channels significantly decreased global heart function shortly after TMR in healthy porcine myocardium (Lutter et al., 1999b). However, unlike the study by Mueller, no recovery of myocardial function was noted at 6 hours after treatment. The major difference between the two studies was the presence of ischemia in the former model and the absence of ischemia in the model that did not have evidence of recovery. Thus, as in other examples of myocardial injury, preconditioned tissue may be more resistant to subsequent further ischemia. This and other aspects of this complex picture warrant further evaluation (see below).

In a chronic pig model of ischemia treated with TMR further improvement in function was noted. Lutter et al. (2000) demonstrated that laser channels significantly improved microperfusion and regional contractility at rest after 3 months of chronic ischemia. In contrast, transmural perfusion and left ventricular function at rest and with stress were not altered by TMR. They also demonstrated that transient decrease in left ventricular function after lasing recovered at 3 months after treatment.

In the clinical setting, Kaul et al. observed that in patients with intractable ischemic symptoms and reduced left ventricular function there was no worsening of regional wall after PMR (Kaul et al., 1999). These patients obtained symptom relief at 6-month follow-up after the procedure.

Laser treatment with TMR is thought to target hibernating myocardium as its primary site of improving myocardial function by enhancing blood supply. However, during TMR some myocardium is irreversibly damaged. Thus the exact number of laser channels needed to achieve beneficial clinical effects with the least amount of myocardial damage has not been defined. At present, the number of laser channels created during TMR has been chosen randomly. This could contribute to the wide variation among studies. Other confounding factors are the laser wavelength and methods of laser delivery (i.e., direct laser beam vs. optical fiber). To examine some of this variability, we proposed to evaluate the effect of the number of laser channels on myocardial contractility.

In an isolated rat heart muscle preparation, Frank-Starling mechanics were used to evaluate the early effect of increasing numbers of TMR channels on myocardial function (Hage-Korban et al., 2001). This was performed by dissecting the left ventricles from Sprague-Dawley rats after an overdose of anesthetic. The ventricles were suspended in a bath of oxygenated physiologic buffer solution and mounted on a contraction preload system. The myocardium was then stimulated by electrical pulses at 1 Hz, and the resulting muscle contraction was displayed on a strip chart recorder. Four preload conditions were evaluated (0–3 g). Repeat salvos of a Ho:YAG laser energy at 250 mJ/pulse were delivered to create 20 transmyocardial channels. Starling mechanics were evaluated after each application of 20 channels. The preliminary data demonstrated that myocardial contractility was reduced after each treatment. However, after 1.5 h (120 channels) from initial laser treatment, there was recovery of contractility with increasing preloads (Table 6.1). This effect could be related to preconditioning of the muscle and not related to perfusion.

6.6. DENERVATION

Myocardial denervation was proposed as yet another mechanism to explain the potential benefits in patient symptoms (see Chapter 5).

Kwong et al. performed TMR using Ho:YAG laser on adult mongrel dogs to evaluate the effect of denervation (Kwong et al., 1997). These authors found that the function of cardiac afferent nerve fibers as well as their specific enzyme was lost after TMR. They

TABLE 6-1.   Myocardial Contractility (mm/pulse on recorder)

Channels	preload = 0 g	preload = 1 g	preload = 2 g	preload = 3 g	p
0	44.3 ± 23.5	57.2 ± 27.9	64.7 ± 31.9	65.9 ± 30.8	0.03
20	38.6 ± 20.4	44.4 ± 19.0	42.4 ± 19.3	38.0 ± 14.5	0.31
60	22.4 ± 16.5	23.3 ± 17.9	22.4 ± 12.1	22.0 ± 13.5	0.46
120	4.3 ± 3.4	23.2 ± 13.2	28.9 ± 13.6	31.6 ± 6.6	0.05
180	6.8 ± 2.1	8.4 ± 1.9	8.7 ± 1.4	11.1 ± 2.5	0.22
240	4.2 ± 2.2	10.9 ± 4.3	9.6 ± 5.9	12.8 ± 8.8	0.34

concluded that denervation is a possible mechanism for angina relief. They also demonstrated that PMR in a canine model resulted in only partial denervation of the myocardium (Kwong et al., 1998). These findings are crucial in understanding the differences reported between results of PMR and TMR (see Placebo Effect section below).

More recent work by Hirsch et al. has demonstrated that after TMR, stellate ganglion stimulation did not result in attenuation of either chronotropic or inotropic responses (Hirsch et al., 1999). However, the same group has evaluated the intrinsic innervation of the heart, providing additional insights on the effect of TMR (Arora et al., 2000). Thus another approach to understanding the mechanism of angina relief with TMR is the remodeling of the intrinsic cardiac nervous system.

The mammalian heart possesses a complex nervous system that can function independent of inputs from extracardiac neurons to regulate regional cardiac function by reflex action (Ardell et al., 1991; Armour, 1991). This nervous system, known as the intrinsic cardiac nervous system (ICNS), contains afferent neurons (Armour and Hopkins, 1990; Cheng et al., 1997), sympathetic efferent postganglionic neurons (Butler et al., 1990; Gagliardi et al., 1988; Hamos et al., 1985), and parasympathetic efferent postganglionic neurons (Blomquist et al., 1987), a population of local circuit neurons that function to interconnect neurons within and between the separate aggregates of ganglia that form the various intrinsic cardiac ganglionated plexuses (Butler et al., 1990). These plexuses are located in discrete locations, typically in fatty tissue surrounding the heart (Armour et al., 1997; Yuan et al., 1994). It has been proposed by Armour, Ardell, and coworkers that the ICNS is capable of interacting on a beat-to-beat basis to coordinate cardiac regional function (Ardell et al., 1991; Armour, 1991), thereby ensuring an efficient cardiac output (Stevenson et al., 2000). The intrinsic cardiac nervous system is essentially a "little brain" on the heart acting as a "low pass" filter to mitigate potential imbalances in neural control of the heart. This results in an overall smoothing of regional cardiac function from neuronal imbalances such as from extracardiac neuronal inputs to the heart, from pathophysiologic events within the heart (such as myocardial ischemia), or from surgical intervention and therapies.

To demonstrate true denervation, these intrinsic cardiac neurons were examined in situ (Hirsch et al., 1999). The integrity of ventricular afferent and efferent axons assessed immediately after TMR was found to be unaffected. However, the question is whether the ICNS function remained intact chronically after TMR. As in the acute study by Hirsch et al., cardiac afferent neuronal function was intact when stimulated with the topical sodium-ion channel modifier veratridine. Similarly, extracardiac electrical stimulation of sympathetic and parasympathetic nerve function remained intact 4 weeks after TMR (Fig. 6-6).

In the acute setting the ICNS responded normally to nicotine and angiotensin II. However, at 4 weeks after TMR in a nonischemic canine-model, the ICNS was unre-

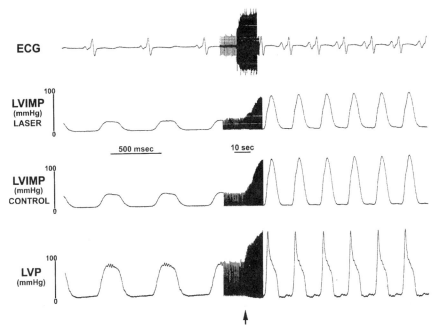

FIGURE 6-6. The effects of stimulating the left stellate ganglion of a dog that had received laser therapy in the ventral region of the left ventricular free wall 1 month previously. When this ganglion was stimulated electrically (4 V, 10 Hz, 5 ms; commencing at arrow below), heart rate, and left ventricular chamber systolic pressure (LVP) were augmented. Left ventricular intramyocardial systolic pressures in the ventricular region previously subjected to TMR (LV IMP laser) as well as an unaffected left ventricular ventral region (LV IMP control) were augmented as well. These data indicate that chronic TMR therapy does not obtund the capacity of sympathetic efferent neurons to enhance ventricular contractility in the affected myocardium (Courtesy of Dr. Rakesh Arora, Dalhousie University.)

sponsive to nicotine or angiotensin II (Fig. 6-7). This lack of effect of nicotine and angiotensin II would indicate that the ICNS (i.e., postganglionic neurons in the fatty tissue directly on the heart) is altered or "remodeled" globally in a delayed fashion by TMR. It has now been shown that remodeling of the ICNS occurs in autotransplanted dogs (Murphy et al., 2000), chronically decentralized dogs (Ardell et al., 1991), and dogs undergoing spinal cord stimulation (Forman et al., 2000). It is therefore becoming apparent that some surgical procedures and therapeutic interventions have the ability to alter the functioning of this important neuronal system. Such remodeling by TMR may represent a novel mechanism whereby this form of therapy imparts symptomatic relief (Arora et al., 2000).

6.7. PLACEBO EFFECT

Placebo effects are commonly observed in patients with cardiovascular diseases who receive either drug or surgical therapies as treatments (Bienenfeld et al., 1996). In 1976, Byerly defined placebo effect as "any change in a patient's symptoms that is the result of the therapeutic intent and not the specific physiochemical nature of a medical procedure" (Byerly, 1976).

Historically this concept has been well validated. It was once thought that internal mammary artery ligation improved angina

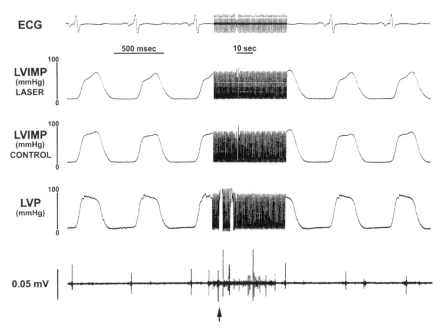

FIGURE 6-7.   Systemic administration of a relatively large dose of nicotine (20 μg/kg iv, arrow below) failed to activate intrinsic neuronal activity (last line of figure). Each deflection indicates an action potential from a single neuronal unit. Normally, nicotine increases neuronal activity, however, in this instance, there was no increase in ICNS activity after its systemic administration. These data indicate that the capacity of nicotine-sensitive cardiac efferent neurons to affect cardiodynamics becomes obtunded after previous exposure of a ventricular region to TMR. This large dose of nicotine is more than sufficient to activate cardiac parasympathetic and sympathetic efferent neurons in normal preparations, thereby inducing considerable changes in these cardiac indices. The symbols used in this figure are the same as those in Fig. 6-6 (Courtesy of Dr. Rakesh Arora, Dalhousie University.)

pectoris until studies showed a similar benefit in patients in whom a sham procedure consisting of skin incision with no ligation was performed. Similar concern has been raised about TMR/PMR procedures. The majority of laser revascularization studies showed a beneficial antianginal effect, but they lacked the inclusion of a placebo control group. The DIRECT study was designed to investigate this issue (Leon et al., 2000). Using the Biosense LV mapping (Johnson & Johnson) system, direct myocardial revascularization (DMR) was performed in 298 patients recruited from 14 centers. DMR was performed using the Ho:YAG laser at 2 J/pulse/site with a 300-μm silica fiber system. This laser catheter was a non tissue-contact system, but the investigators, on the basis of prior animal trials, expected to create 5-mm-depth channels with a 5-mm acoustic shock zone. Treatment was performed in patients randomly assigned to three groups; placebo (LV mapping alone without DMR); low dose (10–15 channels per treatment zone), and high dose (20–25 channels per treatment zone). Treatment was blinded to the patients and all the investigators involved in the assessment of the final endpoints. After 6 months of follow-up, all the three treatment groups showed significant improvement in exercise duration, time to first anginal episode, angina frequency, and quality of life compared with placebo (42% of the placebo group improved by 2 or more angina classes). However, no difference was observed among the three groups, suggesting a robust placebo effect in both laser groups.

The results of the DIRECT trial must be interpreted very cautiously, and generalization of its conclusion to the other systems like the Eclipse system or the TMR methods is still premature.

In fact, previous studies have found an improvement in exercise tolerance of about 100 s with the PMR and TMR systems compared to about 30-s improvement seen in DIRECT. Similarly, 58% of patients treated with the PMR system and about 70% of those with the surgical systems have improved two CCS functional classes or better symptoms, compared to about 30% in DIRECT. This would make the DMR treatment group equivalent to the medically treated groups of most of the other studies that have been performed. Thus, if the DMR did not create a significant channel, this group would be expected to be equivalent to placebo. Also, unless the investigators demonstrated that this noncontact system could penetrate the tissue with the energy parameters used in the abnormal ischemic and scarred human myocardium, the animal studies on normal hearts are would not be an adequate representation of the clinical scenario.

The Biosense™ system is different in a way such that it does not penetrate the myocardium that might or might not be important in the beneficial observed effect compared with the previous studies. It has been previously demonstrated that unless the fiber was in direct tissue contact under some pressure, the presence of blood will greatly attenuate the impact of the laser beam on the tissues (Abela et al., 1982; Fenech et al., 1985). This issue is extremely important because all other PMR studies have been conducted using systems that penetrated the tissue during the procedure. Thus it is difficult to generalize the results of the DIRECT study. However, treatment with other devices continues to demonstrate clinical benefit as seen most recently by the results of the PACIFIC study (Oesterle et al., 2000). This is further supported by a very recent report, the BELIEF trial by Nordrehaug et al. from Norway (Nordrehaug et al., 2001). This was also a double blind study of lased versus placebo treatment that demonstrated a significant improvement with PMR using the tissue-penetrating Eclipse laser system. In this study, 82 patients with mainly class III and IV angina were randomized to PMR (40 patients) or placebo (42 patients). Patient demographics were comparable, and left ventricular ejection fraction was >25%. No crossover of patients was allowed. Two laser catheters were attached to the emission box, and only the technologist was aware of whether the laser actually fired or not. The Ho:YAG laser was synchronized to the EKG during discharge. Patients received an average of 20 channels each. One-half of the patients had anterior wall treatments. Acute events were not significantly different, and on 6 months follow-up 63% of the laser-treated patients had at least one class of angina improvement versus only 38% for the placebo group ($P < 0.006$). For two-angina class improvement, 41% of PMR were improved versus only 13% for placebo. For exercise duration, there was a significant increase in the time to angina in the PMR group, but no difference was noted in total exercise time or oxygen uptake between the two groups. These results were very similar to the outcome of the PACIFIC trial, which randomized patients to laser versus medical therapy. Also, it is worthwhile to note that in addition to the long-term improvement noted in the BELIEF trial there were a few patients who reported immediate improvement in symptoms after PMR. One-year follow-up is pending.

6.8. CONCLUSION

In conclusion, PMR and/or TMR seem to offer to "no option " patients a valuable and unique remedy to their disabling angina. The majority of trials have consistently demonstrated that these techniques are effective in relieving angina in patients who have had longstanding symptoms and for whom all other available therapies have failed. The mechanism behind this beneficial effect is still the center of debate. It is most likely that this is related to a combination of mechanisms, each with different contribution at various times after therapy. This concept deserves further investigation to include the contribution of 1) patent transmyocardial channels, 2) mechanical remodeling conferred by the lasing system, 3) angiogenesis resulting from the thermal and mechanical injury, 4) direct or indirect denervation, 5) remodeling of the intrinsic nervous system, 6) altered myocardial function, as well as 6) the placebo effect. The controversies observed in the literature are most probably due to great variations in different catheter and energy sources used as well as great variability in the coronary circulation of animal models. Further research is needed under comparable conditions to help sort out some of the controversies. Thus far, PMR appears to be an effective procedure. However, time will tell whether it will become a widely accepted method for myocardial revascularization.

References

Abela GS, Normann SJ, Cohen D et al. Effects of carbon dioxide, Nd:YAG and argon laser radiation on coronary atheromatous plaques. *Am J Cardiol* 1982; 50: 1199–1205.

Abela GS, K, Griffin JC, Hill JA, Normann S, Conti CR. Transvascular argon laser-induced atrioventricular conduction ablation in dogs. *Circulation* 1983; 68: 111–145.

Ardell JL, Butler CK, Smith FM et al. Activity of in vivo atrial and ventricular neurons in chronically decentralized canine hearts. *Am J Physiol* 1991; 260: H713–H721.

Armour JA, Hopkins DA. Activity of in situ canine left atrial ganglion neurons. *Am J Physiol* 1990; 259: H1207–H1215.

Armour JA. Anatomy and function of the intrathoracic neurons regulating the mammalian heart. In: Zucker IH, Gilmore JP, eds. *Reflex Control of the Circulation*. CRC Press, Boca Raton, FL, 1991, pp. 1–37.

Armour JA, Murphy DA, Yuan BX et al. Anatomy of the human intrinsic cardiac nervous system. *Anat Rec* 1997; 297: 289–298.

Arora R, Hirsch G, Armour A. Transmyocardial laser revascularization (TMLR) remodels the intrinsic cardiac nervous system in a chronic setting(abstract). *Circulation* 2000; 102: II–765.

Berwing K, Gauer EP, Strasser R et al. Transmural laser revascularization: first proof of perfusion through open laser channels. German Society of Cardiologists, April 1996, Mannheim, Germany.

Bienenfeld L, Frishman W, Glasser S. The placebo effect in cardiovascular disease. *Am Heart J* 1996; 132: 1207–1221.

Blomquist TM, Priola DV, Romero AM. Source of intrinsic innervation of canine ventricles: a functional study. *Am J Physiol* 1987; 252: H638–H644.

Burkhoff D, Fisher PE, Apfelbaum M et al. Histologic appearance of transmyocardial laser channels after 4½ weeks. *Ann Thorac Surg* 1996; 61: 1532–1535.

Butler CK, Smith FM, Cardinal R et al. Cardiac responses to electrical stimulation of discrete loci in canine atrial or ventricular ganglionated plexi. *Am J Physiol* 1990; 259: H1365–H1373.

Byerly H. Explaining and exploiting placebo effects. *Perspect Biol Med* 1976; 19: 423–435.

Cheng Z, Powley TL, Schwaber JS et al. Vagal afferent innervation of the atria of the rat heart reconstructed with confocal microscopy. *J Comp Neurol* 1997; 381: 1–17.

Chiu RC, Scott HJ. The nature of early run-off in myocardial arterial implants. *J Thorac Cardiovasc Surg* 1973; 65: 768–777.

Conger JL, Wilansky S, Moore WH. Myocardial revascularization with laser: preliminary findings. *Circulation* 1995; 92: II-58–II-65

Cooley DA, Frazier OH, Kadipasaoglu KA et al. Transmyocardial laser revascularization. Anatomic evidence of long-term channel patency. *Tex Heart Inst J* 1994; 21: 220–224.

Curtis AB, Abela GS, Griffin JC et al. Transvascular argon laser ablation of atrioventricular conduction in dogs: Feasibility and morphological results. *Pace* 1989; 12: 347–357.

Curtis AB, Vincent GM, Abela GS in GS Abela, ed., *Lasers in Cardiovascular Medicine and Surgery: Fundamentals and Techniques*, Kluwer Academic Publishers, New York, 1990, p.197.

Domkowski PW, Biswas SS, Steenbergen C et al. Histological evidence of angiogenesis 9 months after transmyocardial laser revascularization. *Circulation* 2001; 103: 469–471.

Eckstein FS, Scheule AM, Vogel U et al. Transmyocardial laser revascularization in the acute ischaemic heart: no improvement of acute myocardial perfusion or prevention of myocardial infarction. *Eur J Cardiothorac Surg* 1999; 15: 702–708.

Fenech A, Abela GS, Crea F et al. A comparative study of laser beam characteristics in blood and saline media. *Am J Cardiol* 1985; 55: 1389–1392.

Fisher PE, Kohmoto T, DeRosa CM et al. Histologic analysis of transmyocardial channels: comparison of CO_2 and holium:YAG lasers. *Ann Thorac Surg* 1997; 64: 466–472.

Forman RD, Linderoth B, Ardell JL et al. Modulation of intrinsic cardiac neurons by spinal cord stimulation: implications for its therapeutic use in angina pectoris. *Cardiovasc Res* 2000; 47: 367–375.

Frazier OH, Cooley DA, Kadipasaoglu KA et al. Myocardial revascariztion with laser: preliminary findings. *Circulation* 1995; 92 (*Suppl* II): II-58–II-65.

Gagliardi M, Randall WC, Bieger D et al. Activity of neurons located on the *in situ* canine heart. *Am J Physiol* 1988; 255: H789–H800.

Gassler N, Wintzer HO, Stubbe HM et al. Transmyocardial laser revascularization: histological features in human nonresponder myocardium. *Circulation* 1997; 95: 371–375.

Goldman A, Greenstone SM, Preuss FS et al. Experimental methods for producing a collateral circulation of the heart directly from the left ventricle. *J Thorac Surg* 1956; 31: 364–374.

Hage-Korban EE, Ma H, Huang R et al. Effect of transmyocardial laser on heart function(abstract). *Lasers Med Surg* 2001; 28 (*Suppl* 13):46.

Hamos JE, vanHorn SC, Rackowski D et al. Synaptic connectivity of a local circuit neurone in lateral geniculate nucleus of the cat. *Nature* 1985; 341: 197–211

Hardy RJ, James FW, Millard RW et al. Regional myocardial blood flow and cardiac mechanics in dog hearts with CO_2 laser-induced intramyocardial revascularization. *Basic Res Cardiol* 1990; 85: 179–197.

Hirsch GM, Thompson GW, Arora RC et al. Transmyocardial laser revascularization does not denervate the canine heart. *Ann Thorac Surg* 1999; 68: 460–469.

Horvath KA, Mannting F, Cummings N et al. Transmyocardial revascularization with laser: operative techniques and clinical results at two years. *J Thorac Cardiovasc Surg* 1996; 111: 1047–1053.

Hughes GC, Kypson AP, St. Louis JD et al. Improved perfusion and contractile reserve after transmyocardial laser revascularization in a model of hibernating myocardium. *Ann Thorac Surg* 1999; 67: 1714–1720.

Kaul U, Shawl F, Singh B et al. Percutaneous transluminal myocardial revascularization with a holmium laser system: procedural results and early clinical outcome. *Cathet Cardiovasc Interv* 1999; 47: 287–291.

Kim CB, Kesten R, Javier M et al. Percutaneous method of laser transmyocardial revascularization. *Cathet Cardiovasc Diagn* 1997; 40: 223–238.

Kohmoto T, Fisher PE, Gu A et al. Does blood flow through transmyocardial CO_2 laser channels? *J Am Coll Cardiol* 1996; 27: 13A.

Kohmoto T, Fisher PE, Gu A et al. Physiology, histology, and 20 week morphology of acute transmyocardial channels made with a CO_2 laser. *Ann Thorac Surg* 1997; 63: 1275–1283.

Kwong K, Kanellopoulos GK, Nickols J et al. Trans-myocardial laser treatment denervates canine myocardium. *J Thorac Cardiovasc Surg* 1997; 114: 883–890.

Kwong KF, Schuessler RB, Kanellopoulos GK et al. Nontransmural laser treatment incompletely denervates canine myocardium. *Circulation* 1998; 98: II-67–II-72.

Landreneau R, Nawarawong W, Laughlin H et al. Direct CO_2 laser revascularization of the myocardium. *Lasers Surg Med* 1991; 11: 35–42.

Leon MB, Baim DS, Moses JW et al. A randomized blinded clinical trial comparing percutaneous laser myocardial revascularization (using Biosense LV Mapping) vs. placebo in patients with refractory coronary ischemia(abstract). *Circulation* 2000; 102: II–565.

Lutter G, Martin J, Koster W et al. Analysis of the new indirect revascularization method by determining objective parameters of clinical chemistry and histology. *Eur J Cardi thoracic Surg* 1999a: 709–716.

Lutter G, Martin J, Takahashi N et al. Transmyocardial laser revascularization: experimental studies in healthy porcine myocardium. *Ann Thorac Surg* 1999b; 67: 1708–1713.

Lutter G, Martin J, Dern P et al. Evaluation of the indirect revascularization method after 3 months chronic myocardial ischemia. *Eur J Cardiothorac Surg* 2000; 18: 38–45.

Mirhoseini M, Cayton MM. Revascularization of the heart by laser. *J Microsurg* 1981; 2: 252–260.

Mirhoseini M, Cayton MM, Shelgikar S et al. Clinical report: laser myocardial revascularization *Lasers Surg Med* 1986; 459–461.

Mueller XM, Tevaearai HT, Chaubert P et al. Transmyocardial laser revascularization in acutely ischaemic myocardium. *Eur J Cardiothoracic Surg* 1998: 170–175.

Mueller XM, Tevaearai HT, Chaubert P et al. Mechanism of action of transmyocardial laser revascularization. *Schweiz Med Wochenschr* 1999a; 129: 1889–1892.

Mueller XM, Tevaearai HT, Genton CY et al. Myocardial scarring after transmyocardial laser revascularization: a potential mechanism of clinical improvement? *Lasers Surg Med* 1999b; 25: 79–87.

Murphy DA, Thompson GW, Ardell JL et al. The heart reinnervates after transplantation. *Ann Thorac Surg* 2000; 69: 1769–1781.

Nordrehaug JE, Salem M, Rotevatn S et al. Blinded evaluation of laser (PTMR) intervention electively for angina pectoris (BELIEF) (oral presentation). American College of Cardiology, Orlando, FL, March 19, 2001.

Oesterle SN, Sanborn TA, Ali N et al. Percutaneous transmyocardial laser revascularization for severe angina: the PACIFIC randomized trial. *Lancet* 2000; 356: 1705–1710.

Pifarré R. An experimental evaluation of different procedures to induce ventricular-luminal myocardial circulation. Master of Science Thesis, McGill University, 1962.

Pifarré R, Jasuja ML, Lynch RD et al. Myocardial revascularization by transmyocardial acupuncture. A physiologic impossibility. *J Thorac Cardiovasc Surg* 1969; 58: 424–231.

Sen PK, Udwadia TE, Kinare SG et al. Transmyocardial acupuncture. *J Thorac Cardiovasc Surg* 1965; 50: 181–189.

Spanier T, Smith CR, Burkhoff D. Angiogenesis: a possible mechanism underlying the clinical benefits of transmyocardial revascularization. *J Clin Laser Med Surg* 1997; 15: 269–273.

Stevenson RS, Thompson GW, Wilkinson M et al. Neuronally induced augmentation of cardiac output. *Can J Cardiol* 2000; 15: 1361–1366.

Wearn JT. The role of the thebesian vessels in the circulation of the heart. *J Exp Med* 1928; 47: 293.

Wearn JT, Mettler SR, Klump TJ et al. The nature of the vascular communication between the coronary arteries and the chambers of the heart. *Am Heart J* 1933; 9: 143–164.

Whittaker P, Kloner RA, Przyklenk K. Laser mediated transmural myocardial channels do not salvage acutely ischemic myocardium. *J Am Coll Cardiol* 1993; 22: 302–309.

Whittaker P. Laser-mediated reversal of cardiac expansion after myocardial infarction. *Lasers Surg Med* 1999; 25: 198–206.

Whittaker P, Spariosu K, Ho ZZ. Success of transmyocardial laser revascularization is determined by the amount and organization of scar tissue produced in response to initial injury: results of ultraviolet laser treatment. *Lasers Surg Med* 1999; 24: 253–260.

Yuan BX, Ardell JL, Hopkins DA et al. Gross and microscopic anatomy of canine intrinsic cardiac neurons. *Anat Rec* 1994; 239: 75–87.

7

Biosense NOGA™: Percutaneous Laser Myocardial Revascularization and Gene Transfer

Malcolm T. Foster III, M.D., F.A.C.C.,
Ramon C. Raneses Jr., M.D., F.A.C.C.,
Michael A. Lauer, M.D., and
Tim A. Fischell, M.D., F.A.C.C., F.S.C.A.I.

Heart Institute at Borgess Medical Center
Kalamazoo, Michigan

SUMMARY

The Biosense/NOGA system is an endocardial mapping system that provides a three-dimensional electromechanical image of the left ventricle.

Electromechanical mapping has been shown to be useful in differentiating infarcted myocardium from healthy myocardium.

The Biosense DMR system allows for the precise targeting of myocardial segments that may be appropriate for therapeutic angiogenesis.

NOGA/DMR was tested in the DIRECT trial, a blinded, randomized study design to test the hypothesis that laser injury promotes neovascularization and therapeutic angiogenesis. Active treatment did not appear to be better than placebo. Another study, the BELIEF trial, demonstrated significant improvement using a laser catheter system that penetrated the myocardium.

NOGA guidance is being investigated for use with myocardial gene transfer via percutaneous catheter.

7.1. INTRODUCTION

Biosense NOGA/DMR is an integrated system for mapping the left ventricle and performing laser myocardial revascularization and catheter-based gene transfer. The NOGA diagnostic catheter acquires three-dimensional (3D) electromechanical data that identify viable but ischemic myocardium. The DMR laser catheter creates endomyocardial channels in the target tissue using NOGA guidance. The system is currently in use in the DIRECT trial, a phase II randomized trial of nonrevascularizable patients with documented ischemia. This chapter details the components and procedures of the NOGA/DMR system.

Myocardial Revascularization: Novel Percutaneous Approaches, Edited by George S. Abela.
ISBN 0-471-36166-6   Copyright © 2002 Wiley-Liss, Inc.

7.2. NOGA

The Biosense NOGA system is a nonfluoro-scopic, catheter-based endocardial mapping system that generates a 3D electromechanical image of the left ventricle. The system consists of a flexible catheter connected to a mapping and navigation workstation. Magnetic energy indicates the location and orientation of the catheter while local intracardiac electrograms are simultaneously recorded. The geometry of the left ventricle is constructed in real time. Electrophysiologic information is color coded and superimposed on the electromechanical map.

The navigation and mapping system consists of a passive magnetic field, an external ultra-low magnetic field emitter (locator pad), and a processing unit. The catheter is similar to a standard 8F deflectable-tip pacing catheter composed of tip and ring electrodes, with a location sensor embedded in the tip. The locator pad is positioned beneath the catheterization laboratory table. Three coils in the locator pad generate an ultra-low magnet field that decays as a function of distance from each coil. The location sensor measures the strength of each magnetic field and the distance from each coil. The distances determine the radii of theoretical spheres around each coil. Triangulation of the three spheres determines the location of the sensor in space. The system accurately determines the location and orientation of the catheter in six degrees of freedom (x, y, z, roll, pitch, and yaw) and simultaneously records the local intracardiac electrogram. The 3D geometry of the chamber is reconstructed in real time. Electrophysiologic information is color coded and superimposed on the electromechanical map.

7.2.1. Procedure

The mapping catheter is advanced under fluoroscopic guidance to the thoracic aorta. The catheter tip is deflected to form a J shape and advanced across the aortic valve into the left ventricle. Three initial points are acquired: the left ventricular apex, the high septum/aortic outflow tract, and the high lateral wall below the mitral annulus. The initial points create an elementary (triangular) map. Seventy to one hundred additional points are obtained, using fluoroscopy as needed, to complete a comprehensive 3D map of the left ventricle. The map is created in real time as each point is acquired. Local activation time and unipolar and bipolar intracardiac recordings are simultaneously color coded and superimposed on the 3D map. The electromechanical information obtained during systole and diastole generates functional data including end-diastolic and end-systolic volumes, stroke volume, ejection fraction, local endocardial shortening, electrical activation time, and electromechanical delay.

7.2.2. Results

In-vitro and in-vivo studies have demonstrated catheter location to be reliable and accurate. Investigators performed repeated location measurements of the same site and found the accuracy to be 0.16 ± 0.02 mm (Gepstein et al., 1997). Location accuracy was measured in a test jig by comparing the distances between catheter locations at different sites compared with known distances. A high degree of precision was found with a mean error range of 0.31–0.71 mm and a total mean error of 0.42 ± 0.05 mm (Gepstein et al., 1997). Reproducibility and precision of catheter placement were validated in a porcine model. Reproducibility location accuracy inside the beating heart had a standard deviation of 0.74 ± 0.13 mm and an average maximal range and mean error of 1.26 ± 0.08 and 0.54 ± 0.05 mm, respectively (Gepstein et al., 1997). Catheter location was determined with a high degree of precision (mean relative distance error 0.73 ± 0.03 mm) (Gepstein et al., 1997).

Electromechanical data from the endocardial surface differentiate normal myocardium from infarcted myocardium. Infarcted myocardium is characterized by decreased or absent local shortening and low voltage. Investigators ligated the arteries of canine hearts and compared electromechanical data from control and infarcted tissue at baseline, 24 h, and 3 weeks. Significant reductions in both unipolar (UP) and bipolar (BP) voltages were seen at 24 h (32% reduction UP, 58% reduction BP) and 3 weeks (66% reduction UP, 78% reduction BP) (Gepstein et al., 1998; Kornowski et al., 1998b). The reduction in voltage was associated with impaired mechanical activity in the infarct territory manifested by abnormal local shortening (LS) at 24 h and 3 weeks compared with baseline. Both electrical voltage and mechanical local shortening were normal in the noninfarct territory, demonstrating the ability to distinguish healthy from infarcted myocardium (Kornowski et al., 1998b).

Human studies differentiating infarcted myocardium from healthy myocardium have yielded similar results. Electromechanical mapping of infarcted myocardium was compared with that of noninfarct zones as well as control patients. Bipolar and unipolar voltages were significantly lower in infarcted tissue compared with remote noninfarcted zones and normal controls. Similarly, mechanical activity was impaired in the infarcted tissue compared with healthy myocardium (Kornowski et al., 1998b). Thus, in both animal and human models, electromechanical

mapping has been a useful diagnostic tool for differentiating infarcted myocardium from healthy myocardium (see Chapter 13).

In human studies, electromechanical mapping of ischemic myocardium demonstrated a characteristic pattern different from normal and infarcted myocardium. Unipolar voltage potentials and local endocardial shortening were measured in patients with symptomatic chronic angina with reversible and fixed myocardial perfusion defects by adenosine stress SPECT images. Comparative analysis of the myocardial perfusion images and the electromechanical data showed the highest average voltage and local shortening in the normal perfusion segments (14.0 ± 2.0 mV and 12.5 ± 2.8%, respectively). Fixed perfusion defects had the lowest voltage potentials and local shortening (7.5 ± 3.4 mV and 3.4 ± 3.4%, respectively). Myocardial segments with reversible defects had intermediate values for voltage (12.0 ± 2.8 mV; $P = 0.048$ vs. normal and $P = 0.005$ vs. fixed segments) and local shortening (10.3 ± 3.7%; $P = 0.067$ vs. normal and $P = 0.001$ vs. fixed segments) (Kornowski et al., 1998c). Figure 7-1 demonstrates paired electrical and mechanical maps that define a zone of viable but ischemic myocardium. Additional studies comparing electromechanical NOGA mapping with

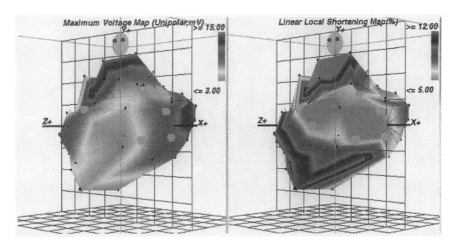

FIGURE 7-1. This figure demonstrates paired electrical and mechanical maps that define a zone of viable but ischemic myocardium in the distribution of the left anterior descending coronary artery.

positron emission tomography (PET) and dobutamine stress echocardiography (DSE) have demonstrated good correlation as well (Kornowski et al., 2000; Van Langenhove et al., 2000).

7.3. DMR

The Biosense DMR system uses a Ho:YAG laser pulse delivered by optical fiber to the catheter tip. NOGA guidance is used to achieve optimal contact between laser and tissue at treatment zones and to prevent repetitive same-site laser firing that may increase the risk of perforation. NOGA identifies and labels ischemic treatment zones and avoids areas of infarction. Figure 7-2 demonstrates 48 laser channels that were targeted to two zones of ischemic but viable myocardium. Note that the channels were fairly evenly dis-

tributed to prevent perforation of the left ventricle. The energy setting is 2 J/pulse, delivered via a 300-μm fiber (Kornowski et al., 1999). Unlike other catheter-based systems, the laser fiber does not penetrate the myocardium. Instead, the catheter tip maintains perpendicular contact with the endocardium, yielding real time electromechanical data (Kornowski et al., 1999). The laser pulse is gated to the cardiac cycle after confirmation of four consistent R-R intervals.

7.3.1. Results

In animal studies, the typical depth of a laser channel is 4–5 mm (Kornowski et al., 1998a). Histologic analysis demonstrated irregular channel borders with a zone of collateral tissue injury. Dissection planes extended into interstitial spaces because of a profound

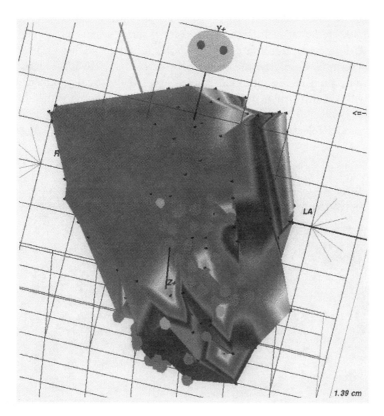

FIGURE 7-2.   This figure demonstrates 48 laser channels that were targeted to 2 zones of ischemic but viable myocardium. Note that the channels were fairly evenly distributed to prevent perforation of the left ventricle.

photoacoustic effect (Kornowski et al., 1998a). Other investigators have demonstrated well-developed capillaries in the laser-treated tissue at 28 days after Ho:YAG therapy. This finding is consistent with the concept that laser injury promotes neovascularization and therapeutic angiogenesis (Lu et al., 1999).

Human data from the phase I clinical trial of the Biosense NOGA/DMR system were encouraging. Procedural success was achieved in 75 of 76 patients (Kornowski et al., 1999). One patient required pericardiocentesis because of perforation of the left ventricle. One patient developed a minor stroke. Ejection fractions did not improve, but angina scores and exercise times increased significantly (Kornowski et al., 1999). These data led to the design of the DIRECT trial, a phase II randomized trial of NOGA/DMR for nonrevascularizable patients with ischemic myocardium. The hypothesis of the trial is that NOGA/DMR will stimulate neovascularization and promote therapeutic angiogenesis. Patients will receive either "high-dose" laser (30–25 channels per zone), "low-dose" laser (10–15 channels per zone), or placebo. The study will be the first clinical trial of any form of laser myocardial revascularization to use a blinded, randomized design to eliminate patient bias and placebo effect. The results of this study presented by Dr. Leon et al. (2000) demonstrated that active treatment did not appear to be better than placebo. However, another study, the BELIEF trial by Nordrehaug et al. (2001), demonstrated significant improvement in angina class but not in total exercise duration. Unlike the DIRECT study with DMR, this study was performed using the Axcis™ system (ECLIPSE, Sunnyvale, CA), a laser catheter system that penetrated the myocardium (see Chapters 6 and 8).

7.3.2. Gene Transfer

A porcine model was used to investigate the feasibility and safety of percutaneous, catheter-based myocardial gene transfer using NOGA guidance (Vale et al., 1999). An injection catheter delivered plasmid using cytomegalovirus promoter/enhancer, encoding a nucleus-specific LacZ gene. Gene transfer was confirmed by measuring peak β-galactosidase activity after 5 days. Subsequently, ameroid constrictors were applied to the left circumflex artery. NOGA mapping was used to target gene transfer to the zone of ischemia. Peak β-galactosidase activity was significantly greater in the left circumflex territory compared with normal control tissue (Vale et al., 1999).

7.4. SUMMARY

Biosense NOGA/DMR is an integrated system for mapping the left ventricle and performing laser myocardial revascularization and catheter-based gene transfer. Electromechanical data from the endocardial surface differentiate normal myocardium from infarcted and ischemic myocardium. The NOGA/DMR system allows precise targeting of myocardial segments that may be appropriate for therapeutic angiogenesis. Results from the phase I clinical trial using NOGA/DMR were encouraging. Preclinical studies of catheter-based gene transfer demonstrated safety and feasibility. However, a blinded, randomized, placebo-controlled, phase II trial (the DIRECT study) showed no significant difference from placebo. Future applications may include the delivery of genes or growth factors in combination with percutaneous laser myocardial revascularization.

References

Gepstein L, Hayam G, Ben-Haim SA. A novel method for nonfluoroscopic catheter-based electroanatomical mapping of the heart. In vitro and in vivo accuracy results. *Circulation* 1997; 95: 1611–1622.

Gepstein L, Goldin J, Lessick G et al. Electromechanical characterization of chronic myocardial infarction in the canine coronary occlusion model. *Circulation* 1998; 98: 2055–2064.

Kornowski R, Hong MK, Leon MB. Current perspectives on direct myocardial revascularization. *Am J Cardiol* 1998a; 81: 44E–48E.

Kornowski R, Hong MK, Gepstein L et al. Preliminary animal and clinical experiences using an electromechanical endocardial mapping procedure to distinguish infarcted from healthy myocardium. *Circulation* 1998b; 98: 1116–1124.

Kornowski R, Hong MK, Leon MB et al. Comparison between left ventricular electromechanical mapping and radionuclide perfusion imaging for detection of myocardial viability. *Circulation* 1998c; 98: 1837–1841.

Kornowski R, Bhargava B, Leon MB. Percutaneous transmyocardial laser revascularization: an overview. *Cathet Cardiovasc Interv* 1999; 47: 354–359.

Kornowski R, Fuchs S, Hendel R et al. Endocardial electromechanical mapping to assess myocardial viability: a comparative ROC analysis with radionuclide perfusion imaging (abstract). *J Am Coll Cardiol* 2000; 35A: 81A.

Leon MB, Baim DS, Moses JW et al. A randomized blinded clinical trial comparing percutaneous laser myocardial revascularization (using Biosense LV Mapping) vs. placebo in patients with refractory coronary ischemia (abstract). *Circulation* 2000; 102: II-565.

Lu CH, Yu TJ, Lai ST. Transmyocardial holmium-YAG laser channels in an animal model: a preliminary morphologic and histologic study. *Chung Hua I Hsueh Tsa (Taipei)* 1999; 62: 614–618.

Nordrehaug JE, Salem M, Rotevatn S et al. Blinded evaluation of laser (PTMR) intervention electively for angina pectoris (BELIEF). American College of Cardiology, Orlando, FL, March 19, 2001.

Vale PR, Losordo DW, Tkebuchava T et al. Catheter-based myocardial gene transfer utilizing nonfluoroscopic electromechanical left ventricular mapping. *J Am Coll Cardiol* 1999; 34: 246–254.

Van Langenhove G, Smits PC, Hamburger JN et al. Hibernating myocardium diagnosis with nonfluoroscopic electromechanical 1 (NOGA™) mapping: a comparison with dobutamine stress echocardiography (abstract). *J Am Coll Cardiol* 2000; 35A: 81A.

III

Current Technology for Percutaneous Myocardial Revascularization

8

Percutaneous Myocardial Revascularization (PMR): Indications and Clinical Experience

Joel D. Eisenberg, M.D., Elie Hage-Korban, M.D.,
Khaled Ghosheh, M.D.,
George S. Abela, M.D., M.Sc., M.B.A.

Department of Medicine/Cardiology
Michigan State University
East Lansing, Michigan

and

Stephen N. Oesterle, M.D.

Department of Medicine/Cardiology
Massachusetts General Hospital
Harvard Medical School
Boston, Massachusetts

SUMMARY

- PMR differs from TMR in both approach (open vs. closed, endocardial vs. pericardial) and in the type of laser used for the procedure (CO_2 vs. excimer, Ho:YAG, and Er:YAG lasers).
- The three types of catheter systems used for PMR all use Ho:YAG lasers; however, they differ in fiber diameter, catheter design, and energy parameters.
- Initial trials have indicated that there is a greater degree of acute thermal damage with the Ho:YAG laser as well suggesting that it may acutely depress left ventricular function.
- The first relatively large randomized trial of PMR to be published in human subjects was the PACIFIC trial. This trial consisted of 221 patients randomized to PMR with medical therapy versus medical therapy only and resulted in a median improvement in exercise duration of 89 s for the PMR group (vs. 12.5 s for the medical therapy group). Angina class was II or lower in 34.1% with PMR patients compared with 13.0% of those medically treated.

Myocardial Revascularization: Novel Percutaneous Approaches, Edited by George S. Abela.
ISBN 0-471-36166-6 Copyright © 2002 Wiley-Liss, Inc.

Mechanisms that have been proposed for potential clinical benefit of PMR (and TMR) include direct reperfusion of the myocardium, denervation, angiogenesis, mechanical remodeling of the heart muscle, and placebo effect.

Initial results of PMR are enticing; however, further trials must be completed to test the actual benefit to patients. Information thus far has been mostly derived from non-randomized studies, and the number of patients is usually small. In addition, the placebo factor cannot be estimated from the present studies.

8.1. THE EVOLUTION OF PMR

Transmyocardial laser revascularization (TMR) is an approved surgically based therapy for patients with advanced coronary disease. Multiple studies have indicated that significant angina relief can be achieved for many patients without options for conventional revascularization strategies (Aaberge et al., 2000; Allen et al., 1999a; Frazier et al., 1999). The development of PMR (percutaneous myocardial revascularization) has followed the trend of utilizing less invasive percutaneous procedures for the treatment of coronary heart disease. The PMR technique was developed to avoid many of the limitations of TMR including thoracotomy and general anesthesia. The goal of PMR is to mitigate attendant morbidity and mortality risks while deriving clinical benefits similar to those noted with TMR (Aaberge et al., 2000; Allen et al., 1999a; Frazier et al., 1999).

In early studies of TMR, perioperative mortality ranged between 9% and 19% with an overall 6-month mortality of 25% (Horvath, 1997). In one study 33% of patients had wound or respiratory infections related to thoracotomy and anesthesia (Schofield et al., 1999).

TMR was first performed in conjunction with bypass surgery by Mirhoseini et al. (1986). Now, except when bypass surgery is performed, a limited left thoracotomy is the usual approach for TMR (Horvath, 1998).

This modified approach has resulted in a less than 2% 30-day mortality in one randomized trial and only 3% in another randomized trial (Burkhoff et al., 1999a; Frazier et al., 1999). However, the morbidity and mortality have been reported higher as noted in one recent review (Verdaasdonk, 2000).

Another issue is the length of hospitalization, which was not reported in the aforementioned trials (Burkhoff et al., 1999a; Frazier et al., 1999). Allen et al., utilizing a Ho:YAG system, reported a perioperative mortality of 12% with a hospital stay that ranged from 1 to 25 days (mean 5.5 days) (Allen et al., 1999b). The experience at Duke University was recently reviewed in 34 consecutive patients, utilizing an 800-W CO_2 laser. There were two perioperative deaths (5.9%). The hospital stay was 9.6 ± 16.4 days (Hughes et al., 1999). In a randomized study the perioperative mortality was 4% with a mean hospital stay of 11.1 days (Aaberge et al., 2000). In a relatively large randomized study the 30-day mortality was 5%, with a 1-year survival of 84% (Allen et al., 1999a).

A thoracoscopic approach may further reduce morbidity and mortality. At least three groups have reported on such an approach (Deguzman et al., 1997; Horvath, 1998; Milano et al., 1999). The merits of these differing operative approaches are confounded by patient selection and preoperative risk factors (Burkhoff et al., 1999b; Hughes et al., 1999). Such issues will also confound results of studies on PMR.

Most of the surgical experience with TMR has been acquired with the PLC Heart-Laser™. This CO_2 laser cannot be delivered via present-day fiberoptics (Verdaasdonk, 2000) and relies on a series of articulated mirrors for hand-held delivery to the epicardial surface. In contrast, excimer (XeCl), Ho:YAG, and Er:YAG laser energy wavelengths can be delivered via flexible fiberoptics, enabling channel creation from the endocardial surface with a percutaneous catheter-based approach.

It is critical to recognize at the onset that the comparison of studies performed with different lasers and approaches to performing TMR or PMR is greatly limited by the different tissue effects of the different laser modalities (Kadipasaoglu and Frazier, 1999). In at least one animal study of TMR Ho:YAG led to a significant decrease in myocardial blood flow to the lased region compared with a CO_2 laser (Hughes et al., 2000). Hughes also reported that, in an animal model, the use of an excimer laser does not lead to neovascularization, which was found with both Ho:YAG and CO_2 laser therapy (Hughes et al., 1998). The difference was attributed to the need to have thermal injury, which is not present with excimer. Yet, despite this, many studies have been reported to have similar outcomes (see Chapters 5 and 6 on mechanisms).

8.2. THE CATHETER SYSTEMS

Three PMR catheter systems have been utilized in humans. All use Ho:YAG laser; however, they differ in the fiber diameter, catheter design, and energy parameters.

8.2.1. CardioGenesis Axcis™ PMR system (Eclipse Surgical Technologies, Sunnyvale, CA)

This coaxial catheter system consists of a 9F guiding catheter that delivers a lasing catheter to reach the endocardial surface. The optical fiber is coupled to a Ho:YAG laser that produces an output wavelength of 2.1 nm. The optical fiber is 400 μm in diameter, and it is capped by a 1,750-μm lens (Fig. 8-1). It delivers 2-J pulses in 350 ms, producing a peak power of 5.7 kW and a fluence of 83 J/cm^2. Pulses are delivered in groups of 2 (a single burst) at a frequency of 17 Hz. Two bursts are delivered to each intended channel site to make a deep but nontransmural channel.

During the procedure, patients are provided with conscious sedation as in other percutaneous cardiac procedures. Femoral arterial and venous accesses are obtained using the standard techniques. Biplane ventriculography and coronary angiography are used to direct the catheter to the targeted

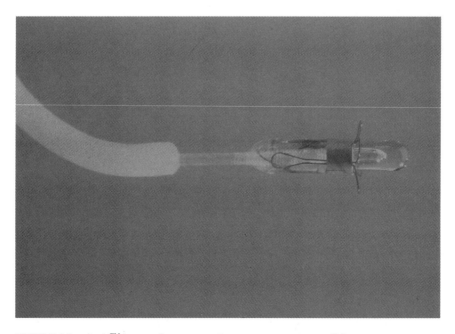

FIGURE 8-1. Axcis™ laser catheter system for percutaneous myocardial revascularization catheter system.

left ventricular segment. The laser catheters are introduced into the left ventricle (LV) across the aortic valve via the 9 F guiding catheter. These catheters have different angulated tips (Fig. 8-2). The combination of the laser and the guiding catheters can be manipulated into different configurations that facilitate access to the different segments of the ventricular wall. Its coaxial design allows different degrees of longitudinal and rotational movements, which also helps in positioning the laser catheters. (Fig. 8-3). The lens (gold markers) is capped by petal-like structures made of nitinol wire to help stabilize the lens on the endocardial surface and to limit penetration into the myocardium (Fig. 8-4). After the catheter is positioned at the intended channel site, the laser fiber is advanced until firm contact has been established between the lens and the endocardium. A channel is formed by bursts of two laser pulses that are usually then repeated after catheter advancement by 1–2 mm. Channels created measure about 5 mm in depth. After a channel is created, the laser catheter tip is retracted and repositioned to establish contact at the next intended channel site. Approximately one channel is made in every 1 cm^2 of ischemic myocardium. The size and the total number of ischemic areas, usually determined at screening, determine the total number of channels required. Ventriculography is repeated at the end of the

laser procedure to confirm the nontransmural placement of the channels. The entire procedure is usually accomplished in 60–90 min. In 1999, the total number of procedures performed using the CardioGenesis system was reported to be more than 300 worldwide. The CardioGenesis Axcis™ catheter remains an investigational device, currently being considered by the FDA for premarket approval.

8.2.2. Eclipse System (Eclipse Surgical Technologies, Sunnyvale, CA)

This PMR system couples a pulsed Ho:YAG laser with a flexible multi-fiberoptic delivery system located in an 8.3 F catheter. Laser energy is delivered at 0.7 J per pulse given in three pulses. The system uses fluoroscopic guidance for orientation inside the LV. Femoral arterial and femoral venous accesses are obtained with 9 F and 8 F introducers, respectively, using the standard techniques. Heparin 5,000 IU is administered intravenously to achieve an activated clotting time ≥280 s. A 6 F pigtail catheter is advanced into the LV, and ventriculography is performed in the 30° right anterior oblique (RAO) projection. A 45° left anterior oblique (LAO) ventriculogram is performed if the wall to be lased is the posterolateral wall. A 90°-left lateral view is obtained if the anterior wall is to be lased. The pigtail catheter is then

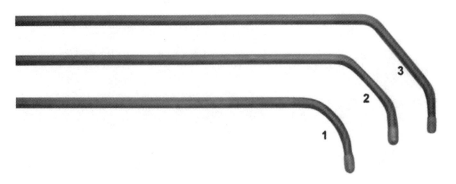

FIGURE 8-2. Guiding laser catheter system that allows for various positionings. These catheters have different angulated tips that help manipulate into configurations and access different segments of the ventricular wall.

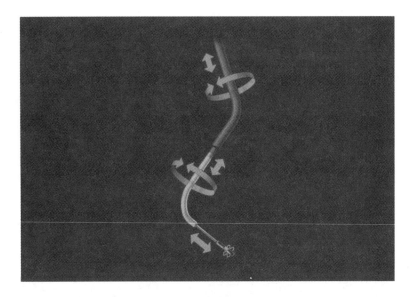

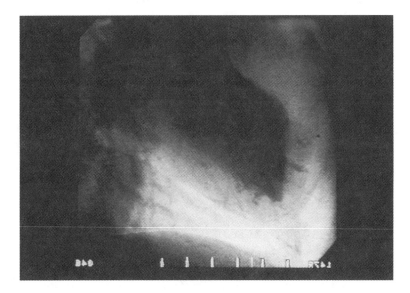

FIGURE 8-3. (Top) Percutaneous myocardial revascularization catheter system consisting of a guiding catheter and the laser catheter. Various manipulations and rotational angles are displayed (Reprinted with permission of the American College of Cardiology, *J Am Coll Cardiol* 1999; 34: 1663–1670.) (Bottom) Left ventricular angiogram from a dog model treated with the above catheter. Channels made by the laser fill with contrast during systole (Kim C, Kasten R, Javier M et al. Percutaneous method of laser transmyocardial revascularization. *Cathet Cardiovasc Diagn* 1997; 40: 223–228. Reprinted by permission of Wiley-Liss, Inc., a subsidiary of John Wiley & Sons, Inc.)

replaced with a 5- or 7-cm PMR catheter over a 0.038-in. curved, coated Amplatz extra-stiff guidewire. The PMR catheter is shaped to conform on the left ventricular wall. The guidewire is then removed, and the PMR catheter is aspirated, flushed, and attached to a Touhy-Borst Y-adapter. The other end of the Y-adapter is attached to a continuous

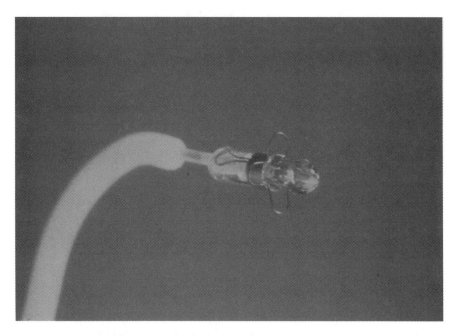

FIGURE 8-4. Axcis™ laser catheter system for percutaneous myocardial revascularization catheter system. The laser fiber tip with lens and nitinol petals is shown. (Reprinted with permission of the American College of Cardiology, *J Am Coll Cardiol* 1999; 34: 1663–1670.)

heparin flushing system. The SlimFlex laser fiber (Eclipse Surgical Technologies) is introduced into the PMR catheter and advanced under fluoroscopic guidance to the LV (Fig. 8-5). The PMR catheter is advanced to the apex and then deflected toward the wall intended to be lased. The PMR catheter and the SlimFlex fiber are aligned. A distal marker band on the SlimFlex fiber is advanced to a position slightly distal to the marker of the PMR catheter. Laser energy (3.5 W) is delivered in a series of three pulses through the 1-mm-diameter optical fiber. The channels are created starting at the most apical portion of the target myocardium, and then the catheter is gradually retracted basally. The channels are 1 cm apart. The catheter position is verified using both RAO and the LAO ventriculography before laser activation. After all the channels are created, the laser fiber and the PMR catheter are removed. The 0.038-in. guidewire is then advanced and the PMR catheter is exchanged for a pigtail catheter. Final hemodynamics and left ventriculography are then performed utilizing the original projection angles.

8.2.3. DMR Using the Biosense Guidance System

This is a nonfluoroscopic platform for PMR that uses a Ho:YAG system (Fig. 8-6). Biosense developed this three-dimensional guidance system, which is an electroanatomic mapping system (Fig. 8-7). The navigation and mapping rely on low-intensity electromagnetic field energy source for three-dimensional reconstruction of the LV. This system minimizes the need for fluoroscopy or contrast administration. Because of the ability of the system to collect the endocardial electrical data with unipolar and bipolar voltages, the status of the myocardial viability can be assessed depending on the presence of normal or reduced endocardial voltage potential. The mechanical map with the local

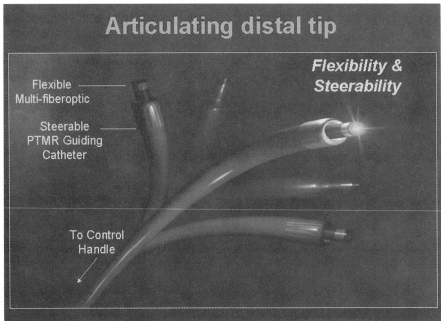

FIGURE 8-5. (A) Steerable percutaneous guiding catheter system (Eclipse Surgical Technologies, Sunnyvale, CA). (B) Steering device handle to manipulate catheter tip (Courtesy of Eclipse Surgical Technologies, Sunnyvale, CA.)

endocardial shortening can provide global and regional data on the contractility of the LV. This system uses a single fiber laser integrated within an 8 F mapping catheter. It delivers 2 J for a single pulse. The laser fiber does not penetrate the myocardium, but instead it maintains contact with the endocardium during laser activation.

Biosense DMR

An Electromechanical Mapping and Guidance System for Direct Myocardial Revascularization

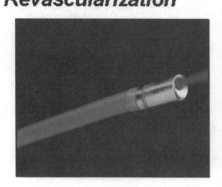

Laser catheter

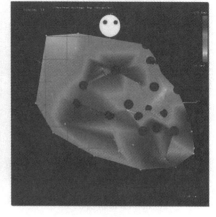

Noga Map

FIGURE 8-6. DMR laser catheter system (left) and the Noga™ navigation (right) used in the DIRECT Trial (Courtesy of Cordis, J&J, Miami, FL.) (See color plates.)

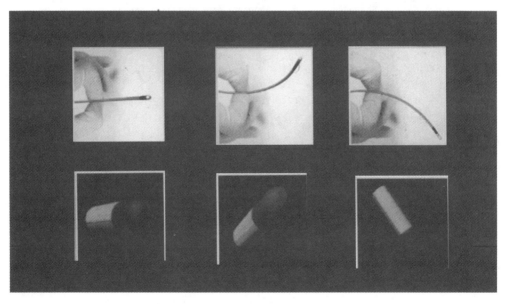

FIGURE 8-7. Real time catheter tip localization and orientation in space demonstrating real time with computer simulation (Courtesy of Cordis, J&J, Miami, FL.)

8.3. TRIAL RESULTS (ANIMAL AND HUMAN)

8.3.1. Animal Trials

The first use of a transvascular approach for direct delivery of laser irradiation to the myocardium via an optical fiber was reported by Abela et al. in 1983 in a canine model (Abela et al., 1983). This approach was performed to induce intramyocardial lesions to interrupt A-V conduction pathways with an argon laser. Histologic analysis of the lased myocardium demonstrated channels with areas of surrounding thermal injury. Using a similar approach via the left atrium. Jeevanandam et al. reported the use of a thulium-holmium-chromium:YAG (THC:-YAG) laser in a canine model (Jeevanandam et al., 1990). Nontransmural channels (4 channels/cm^2) were created, each measuring 600 μm in diameter. These channels were placed in a left ventricular wall segment rendered ischemic by prior ligation of the left anterior descending (LAD). The laser was fired until blanching was seen on the epicardial surface. Energy was delivered in pulses of 800 mJ at a frequency of 3 Hz. At 6 weeks, laser-treated animals were found to have significantly smaller infarcts compared to nontreated controls. Contrast ventriculography showed patent myocardial channels perfusing the ventricular wall in systole.

Yano et al. used the same technique to assess the effect of nontransmural channels on myocardial contractility in acute ischemia (Yano et al., 1993). A Ho:YAG laser with a wavelength of 2.1 μm was used to create channels in the distribution of the LAD. An average of 3 channels/cm^2 was created using laser energy of 600 mW/pulse at a frequency of 10 Hz. An average of 20 repetitions were required to create one channel (about 12 J). An average of 40 channels were created in each animal. Myocardial contractility was assessed utilizing ultrasonic transducers implanted in the myocardium and by two-dimensional echocardiography. The LAD was occluded for 90 min in the treatment and control groups. Myocardial contractility during acute ischemia and reperfusion was analyzed. There was limited preservation of regional contractility in the treatment group, whereas immediate and sustained akinesis or dyskinesis was noticed in the involved area of the control group. It was because of these results that laser revascularization using Ho:YAG laser via a percutaneous approach was felt to be potentially applicable to human subjects.

Laser catheters were then developed for PMR. Kim et al. (1997) reported the first true PMR study on the canine model using Ho:YAG laser fiberoptic catheters delivered via 9 F catheters. With a femoral arterial approach, the catheter was directed using biplane coronary angiography, left ventriculography, and transesophageal echocardiography (TEE). The catheters were directed to anterior, lateral, inferoposterior, or septal regions of the LV by selecting different guiding and lasing catheters. Small manipulations were required for a refinement in the position of the catheter. Laser firing was synchronized to the QRS complex to deliver energy during systole 100–150 ms after the QRS complex. Channels measured 1 mm in diameter and 5 mm in depth. They were visualized with contrast ventriculography showing diastolic filling of multiple channels originating from the endocardial surface. After initial experiments, two bursts of 12 J each were used to produce channels 5–8 mm in depth. The procedure was well tolerated with no hemodynamic compromise, sustained ventricular arrhythmias, or abnormalities of ventricular wall motion. The number of channels found on gross examination was 70–90% of the number of channels attempted. On gross and microscopic examinations, these channels appeared similar to those created by CO_2 laser in TMR. However, there is a greater degree of acute thermal damage surrounding Ho:YAG channels (Fig. 8-8). Other laser wavelengths such as the Er:YAG laser (λ = 2,940 nm) are better absorbed by the water in the tissue and create a channel with shaper edges and less thermal damage (Fig. 8-9).

The latter observation of a greater degree of lateral thermal damage with Ho: YAG is

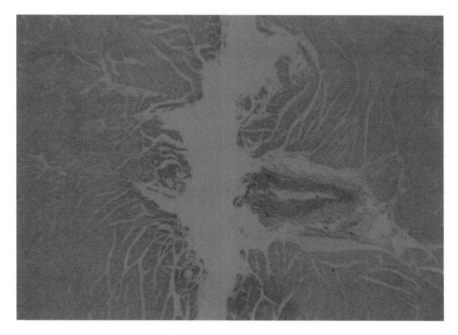

FIGURE 8-8.   Myocardial channel made by a Ho:YAG laser using a 600-mm core fiber under a saline solution. Both shock wave and some thermal injury are seen. The laser has cut through the edge of an intramyocardial artery (hematoxylin and eosin, original magnification ×25) (Abela et al., 1999. Published with permission of Kluwer Academic Publishers.)

supported by the work of Hughes et al. (2000). Using a swine model, they compared Ho:YAG and CO_2 lasers. The Ho:YAG laser resulted in a decrease in myocardial blood flow not seen with the CO_2 laser. Furthermore, depressed contractility was noted only in the Ho:YAG-treated group. The authors hypothesized that the longer wavelength of CO_2 lasers results in less collateral thermal necrosis of nearby arterioles and capillaries.

The suggestion that Ho:YAG laser may depress LV function acutely is also supported by an endovascular approach similar to that utilized in PMR. Kanellopoulos et al. used such an approach in the swine model (Kanellopoulos et al., 1999). Flow in the LAD was reduced to 70% of normal and maintained for 30 min before the delivery of endocardial nontransmural laser with a Ho:YAG system. Both dp/dt and stroke volume were noted to decline after delivery of the laser pulses. This group felt that their results called for caution in the use of Ho:YAG laser in humans.

8.3.2. Human Trials

The performance of PMR in humans followed initial favorable results with TMR utilizing Ho:YAG laser. Among the first to report were Sundt et al. (1996). The CardioGenesis TMR system was used to create intraoperative channels in seven patients with varying severity (Class II–IV) of angina. An average of 18.7 channels were created in each patient. Transient ECG changes with ST segment elevation were noted in one patient. Only a modest rise in cardiac enzymes (CK-MB) was noted, with a range of 6–30 IU/L. After a mean follow up of 9.2 weeks, all the patients had class I–II angina. There were no reported deaths.

In 1998, Oesterle et al. published the initial human experience with PMR using the CardioGenesis (Ho:YAG) Axsis™ system (Oesterle et al., 1998). This feasibility study included 30 patients with Canadian class III–IV angina with disease by coronary

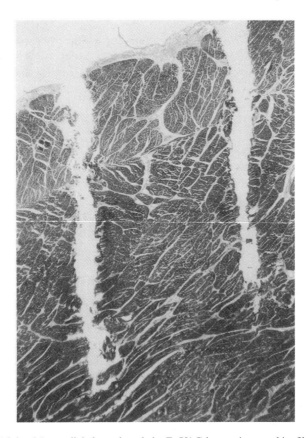

FIGURE 8-9. Myocardial channel made by Er:YAG laser using sapphire fiberoptics. The energy density was 250 mJ/pulse for 60 s. This was done while flushing a solution of normal saline. Minimal thermal injury is noted in the myocardium adjacent to the channel lumen, and channel edges are sharp with a few lateral dissection planes from shock wave effects (Abela et al., 1999. Published with permission of Kluwer Academic Publishers.)

angiography not felt to be amenable to conventional revascularization. All patients had objective evidence of reversible ischemia by thallium scanning. They excluded patients with myocardial wall thickness of under 8 mm and patients with an ejection fraction of under 30%. An average of 10–15 channels were created in each patient. The results showed that the PMR procedure was safe, and the initial short-term results were encouraging. In this study, there were no periprocedural deaths. One case of pericardial tamponade occurred and was relieved by percutaneous drainage. Arrhythmias were all nonsustained. On limited follow-up, most patients had improvement in angina class and exercise capacity.

Shawl et al. enrolled 27 patients in a phase I study of the Eclipse PTMR system. This study was conducted between June 1997 and February 1998 (Shawl et al., 1999) at two hospitals [Batra Hospital, India (16 patients) and Washington Adventist Hospital, Maryland (11 patients)]. Inclusion criteria mandated that the left ventricular wall thickness be greater than 9 mm (as seen on echocardiography) and that the left ventricular ejection fraction be >25%. All patients were symptomatic before the procedure (10 patients in CCS functional class III and 17 in class IV). Fifteen patients had a positive exercise stress test, whereas twelve patients could not undergo the test because intravenous nitroglycerin could not be weaned. An average of

17 ± 4 channels were created in each patient. Postoperatively, patients were observed with telemetry for 24 h. Two-dimensional echocardiography was performed in the first 24 h after the procedure. A 12-lead EKG was done, and the creatinine kinase (CK) was measured to evaluate myocardial necrosis. TEE was used in 11 patients, and left ventriculography was used in 16 patients to evaluate left ventricular function. An exercise test was performed on all the patients after 6 months. There were no procedure-related deaths or deaths at 30 days. Regional wall motion either remained stable or improved. CK increased in one patient. The hospital stay was 1.8 ± 1.5 days. The mean CCS functional class improved from 3.6 ± 0.5 to 0.65 ± 0.8 ($P < 0.01$) at 1 month and was 0.94 ± 0.97 at 6 months postprocedure. Stress test results were available only in 12 patients at 6 months, 9 of whom had no ECG evidence of ischemia or angina.

Whitlow et al. published encouraging phase I results with the Eclipse PMR system (Whitlow et al., 1999). Forty-one patients were enrolled at seven centers. They reported a procedure time of 61 ± 21 min. The number of channels created varied from 9 to 33. Acute complications included one cardioversion for ventricular tachycardia, placement in one hypotensive patient of an intra-aortic balloon pump, and transient heart block and a transient ischemic attack in another patient. At 3 months there were two deaths, one after CABG and one 8 days after repeated PMR. However, 90% of patients improved their anginal status to Class II or less, and the time on the treadmill with a Naugton protocol doubled at 6 months.

In 1999, Lauer et al. reported their single-institution experience with the CardioGenesis PMR system (Lauer et al., 1999). They successfully treated 34 patients, creating 8–15 channels in each subject. Left ventricular wall thickness had to be at least 8 mm, and the left ventricular ejection fraction was at least 35% in all enrollees. There were no periprocedural deaths. The length of hospital stay was 3.5 ± 2.9 days. At 3 months postprocedure, there was improvement in anginal symptoms and exercise capacity but not in myocardial perfusion as assessed by dipyridamole stress thallium perfusion. Follow-up data at 6 months were limited to only 17 patients. These patients had improvement in their angina class at 6 months from a mean of 3.0 ± 0.0 to a mean of 1.3 ± 0.8 ($P < 0.01$). They also had an increase in exercise time on bicycle ergometry from 384 ± 141 s before PMR to 514 ± 158 s ($P < 0.005$). Disappointingly, there was no improvement either in myocardial perfusion or in left ventricular function at 6 months.

The PACIFIC trial was the first human randomized trial to be published (Oesterle et al., 2000). A multicenter study, it consisted of 221 patients randomized to PMR with the CardioGenesis Axcis™ system coupled to a Ho:YAG laser plus medical therapy versus medical therapy only. All patients had class III–IV angina and a recent coronary angiogram. To be eligible for enrollment, patients had to have at least two of four treadmill stress tests with similar exercise durations, with one of these resulting in exercise-induced angina. Exclusions included poor left ventricular function (LVEF <30%) or left ventricular wall thickness on echocardiography of <8 mm. The primary end point of the study was improved exercise duration at 12 months. This was achieved with a median increase in exercise duration of 89 s in the PMR group and only a 12.5-s median increase in the medical therapy-only group ($P < 0.008$). Anginal class by the Seattle Angina Questionnaire improved to Class II or less 34.1% of the time in the PMR group and only 13.0% in the medical treatment-only arm. Although the study was not powered to detect mortality differences, there were eight deaths in the group assigned to PMR and three deaths in the medical treatment-only arm. None of these deaths occurred during or within 24 h of the procedure. There were no differences in the use of antianginal medications. There was no study of myocardial perfusion, and left ventricular function remained similar in both groups.

Kornowski et al. performed successful DMR in 76 of 77 patients using the BioSense system (Kornowski et al., 2000). Eleven to fifty channels were created in each patient (average 26 ± 10). One patient developed pericardial effusion requiring pericardiocentesis. Another patient developed a minor stroke. There was no immediate effect on the EKG. However, 18% of patients had CK-MB elevation three times normal and 3% of the patients had an increase of three to eight times normal. Left ventricular ejection fractions were unchanged in the immediate postoperative period or after 1 month of follow-up. A significant increase was noticed in exercise times before and 6 months after PMR from 387 ± 178 to 493 ± 162 s and in times on the treadmill to ST depression >1 mm from 327 ± 177 to 440 ± 178 s (both $P = 0.0001$). At 6 months, the anginal class improved in from 3.3 ± 0.5 to 2.0 ± 1.2 ($P < 0.001$).

Leon et al. reported preliminary results of the BioSense "DIRECT trial" at the Transcatheter Cardiovascular Therapeutics 2000 Conference (Leon et al., 2000a). Two hundred and ninety-eight patients at 14 centers were randomized to an active PMR arm utilizing the BioSense system versus medical therapy. Patients were blinded to treatment assignment. Those patients assigned to medical therapy underwent intraventricular mapping with the BioSense NOGA system, without channel creation (Leon et al., 2000b). The placebo-assigned patients experienced clinical benefits similar to those in the laser arm, including improvement in exercise capacity of nearly 30%. The clinical improvements in the placebo group were similar to those of treated patients in previous PMR and TMR trials. Dr. Leon concluded, "The blinding process clearly demonstrates a profound placebo effect in 'no-option' patients with severe angina when exposed to a new, innovative technology with presumed therapeutic actions." He added, "I believe that all other clinical trials in this field should be viewed with caution and skepticism unless proper attention is taken to account for placebo effects of experimental therapies" (Leon et al., 2000a). This group had earlier reported encouraging preliminary results in humans (Kornowski et al., 1999, 2000) and had docu-

mented the creation of laser channels with this system in an animal model (Kornowski et al., 1998). As previously mentioned, PMR and TMR systems use different devices and laser energies. The failure of the DIRECT trial does not necessarily imply a class failure for PMR or TMR. This may only reflect a device failure for the BioSense system. Further investigation is required to resolve these ambiguities. In fact, a recent report, the BELIEF Trial from Norway by Nordrehaug et al. using the Acsis system by Eclipse, demonstrated in a similarly designed study a significant difference with major benefit with respect to reduction of one and two angina classes as in patients undergoing PMR (Nordrehaug et al., 2001). Eighty two patients were randomized, with all patients undergoing catheter placement, but only 40 patients actually having the creation of laser channels (averaging 20 each). Although the placebo group showed improvements by one anginal class in 38% and by two anginal classes in 13%, this was markedly less than the active treatment group, with 63% and 41%, respectively at 6 months, which was highly significant. Exercise tolerance also improved more in the laser-treated group.

8.4. POTENTIAL MECHANISMS FOR BENEFIT

Several mechanisms have been proposed for the putative clinical benefits of PMR/TMR. These include: (1) direct reperfusion of the myocardium (Cooley et al., 1994). (2) angiogenesis (Burkhoff et al., 1996). (3) denervation (Al-Sheikh et al., 1999). (4) placebo (Leon et al., 2000a), and (5) mechanical remodeling of the heart muscle. For a more extensive review of these potential mechanisms the reader is referred to Chapter 6. Suffice it to say that there is controversy and conflicting evidence regarding either a direct or indirect mechanism of improvement in perfusion (Allen et al., 1999a; Frazier et al., 1999). Limited pathologic studies suggest that there is no permanence to the laser-created channels (Cooley et al., 1994; Gassler et al., 1997; Summers et al., 1999). The latter reference, although limited to one patient, is of interest in that the patient was asymptomatic before death and died as a result of an automobile accident. The findings were pertinent not only for a lack of permanent laser-created channels but also for a paucity of any neovascularization in the dense scar tissue at the sites of laser therapy (Summers et al., 1999). The concept of denervation might explain clinical relief of angina, without improvement in perfusion. With the use of positron emission tomographic (PET) imaging with [^{11}C]hydroxyephedrine (HED), this concept was assessed after and after TMR (Ho-YAG) in eight patients (Al-Sheikh et al., 1999). Perfusion with [^{13}N]ammonia was also assessed. Approximately 2 months after TMR, repeat imaging was obtained. Anginal class had improved from Class IV to Classes I and II in all patients. In six of eight patients sympathetic denervation was noted to increase by $27.5 \pm 15.9\%$ whereas perfusion remained unchanged. In two patients perfusion improved, and in these patients denervation decreased. Recently a much more variable response to denervation was noted in seven patients undergoing PMR, but perfusion was not reported, only the uptake of HED by PET (Stahl et al., 2000). The experience at William Beaumont Hospital suggests that neither improved perfusion nor mechanical remodeling occurs, as judged by dobutamine echocardiography (George et al., 2000). When both lased (Eclipse holmium laser) and nonlased segments were examined, neither showed an improvement in function. Thus it appears that the mechanism of angina relief may vary from patient to patient and may possibly be due to one or more of these mechanisms including placebo effect.

8.5. INDICATIONS AND PATIENT SELECTION

Advances in medical therapy, CABG, and PTCA have improved the outcome of patients with coronary artery disease. However, because of the success of these therapies, an increasing number of these patients with disease progression will be prone to develop

recurring severe or lifestyle-limiting anginal symptoms not amenable to a repeat standard procedure. These patients are considered "refractory" or "no-option" patients, because no other therapeutic measure can be utilized. The only other option for these patients, if they meet the selection criteria, is cardiac transplantation. Over the last two decades, novel revascularization strategies have been proposed for these patients. The techniques include TMR, the newly developed PMR, and the use of angiogenic growth factors. Patients who should be considered for these novel revascularization techniques include subjects with Class III–IV angina and:

1. Ischemic territories not amenable to traditional revascularization techniques:
   A. Patients with diffuse coronary artery disease
   B. Patients with small target coronary arteries
   C. Chronic total occlusions
2. Repetitive CABG and/or PTCA failures:
   A. Patients with recurrent graft occlusions/restenosis
   B. Patients who are considered poor candidates because of comorbidities.
3. No previous CABG/PTCA, but are poor surgical candidates (not applicable to TMR).

Mukherjee and colleagues (1999) have suggested that 5% of patients admitted for cardiac catheterization at tertiary centers exhibit these characteristics and may be candidates for some attempt at percutaneous myocardial revascularization or gene therapy (George et al., 2000) (see Chapter 19). In an extensive chart review, they determined that these so-called "no-option" patients were of similar age and risk factor distribution as those of conventional coronary patients. They were noted to be much more likely to have undergone previous CABG (76% vs. 31%), have more diseased vessels (3 vs. 2), have a lower ejection fraction (43% vs. 60%), and to suffer from renal insufficiency (10% vs. 3%). These patients were turned down for CAGB/PTCA for the following reasons:

(1) chronic total occlusions (64.4%), (2) poor target (74.5%), (3) multiple stenoses (1.6%), (4) degenerated saphenous vein graft (23.7%), (5) no conduit (5.0%), and (6) comorbidities (3.3%).

In summary, candidates for PMR must have disabling angina and must not be candidates for PTCA or CABG. However, they must have enough myocardial reserve, with an ejection fraction of at least 30%, to tolerate the procedure and a wall thickness by echocardiography of at least 8 mm in the targeted area.

8.6. MONITORING OF EFFICACY

8.6.1. Indicators of Intraoperative Delivery of Laser Energy

Several criteria are used as evidence of successful laser treatment of myocardium. These include:

1. Premature ventricular contraction
2. Evidence of the laser fiber protruding from the PMR catheter and touching the left ventricular wall
3. Audible laser discharge from the machine
4. Evidence of bubbles in the left ventricular cavity while monitoring with TEE
5. If the patient is awake, as in the case of PMR, the patient reports a "hot" sensation in the heart.

8.6.2. Postoperative Evaluation

Different measures are used to evaluate patients postoperatively. These include the following subjective and objective measures:

1. Anginal status
2. Exercise duration
3. Nuclear perfusion scans
4. Stress-contrast echocardiography
5. Positron emission tomography (PET)
6. MRI perfusion imaging
7. Coronary angiography

Larger trials typically rely on clinical parameters that may be less than objective relative to a placebo effect (angina class and exercise duration). When more sensitive techniques such as PET or MRI scanning are utilized, the numbers of patients studied have been too small to reach meaningful conclusions as to efficacy.

8.7. CONCLUSIONS

The information available on PMR is mostly derived from uncontrolled studies, and the number of subjects has usually been small (Lauer et al., 1999; Kornowski et al., 1999, 2000; Oesterle et al., 1998; Shawl et al., 1999). To date, we have only one published randomized non-placebo-controlled trial with encouraging results (Oesterle et al., 2000). However, the initial results of PMR are enticing, with improvement in the symptomatic status of angina and in exercise capacity. This is achieved at a decreased length of hospitalization compared with TMR. More randomized phase II and III clinical trials are needed for better evaluation of this therapeutic modality for patients with "no-option" heart disease.

There have been no clinical trials comparing PMR with TMR. To date, there has been only one placebo-controlled trial comparing PMR with the standard medical therapy (Leon et al., 2000a, 2000b). Current comparative data are from studies done in different clinical settings. As might be expected, patients often cannot be blinded to the modality of treatment. The placebo factor cannot be estimated from many of the present studies, with the possible exception of two recent studies that have yet to be published in detail (Leon et al., 2000b; Nordrehaug et al., 2001). However with PMR as a less invasive technique, a placebo arm now seems justified in all new larger randomized trials. Further trials should be continued before widespread clinical dissemination of this technology. Given the expense and controversy surrounding heart laser therapy, and the promise that it offers, we strongly recommend such trials.

References

Aaberge L, Nordstrand K, Dragsund M et al. Transmyocardial revascularization with CO_2 laser in patients with refractory angina pectoris. Clinical results from the Norwegian randomized trial. *J Am Coll Cardiol* 2000; 35: 1170–1178.

Abela GS, Griffin JC, Hill JA et al. Transvascular argon laser-induced atrioventricular conduction ablation in dogs. *Circulation* 1983; 68: 111–145.

Allen KB, Dowling RD, Fudge TL et al. Comparison of transmyocardial revascularization with medical therapy in patients with refractory angina. *N Eng J Med* 1999a; 341: 1029–1036.

Allen KB, Dowling RD, Heimansohn DA et al. Transmyocardial revascularization utilizing a holmium:YAG laser. *Eur J Cardiothorac Surg* 1999b; 14: 100–104.

Al-Sheikh T, Allen KB, Straka SP et al. Cardiac sympathetic denervation after transmyocardial laser revascularization. *Circulation* 1999; 100: 135–140.

Burkhoff D, Fisher PE, Apfelbaum M et al. Histologic appearance of transmyocardial laser channels after 4.5 weeks. *Ann Thorac Surg* 1996; 61: 1532–1535.

Burkhoff D, Schmidt S, Schulman SP et al. Transmyocardial laser revascularization compared with continued medical therapy for treatment of refractory angina pectoris: a prospective randomized trial. *Lancet* 1999a; 354: 885–890.

Burkhoff D, Wesley MN, Resar JR et al. Factors correlating with risk of mortality after transmyocardial revascularization. *J Am Coll Cardiol* 1999b; 34: 55–61.

Cooley DA, Frazier OH, Kadipasaoglu KA et al. Transmyocardial laser revascularization: anatomic evidence of long-term channel patency. *Tex Heart Inst J* 994; 21: 220–224.

DeGuzman BJ, Lautz DB, Chen FY et al. Thorascopic transmyocardial laser revascularization. *Ann Thorac Surg* 1997; 64: 171–174.

Frazier OH, March RJ, Horvath KA. Transmyocardial revascularization with a carbon dioxide laser in patients with end-stage coronary artery disease. *N Engl J Med* 1999; 341: 1021–1028.

Gassler N, Wintzer HO, Stubbe HM et al. Transmyocardial laser revascularization: histological features in human nonresponder myocardium. *Circulation* 1997; 95: 371–375.

George PB, O'Neill WW, Henry R et al. Dobutamine stress echocardiography demonstrates no improvement in left ventricular function after PMR (abstract). *Circulation* 2000; 102: II-382.

Horvath KA, Cohn LH, Cooley DA et al. Transmyocardial laser revascularization: results of a multicenter trial with transmyocardial laser revascularization used as sole therapy for end stage CAD. *J Thorac Cardiovasc Surg* 1997; 113: 645–654.

Horvath KA. Thoracoscopic transmyocardial laser revascularization. *Ann Thorac Surg* 1998; 65: 1439–1441.

Hughes GC, Landolfo KP, Lowe JE et al. Perioperative morbidity and mortality after transmyocardial laser revascularization: incidence and risk factors for adverse events. *J Am Coll Cardiol* 1999; 33: 1021–1026.

Hughes GC, Lowe JE, Krypson AP et al. Neovascularization after transmyocardial laser revascularization in a model of chronic ischemia. *Ann Thorac Surg* 1998; 66: 2029–2036.

Hughes GC, Shah AS, Yin B et al. Early postoperative changes in regional systolic and diastolic left ventricular function after transmyocardial laser revascularization: a comparison of holmium:YAG and CO_2 lasers. *J Am Coll Cardiol* 2000; 35: 1022–1030.

Jeevanandam V, Auteri JS, Oz MC et al. Myocardial revascularization by laser-induced channels. *Surg Forum* 1990; 41: 225–227.

Kadipasaoglu KA, Frazier OH. Transmyocardial laser revascularization: effect of laser parameters on tissue ablation and cardiac perfusion. *Semin Thorac Cardiovasc Surg* 1999; 11: 4–11.

Kanellopoulos GK, Svindland A, Ilebekk A et al. Transventricular non-transmural laser treatment of hypoperfused porcine myocardium acutely reduces left ventricular contractile function. *Eur J Cardiothoracic Surg* 1999; 16: 135–143.

Kim C, Kasten R, Javier M et al. Percutaneous method of laser transmyocardial revascularization. *Cathet Cardiovasc Diagn* 1997; 40: 223–228.

Kornowski R, Baim DS, Moses JW et al. Sustained symptomatic and exercise improvements at 6 months following percutaneous direct myocardial revascularization guided by Biosense left ventricular mapping in patients with refractory ischemic syndromes (abstract). *J Am Coll Cardiol* 2000; 35 (Suppl A): 546A.

Kornowski R, Hong MK, Haudenschild CC et al. Feasibility and safety of percutaneous laser revascularization using the Biosense System in porcine hearts. *Coronary Artery Dis* 1998; 9: 535–540.

Kornowski R, Moses J, Baim DS et al. Percutaneous direct myocardial revascularization guided by biosense left ventricular mapping in patients with refractory coronary ischemia (abstract). *J Am Coll Cardiol* 1999; 33 (*Suppl A*): 334A.

Lauer B, Junghans U, Strahl F et al. Catheter-based percutaneous myocardial laser revascularization in patients with end-stage coronary artery disease. *J Am Coll Cardiol* 1999; 34: 1663–1670.

Leon MB and the Direct Trial Investigators. DMR in regeneration of endomyocardial channels trial (oral presentation). Presented at Transcatheter Cardiovascular Therapeutics Meeting, Washington D.C., October, 2000a.

Leon MB, Baim DS, Moses JW et al. A randomized blinded clinical trial comparing percutaneous laser myocardial revascularization (using Biosense LV mapping): vs. placebo in patients with refractory coronary ischemia (abstract). *Circulation* 2000b; 102: II-565.

Milano A, Stefano P, DeCarlo M et al. Transmyocardial holmium laser revascularization: feasibility of a thoracoscopic approach. *J Thorac Cardiovasc Surg* 1999; 14: 105–110.

Mirhoseini M, Cayton MM, Shelgikar S et al. Laser myocardial revascularization. *Lasers Surg Med* 1986; 6: 459–461.

Mukherjee D, Bhatt DL, Roe MT et al. Direct myocardial revascularization and angiogenesis—How many patients might be eligible? *Am J Cardiol* 1999; 84: 598–600.

Nordrehaug JE, Salem M, Rotevatn S et al. Blinded evaluation of laser (PTMR) intervention electively for angina pectoris (BELIEF) (oral presentation). American College of Cardiology, Orlando, FL, March 19, 2001.

Oesterle SN, Reifart NJ, Meier B et al. Initial results of laser-based percutaneous myocardial revascularization for angina pectoris. *Am J Cardiol* 1998; 82: 659–662.

Oesterle SN, Sanborn TA, Ali N et al. Percutaneous transmyocardial laser revascularization for severe angina: the PACIFIC randomized trial. *Lancet* 2000; 356: 1705–1710.

Schofield PM, Sharples LD, Caine N et al. Transmyocardial laser revascularization in patients with refractory angina: a randomized control trial. *Lancet* 1999; 353: 519–524.

Shawl FA, Domanski MJ, Upendra K et al. Procedural results and early clinical outcome of percutaneous transluminal myocardial revascularization. *Am J Cardiol* 1999; 83: 498–501.

Stahl F, Lauer B, Bengel F et al. Myocardial innervation after percutaneous myocardial laser revascularization (abstract). *J Am Coll Cardiol* 2000; 35 (Suppl A): 408A.

Summers JH, Henry AC, Roberts WC. Cardiac observations late after operative transmyocardial laser "revascularization". *Am J Cardiol* 1999; 84: 489–490.

Sundt TM, Carbone KA, Oesterle SN et al. The holmium:YAG laser for transmyocardial laser revascularization: initial clinical experience (abstract). *Circulation* 1996; 94 (*Suppl* I): I-295.

Verdaasdonk R. Transmyocardial revascularization: the magic of drilling holes in the heart. *SPIE (Proceedings of the International Society for Optical Engineering) Critical Review Papers* 2000; 75: 99–135.

Whitlow PL, Knopf WD, O'Neill WW et al. Six-month follow-up of percutaneous transmyocardial revascularization in patients with refractory angina (abstract). *J Am Coll Cardiol* 1999; 23: 29A.

Yano OJ, Bielefeld MR, Jeevanandam V et al. Prevention of acute regional ischemia with endocardial laser channels. *Ann Thorac Surg* 1993; 56: 46–53.

9

Novel Revascularization Strategies: PMR, TMR, and Percutaneous In Situ Coronary Venous Arterialization

Peter J. Fitzgerald, M.D., Ph.D., and Alan C. Yeung, M.D.

Division of Cardiovascular Medicine
Stanford University Medical Center
Stanford, California

and

William B. Abernethy III, M.D., and Stephen N. Oesterle, M.D.

Division of Cardiology
Massachusetts General Hospital
Harvard Medical School
Boston, Massachusetts

SUMMARY

Although TMR appears to improve symptoms of coronary insufficiency, it carries significant perioperative morbidity risks. This inherent risk led to the development of less invasive techniques, including percutaneous catheter-based methods such as PMR.

PMR appears to be safer and better tolerated than TMR and seems to have produced significant improvements in anginal symptoms. However, there have been problems in demonstrating objective improvement, and results have been variable.

Evidence has suggested that in situ coronary vascular bypass may be beneficial to patients in relieving angina via venous arterialization.

Percutaneous in situ coronary venous arterialization (PICVA) and percutaneous in situ coronary artery bypass (PICAB) are two new methods that are being developed to make arterialization of the venous system via a percutaneous approach possible. Using stents to form an arteriovenous shunt and then sealing off the proximal and distal venous system, it is possible to perform an in situ arterial bypass.

If studies using PICVA and PICAB are successful, patients who might benefit from these procedures in the future would include those with chronic total occlusions,

Myocardial Revascularization: Novel Percutaneous Approaches, Edited by George S. Abela.
ISBN 0-471-36166-6 Copyright © 2002 Wiley-Liss, Inc.

diffuse small vessel disease, and repetitive stenosis and candidates for re-do bypass.

9.1. INTRODUCTION

Despite the success of medical therapy, percutaneous coronary interventions (PCI), and coronary artery bypass grafting (CABG) in relieving symptoms of myocardial ischemia, many patients with advanced coronary disease are not treatable with these therapies. These patients with severe refractory angina are often felt to have no options. They typically include patients with diffusely diseased and small-caliber vessels; chronic total occlusions; and recurrent restenoses after PCI with no surgical alternatives. "No-option" patients also include those with saphenous vein graft degeneration or absent arterial conduits; patients with transplant vasculopathy; and patients with severe comorbidities that may preclude CABG. Although the number of such patients is not clear, one analysis from a large single-center study estimated that up to 12% of patients with symptomatic coronary disease may fall into this category (Mukherjee et al., 1999). Perhaps more than 100,000 such patients emerge each year in the U.S. alone. Two promising techniques have evolved as potential therapies for many of these "untreatable" patients: percutaneous myocardial laser revascularization (PMR) and in situ coronary bypass or venous arterialization.

9.2. PERCUTANEOUS TRANSMYOCARDIAL LASER REVASCULARIZATION (PMR)

Transmyocardial laser revascularization (TMR) was proposed by Mirhoseini in 1981 (Mirhoseini et al., 1981) as a method to potentially improve the blood supply of severely ischemic myocardium. Mirhoseini postulated that oxygenated blood could be delivered directly from the left ventricle to the muscle by laser channels bored through the myocardium to the endocardial surface. His concept stemmed from a belief that reptilian physiology could be recapitulated in humans. Reptiles have a poorly defined coronary circulation, with oxygenated blood percolating directly from the ventricular cavity into myocardial sinusoids and bathing the contractile myocardium. In the 1930s, Wearn suggested that remnants of such myocardial sinusoids existed in humans and could serve a similar purpose in the absence of coronary circulation (Wearn et al., 1933).

Mirhoseini's concepts for TMR were based on techniques performed in the early 1960s (Sen et al., 1965, 1968). TMR is performed by activating a laser probe on the epicardial surface of the ischemic heart to form transmural channels into the left ventricular cavity. In an initial uncontrolled trial of TMR in patients with intractable angina, three-quarters of patients reported an improvement in symptoms of two angina classes (Horvath et al., 1997). Several randomized trials of TMR have also shown symptomatic improvement in anginal symptoms in treated patients, although increases in exercise capacity have been less consistent (Allen et al., 1999; Burkoff et al., 1999; Frazier et al., 1999; Schofield et al., 1999).

The performance of TMR can be accompanied by a significant mortality and morbidity. TMR requires an open thoracotomy and is often performed in patients with significant comorbidities. The initial nonrandomized trial and an uncontrolled registry involving over 900 patients, reported an in-hospital mortality of 9% (Horvath et al., 1997) and 9.7% (Burns et al., 1999), respectively. Subsequent randomized trials from the United States and the United Kingdom demonstrated a lower perioperative mortality (5%), but the procedure has also been associated with considerable morbidity (Burkoff et al., 1999; Schofield et al., 1999). In the UK trial (Schofield et al., 1999), morbidity associated with TMR included wound and respiratory infections (33%), transient arrhythmias (typically atrial fibrillation) (15%), and left ventricular failure (12%).

In summary, TMR seems to markedly improve the symptoms of coronary insufficiency but carries a periprocedural mortality between 3 and 10%, as well as a substantial morbidity. The clinical benefit of surgical

TMR, mitigated by significant perioperative morbidity, led to the development of less invasive techniques using thorascopy (DeGuzman et al., 1995) and percutaneous catheter-based methods.

Flexible fiberoptic catheter designs allow a percutaneous approach of laser myocardial revascularization. Working from the transaortic endocardial surface, catheter-based systems can create nontransmural channels from the endocardial surface. The channels are smaller in size but potentially with a tissue effect and clinical response similar to those of the surgical TMR procedure. Nontransmural channels from the endocardial surface are likely to be placed in the area of greatest ischemia: the subendocardium. Moreover, a percutaneous approach facilitates treatment of areas less accessible by surgical TMR (the septum and posterior walls of the left ventricle) and permits the possibility of multiple treatment sessions with lower morbidity and mortality than surgical TMR.

A percutaneous method of myocardial laser revascularization (PMR) was first performed in a canine model (Kim et al., 1997). Working with a similar prototypical PMR catheter (CardioGenesis PMR™, Eclipse Surgical Systems, Sunnyvale, CA), Oesterle reported a pilot study of 30 human subjects (Oesterle et al., 1998). The PMR procedure is carried out under local anesthesia. A 9 Fr guiding catheter is advanced retrograde across the aortic valve into left ventricle to allow steering of the laser catheter to ischemic areas of the myocardium. The laser catheter is then placed on the endocardial surface, and a specified energy is delivered that creates a channel approximately 6 mm deep into the myocardium. Two similar PMR systems utilizing a Ho:YAG laser rely on simple navigation strategies. The Eclipse systems are used with biplane fluoroscopy to guide the operator toward areas of known ischemic myocardium. A third Ho:YAG system (Biosense, Johnson & Johnson) utilizes a low-intensity electromagnetic field to locate and track catheter position within the ventricle. Electrical sensors on the tip of the catheter allow cardiologists to assess areas of myo-cardium that are viable (with normal or reduced endocardial voltage potential) but with impaired mechanical activity (endocardial shortening). These systems are detailed further in Chapters 6 and 13.

PMR has been performed in more than 1,000 patients worldwide. The result of one multicenter, randomized prospective trial comparing PMR with maximal medical therapy in no-option patients has now been published (Oesterle et al., 2000). The PACIFIC study consisted of 221 patients with refractory angina (class III and IV) not suitable for revascularization and randomized to PMR with the CardioGenesis system or continued medical therapy (Oesterle et al., 2000). The primary end points of the trial were improvements in exercise tolerance and angina class. At 1-year, total exercise tolerance increased by a median of 89 s in the PMR group compared with 12.5-s median increase in the medication-only group ($P = 0.008$). Blinded assessment of CCSAS was class II or lower in 34% of PMR patients compared with 13% in the medication-only group ($P = 0.0017$). Other aspects of PMR compared favorably with surgical TMR. There were no in-hospital deaths in the PMR group. The morbidity was also quite low, with only one patient developing tamponade (responsive to pericardiocentesis) and one patient developing heart block requiring a permanent pacemaker. Moreover, the costs of PMR were much less than those of surgical TMR, primarily because of shorter lengths of hospital stay. Patients undergoing PMR are usually discharged home the day after the procedure; however surgical TMR patients may be in the hospital for up to 10 days (Schofield et al., 1999). Therefore, the risk-benefit ratio of PMR may be more favorable than for surgical TMR. Persistent skepticism toward laser myocardial revascularization has limited its widespread use.

9.3. CONTROVERSIES AND CRITICISMS OF PMR

Although the percutaneous approach of laser revascularization ensures a very safe, well-tolerated procedure and seems to produce dramatic symptomatic improvements in anginal symptoms, there has been a less convincing demonstration of objective improvements. Changes in exercise capacity and myocardial perfusion after laser revascularization have been variable (Schofield et al., 1999). Although treadmill exercise time was improved with the largest PMR study (Oesterle et al., 2000), a lack of increase in exercise time in some of the TMR trials may be caused in part by the adverse effects of a thoracotomy.

The effect of laser therapy on myocardial perfusion has been particularly controversial. It has been difficult to demonstrate decreased ischemia after TMR or PMR, and exercise perfusion thallium scanning after the procedure has provided inconsistent findings (Allen et al., 1999; Frazier et al., 1999; Schofield et al., 1999). Although this may be caused by inadequately sensitive tools to assess changes in endocardial blood flow, the controversy partly reflects our poor understanding of the actual mechanism of benefit of laser revascularization. The initial belief that the myocardium would be perfused by passive diffusion of oxygenated blood into the newly formed channels has been invalidated, as most laser-produced channels close soon after the procedure (Hardy et al., 1987; Kohmoto et al., 1996; Krabatsch et al., 1996; Mueller et al., 1998). Thus chronically patent sinusoids supplying myocardial blood flow cannot explain the symptomatic benefit. Laser-induced denervation may potentially contribute to reduction in anginal pain and has been demonstrated in animal models of TMR (Kwong et al., 1997). However, simply attenuating the body's warning system of myocardial ischemia is an unsatisfying mechanism and could feasibly make physical effort more dangerous in such patients. Growing evidence supports laser-induced angiogenesis as the most likely explanation for patient improvement after PMR (Hughes et al., 1998; Kohmoto et al., 1998; Yamamoto et al., 1998), but the angiogenesis effect is relatively small and perhaps is simply a nonspecific response of the myocardium to injury

(Malekan et al., 1998). Although PMR and TMR may stimulate angiogenesis, inflow to these new blood vessels is unpredictable. One can speculate that we are simply creating islet hemangiomas in diffusely ischemic myocardium without reliable inflow. The variable access to inflow may explain the nonuniform response to these strategies for promoting angiogenesis. Moreover, a frequent criticism of TMR and PMR studies is the subjective nature of assessing angina. It is difficult to exclude a potentially powerful placebo effect for patients undergoing laser revascularization. There are many desperate patients and physicians looking for a viable treatment in an otherwise "no-option" circumstance.

Uncertainty over the true benefit of PMR has grown with the report of a recent placebo-controlled, blinded assessment of PMR (Leon et al., 2000). Presented in abstract form, the DIRECT trial (DMR in regeneration of endomyocardial channels trial) involved 298 patients with drug-refractory angina who were not good candidates for revascularization. These patients were randomized to low- or high-dose treatment with the Biosense DMR system or a sham procedure in which all patients were sedated and catheterized but did not receive actual laser treatment. At 6 months, there was no difference between the groups in exercise duration, time to symptom onset, and time to ST segment changes on exercise testing. Similarly, there was no difference in angina frequency or quality of life assessment parameters that would indicate subjective clinical benefit. Although there has been debate over how comparable the different laser systems are in creating sufficient myocardial channel depths, the negative results of the DIRECT trial did fuel more skepticism about the utility of PMR.

The inability to predict which patients will have symptomatic benefit, inconsistent myocardial perfusion findings, and lack of a sound theory explaining the mechanism of benefit with laser myocardial revascularization have tempered some of the initial enthusiasm for the technique (Petre, 1999).

9.4. IN SITU VENOUS ARTERIALIZATION AND CORONARY ARTERY BYPASS

Surgeons have traditionally limited coronary bypass conduits to the saphenous veins, internal mammary arteries, and other arterial vessels (gastroepiploic and radial). The epicardial coronary veins offer another potential conduit of revascularization through either retrograde venous perfusion or the creation of an in situ coronary vascular bypass. Evidence suggests that patients may experience relief of angina with venous arterialization, and the advent of specialized designed catheters offers the possibility of performing venous arterialization or in situ bypass without a thoracotomy (Fitzgerald et al., 1999). Moreover, there are potential benefits on vessel morphology of using in situ venous arterial conduits. Epicardial veins do not contain atheroma, even when the arterial circulation is severely affected. Also, removing and arterializing a peripheral vein generally results in both medial fibrosis and intimal lesions, whereas with in situ vein usage (thereby not disrupting the vessel's vasa vasorum) the medial fibrosis is markedly attenuated (Brody et al., 1972).

9.4.1. Venous System of the Heart

The venous drainage of the myocardium occurs through two complementary systems, the epicardial and the thebesian veins. The epicardial venous system consists primarily of the coronary sinus and its tributaries (Fig. 9-1). In general, these coronary veins run next to the coronary arteries, with branch vessels of the artery being paralleled by correlating branches of the venous tree. The right coronary artery differs from the left coronary artery in that the veins run perpendicular to the artery in the more proximal portion before becoming more parallel in the posterior descending and posterolateral arteries. This frequent disparity between the vein and artery in the proximal to mid-right coronary artery may make this portion of the coronary tree less suitable for in situ arterial bypass.

A less well-understood but equally important system of myocardial venous drainage is the thebesian network of channels that allow the coronary arterioles, capillaries, and venules to drain directly into the cardiac chambers. The physiologic role that the thebesian system plays is unclear, although they have been shown to effectively provide an alternative route of venous drainage when the epicardial veins no longer participate in this function.

Experiments obstructing the outflow of the cardiac veins demonstrate that numerous interconnections, anastomoses, and the double venous systems result in important alternative drainage patterns and ensure that flow is not markedly diminished (Gree et al., 1947; Nakamure et al., 1990; Nakazawa et al., 1978). This redundant aspect of the coronary venous drainage system, along with the anatomic location of epicardial veins paralleling the coronary arteries across much of the heart, support the possibility of using the venous system to provide arterial blood to the myocardium.

9.4.2. Use of the Coronary Venous System in Myocardial Revascularization

Beginning in the 1930s, researchers began exploring the possibility of improving myocardial arterial flow through alterations of the coronary veins. Initially, the hypothesis was that by simply prolonging contact with venous blood, myocardial ischemia or infarction could be attenuated. Experimental studies progressed through several phases, beginning with simple coronary venous occlusion. Interest in the coronary veins waned with the development of cardiopulmonary bypass and surgical coronary artery bypass, but the potential use of the coronary veins has been reexplored over the past 30 years.

Animal studies first demonstrated that, despite the deleterious effects of complete coronary sinus blockage, the procedure seemed to offer improved mortality and limit infarct size after acute occlusion of the left anterior descending artery (LAD) (Gross et al., 1937; Robertson, 1935, 1941). Several

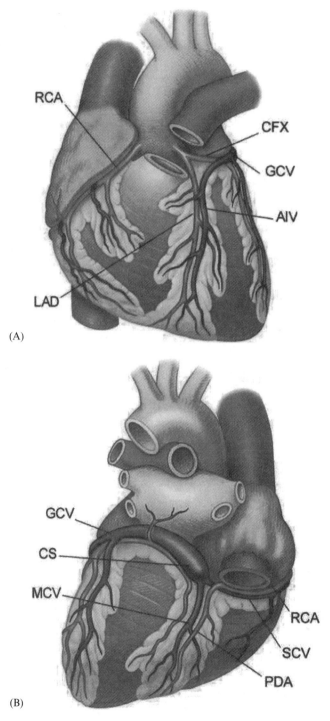

FIGURE 9-1. Arterial and venous anatomy. (A) An anterior projection demonstrating the close relationship between the left anterior descending artery (LAD) and the anterior interventricular vein (AIV) and between the circumflex artery (CFX) and the great cardiac vein (GCV). (B) Posterior view showing the coronary sinus (CS), the oblique vein of Marshal (OVM), and the middle cardiac vein (MCV), which runs close to the posterior descending artery (PDA). Note from the anterior view that the epicardial veins run perpendicular to the right coronary artery (RCA). (Reprinted with permission from Fitzgerald et al., 1999.)

possible explanations for this effect have been put forward. It is possible that ligation of the epicardial venous outflow creates pressure in the coronary circuit that forces arterial blood through alternative channels. This redirection of arterial blood might then supply relatively underperfused myocardium. Efforts were thus made toward directly perfusing the coronary sinus, and after extensive animal experiments, Beck developed a staged procedure to graft a vessel directly from the aorta to the coronary sinus of a beating heart. To lessen an arteriovenous fistula, weeks later the proximal portion of the coronary sinus would be ligated or partially occluded. The surgery was performed in over 200 patients whose chest pain was believed to be caused by ischemic heart disease (although there were severe limitations in diagnostic testing to determine the cause of chest pain) and was associated with improved anginal symptoms in the majority of patients (Beck, 1948a, 1948b). A high perioperative morbidity and mortality dampened enthusiasm for the procedure, and, by the 1960s, efforts had shifted to establishing direct coronary arterial bypass grafting (CABG).

9.4.3. Selective Venous Arterialization

Despite success in developing and refining CABG and percutaneous transluminal coronary angioplasty procedures, a large number of patients with diffuse disease and small vessels remained unamenable to such therapies. This problem prompted investigators to again consider arterialization of the coronary venous system. This revived interest in the coronary veins during the late 1970s focused on selective venous arterialization. Unlike Beck's technique of global arterialization, these studies attempted to limit the degree of arterialization to branches of the venous system that were associated with ischemic myocardium and allowed normal venous drainage of the remainder of the myocardium.

Studies in canine and sheep models demonstrated that segmental venous arterialization (generating coronary flow rates of 20-ml/min)

effectively attenuated or even prevented ischemia in response to arterial occlusion (Bhayana et al., 1974; Chiu et al., 1975; Kay et al., 1975). Extensive canine experiments of the procedure demonstrated that retrograde perfusion would restore more than 30% of normal coronary arterial flow to all layers of the myocardium and was able to reverse ischemic ECG changes (Hochberg, 1977). Left internal mammary artery (LIMA) grafting to the anterior interventricular vein in humans unsuitable for CABG was reported in 1975 (Park et al., 1975). A subsequent survey of 55 American cardiac surgeons reported on the outcome of 117 patients with bypass grafts to a coronary vein, many of which were inadvertent (Hochberg et al., 1979). Survival was nearly 93%, and among patients who underwent repeat cardiac catheterization 92% had patent grafts. Despite these studies showing the feasibility and encouraging results of selective venous coronary bypass grafting, the procedure was not widely adopted, likely in large part because of the greater effort focused on further refining direct CABG.

9.4.4. Percutaneous In Situ Coronary Venous Interventions

New methods and devices are being developed that make possible arterialization of the venous system through a percutaneous approach. Percutaneous cannulation of the coronary sinus is generally straightforward and offers easy access to the coronary venous system. Conduits between the coronary vein and artery form the basis of both percutaneous in situ coronary venous arterialization (PICVA) or percutaneous in situ coronary artery bypass (PICAB).

These procedures begin with standard arterial coronary angiography, usually with longer cine runs and enough contrast to visualize approximate epicardial venous location during the follow-through phase. From a femoral vein approach, a catheter is then positioned in the coronary sinus to allow passage of a guidewire into the more distal vein. A specialized guiding catheter, usually with side holes to allow easy venous out-flow, is then advanced to the coronary sinus ostium. Retrograde dye injections help further delineate sites of close approximation between the target coronary vein and coronary artery segment. A novel over-the-wire catheter [TransVascular (Menlo Park, CA)] is then advanced through the coronary vein to a site in close approximation of the target coronary artery. Guided by intracoronary ultrasound imaging, this catheter is used to puncture from the vein to the coronary artery to form a channel. The channel is made in a proximal portion of the artery, before the severe stenosis or occlusion. A guidewire is then passed between the vein and the artery, and subsequent devices are placed to produce a permanent conduit between the two vessels. This forms an arteriovenous fistula proximal to the diseased portion of the artery, and blood flow through this channel may approach the flow rate of a normal coronary artery.

In the PICVA procedure, a complete or partial blockage is produced beyond the coronary sinus to prevent shunting of the arterial blood (Fig. 9-2). Animal studies have shown the that procedure provides protection from both death and ischemia in the setting of an acute LAD occlusion (Oesterle et al., 2000). The technique can be performed with low morbidity, and continued development in the technology may allow the procedure to be performed in a standard cardiac catheterization laboratory.

In the PICAB procedure, a segment of coronary vein is used to form a bypass of an arterial blockage. Similar to the PICVA procedure, intravascular ultrasound is used to guide a specialized catheter to form a connection between the target artery and parallel vein. In the PICAB procedure, a second connection is then made in the more distal segment of artery such that an inflow and outflow bypass around an obstruction is created. Blocking devices then placed in the upstream and downstream sections of vein to isolate the segment form a bypass of the arterial obstruction (Fig. 9-3). A comparable technique has been successfully used in peripheral arterial disease, showing a long-term patency similar to open surgery

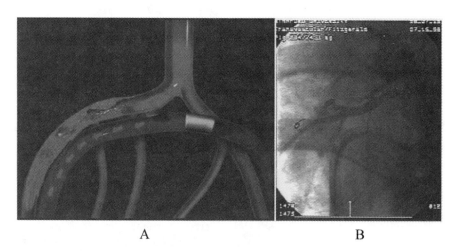

A   B

FIGURE 9-2. The percutaneous in situ coronary venous arterialization procedure.
A. Schematic of procedure showing diversion of arterial blood from the left anterior descending artery to the anterior interventricular vein and a proximal venous occluder.
B. An angiogram from an animal study showing arterial diversion from the left anterior descending artery (LAD) (solid arrow) into the interventricular vein (AIV) (open arrows) with proximal blockage. CX, circumflex artery; GCV, great cardiac vein; LM, left main. (Reprinted with permission from Fitzgerald et al., 1999.)

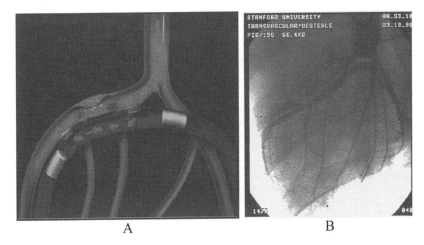

FIGURE 9-3. The percutaneous in situ coronary artery bypass procedure. A. Schematic of procedure showing a proximal diversion of arterial blood from the left anterior descending artery to the anterior interventricular vein, with a second connection bringing the blood back into the left anterior descending artery. Distal and proximal aspects of the vein are occluded. B. Angiogram from an animal study showing segmental arterial bypass from the left anterior descending artery (LAD) (solid arrow) through the interventricular vein (AIV) (open arrows) with reconstitution in the distal LAD (solid arrows). This procedure requires both proximal and distal venous blockage. CX, circumflex artery; GCV, great cardiac vein; LM, left main. (Reprinted with permission from Fitzgerald et al., 1999.)

and avoiding much of the perioperative morbidity (Leor et al., 1992; Rosenthal et al., 1994).

The techniques of PICVA and PICAB are now entering clinical studies. The first successful PICVA procedure in a human was reported by Oesterle and Colleagues in 2001(Oesterle et al., 2001) Although the long-term effects are not yet clear, the procedures have been demonstrated to effectively restore coronary blood flow and may prove to be an effective alternative therapeutic approach in patients who are poor candidates for traditional revascularization approaches. Potential patients for PICVA and PICAB include those patients with chronic total occlusions, repetitive restenosis, or diffuse small vessel disease or those who are candidates for re-do bypass. Further refinements in the techniques of PICAB and PICVA may expand these procedures to those groups of patients now undergoing open surgical bypass, and they may not simply be reserved for the limited-option patient.

9.5. SUMMARY

In summary, PMR and TMR offer patients without revascularization options the possibility of angiogenesis. As will be true with gene therapy, new blood vessels in an ischemic zone will require significant inflow for functional relevance. The novel strategy of percutaneous venous arterialization and bypass offer mechanical solutions to ischemia, relying on the unique potential for retroperfusion in PICVA and the possibility of significant inflow in both PICVA and PICAB.

References

Allen KB, Dowling RD, Fudge TL et al. Comparison of transmyocardial revascularization with medical therapy in patients with refractory angina. *N Engl J Med* 1999; 341: 1029–1036.

Beck CS et al. Nourishment of the myocardium by way of the coronary veins. *Fed Proc* 1948a; 2: 90.

Beck CS et al. Revascularization of the heart by graft or systemic artery into the coronary sinus. *JAMA* 1948b; 137: 436–442.

Bhayana JN, Olsen DB, Byrne JP et al. Reversal of myocardial ischemia by arterialization of the coronary vein. *J Thorac Cardiovasc Surg* 1974; 67: 125–132.

Brody WR, Kosek JC, Angell WW. Changes in vein grafts following aorto-coronary bypass induced by pressure and ischemia. *J Thorac Cardiovasc Surg* 1972; 64: 847–854.

Burkhoff D, Schmidt S, Schulman SP et al. Transmyocardial laser revascularisation compared with continued medical therapy for treatment of refractory angina pectoris: a prospective randomised trial. *Lancet* 1999; 354: 885–890.

Burns SM, Sharples LD, Tait S et al. The transmyocardial laser revascularization international registry report. *Eur Heart J* 1999; 20: 31–37.

Chiu DJ, Mulder DS. Selective arterialization of coronary veins for diffuse coronary occlusion. An experimental evaluation. *J Thorac Cardiovasc Surg* 1975; 70: 177–182.

DeGuzman BJ et al. Thorascopic transmyocardial laser revascularization(abstract). *Circulation* 1995; 92 (*Suppl* 1): I-176.

Fitzgerald PJ et al. New approaches and conduits: *in situ* venous arterialization and coronary artery bypass. *Curr Interv Cardiol Rep* 1999; 1: 127–137.

Frazier OH, March RJ, Horvath KA. Transmyocardial revasculatization with a carbon dioxide laser in patients with end-stage coronary artery disease. *N Engl J Med* 1999; 341: 1021–1028.

Gree DE, S. RE. Studies of the venous drainage of the heart. *Am J Physiol* 1947; 155: 13–25.

Gross L, Blum L, Silverman G. Experimental attempts to increase the blood supply to the dog's heart by means of coronary sinus occlusion. *J Exp Med* 1937; 65: 91–108.

Hardy RI, Bove KE, James FW et al. A histologic study of laser-induced transmyocardial channels. *Lasers Surg Med* 1987; 6: 563–573.

Hochberg MS, Roberts WC, Morrow AG et al. Selective arterialization of the coronary venous system. Encouraging long-term flow evaluation utilizing radioactive microspheres. *J Thorac Cardiovasc Surg* 1979; 77: 1–12.

Hochberg M. Hemodynamic evaluation of selective arterialization of the coronary venous system. *J Thorac Cardiovasc Surg* 1977; 74: 774–783.

Horvath KA, Cohn LH, Cooley DA et al. Transmyocardial revascularization: results of a multicenter trial with transmyocardial laser revascularization used as a sole therapy for end-stage coronary artery disease. *J Thoracic Cardiovasc Surg* 1997; 113: 645–654.

Hughes GC, Lowe JE, Kypson AP et al. Neovascularization after transmyocardial laser revascularization in a model of chronic ischemia. *Ann Thorac Surg* 1998; 66: 2029–2036.

Kay EB, Suzuki A. Coronary venous retroperfusion for myocardial revascularization. *Ann Thorac Surg* 1975; 19: 327–330.

Kim CB, Kesten R, Javier M et al. Percutaneous method of laser transmyocardial revascularization. *Cathet Cardiovasc Diagn* 1997; 40: 223–228.

Kohmoto T, Fisher PE, Gu A et al. Does blood flow through holmium: YAG transmyocardial laser channels? *Ann Thorac Surg* 1996; 61: 861–868.

Kohmoto T, DeRosa CM, Yamamoto N et al. Evidence of vascular growth associated with laser treatment of normal canine myocardium. *Ann Thorac Surg* 1998; 65: 1360–1367.

Krabatsch T, Schaper F, Leder C et al. Histological findings after transmyocardial laser revascularization. *J Card Surg* 1996; 11: 326–331.

Kwong KF, Kanellopoulos GK, Nickols JC et al. Transmyocardial laser treatment denervates canine myocardium. *J Thorac Cardiovasc Surg* 1997; 114: 883–889.

Leon MB, Baim DS, Moses JW et al. A randomized blinded clinical trial comparing percutaneous laser myocardial revascularization (using Biosense LV mapping) vs. placebo in patients with refractory coronary ischemia. *Circulation* 2000; 102: II-565.

Leor J, Battler A, Har-Zahav Y et al. Iatrogenic coronary arteriovenous fistula following percutaneous coronary angioplasty. *Am Heart J* 1992; 123: 784–786.

Malekan R, Reynolds C, Narula N et al. Angiogenesis in transmyocardial laser revascularization: a nonspecific response to injury. *Circulation* 1998; 98 (*Suppl* 19): II-62–II-66.

Mirhoseini M, Cayton MM. Revascularization of the heart by laser. *J Microsurg* 1981; 2: 253–260.

Mueller XM, Tevaearai HH, Genton CY et al. Transmyocardial laser revascularization in acutely ischemic myocardium. *Eur J Cardiothorac Surg* 1998; 13: 170–175.

Mukherjee D, Bhatt DL, Roe MT et al. Direct myocardial revascularization and angiogenesis-how many patients might be eligible? *Am J Cardiol* 1999; 84: 598–600.

Nakamura Y, Iwanaga S, Ikeda F. Venous flow in the great cardiac vein of the dog. *Jpn Heart J* 1990; 31: 99–108.

Nakazawa HK, Roberts DL, Klocke FJ. Quantitation of anterior descending versus circumflex venous drainage in the canine great cardiac vein and coronary sinus. *Am J Physiol* 1978; 324: H163–H166.

Oesterle SN, Reifart NJ, Meier B et al. Initial results of laser-based percutaneous myocardial revascularization for angina pectoris. *Am J Cardiol* 1998; 82: 659–662.

Oesterle SN, Yeung AC, Lo S et al. Percutaneous in-situ coronary venous arterialization (PICVA) improves survival in response to acute ischemia in the porcine model(abstract). *J Am Coll Cardiol* 2000; 35: 61A.

Oesterle SN Sanborn TA, Ali N, et al. Percutaneous myocardial laser revascularization: final results from the PACIFIC randomized trial. *Lancet* 2000; 356: 1705–1710.

Oesterle SN, Reifart N, Hauptmann E, Hayase M, Yeung A. Percutaneous *in situ* coronary venous arterialization: Report of the first human catheter based coronary artery bypass. *Circulation* 2001; 103: 2591–2597.

Park SB, Magovern GJ, Liebler GA et al. Direct selective myocardial revascularization by internal mammary artery coronary vein anastomosis. *J Thorac Cardiovasc Surg* 1975; 69: 63–72.

Petre R. Laser to the heart: magic but costly or only costly? *Lancet* 1999; 353: 512–513.

Robertson H. The physiology, pathology, and clinical significance of experimental coronary sinus obstruction. *Surgery* 1941; 9: 1–24.

Robertson H. The re-establishment of cardiac circulation during progressive coronary occlusion. *Am Heart J* 1935; 10: 533–541.

Rosenthal D, Dickson C, Rodriguez FJ et al. Intrainguinal endovascular in situ saphenous vein bypass: ongoing results. *J Vasc Surg* 1994; 20: 389–395.

Schofield PM, Sharples LD, Caine N et al. Transmyocardial laser revascularization in patients with refractory angina: a randomized controlled trial. *Lancet* 1999; 353: 519–524.

Sen PK, Daulatram J, Kinare SG et al. Further studies in multiple transmyocardial acupuncture as a method of myocardial revascularization. *Surgery* 1968; 64: 861–870.

Sen PK, Udwadia TE, Kinare SG et al. Transmyocardial acupuncture: a new approach to myocardial revascularization. *J Thorac Cardiovasc Surg* 1965; 50: 181–189.

Wearn JT, Mettler SR, Klumo TJ et al. The nature of the vascular communications between the coronary arteries and the chambers of the heart. *Am Heart J* 1933; 9: 143–170.

Yamamoto N, Kohmoto T, Gu A et al. Angiogenesis is enhanced in ischemic canine myocardium by transmyocardial laser revascularization. *J Am Coll Cardiol* 1998; 31: 1426–1433.

IV

Other Methods of Myocardial Revascularization

10

Transmyocardial and Percutaneous Myocardial Revascularization: Nonlaser Approaches

Birgit Kantor, M.D., Paul C. Keelan, M.D.,
David R. Holmes Jr., M.D., and Robert S. Schwartz, M.D.

Division of Cardiovascular Diseases and Internal Medicine
Mayo Clinic and Foundation
Rochester, Minnesota

SUMMARY

Initial clinical studies evaluating the feasibility and safety of both percutaneous laser revascularization (PMR) and transmyocardial laser revascularization (TMR) have shown promising results in improving ischemic symptoms in patients with end-stage coronary artery disease not amenable to bypass surgery or percutaneous interventions.

It was initially assumed that different laser systems or would affect procedural outcome. However, it now appears likely that neovascularization can be stimulated by other energy sources with similar success as the laser.

In all new proangiogenic therapies, imaging and measuring the efficacy of the intervention is a common problem. There have been conflicting results with attempts to show increased perfusion late after TMR.

Focused ultrasound and radio frequency are experimental methods of generating channels by vaporizing myocardium. This is potentially important in that it will allow for channel generation as well as being less expensive than a laser system.

Mechanical revascularization via acupuncture needles has been undertaken; however, clinical trials are necessary to investigate whether these will translate into clinical benefits for human patients.

With increasing evidence that chronic angiogenesis is a key factor in clinical success of treating patients with intractable ischemic symptoms, future studies are needed to assess the efficacy and durability of the clinical benefit of TMR and PMR.

10.1. INTRODUCTION

Current therapy for myocardial ischemia relies on invasive revascularization procedures of the epicardial coronary arteries or on drugs to reduce myocardial oxygen demand. There is an increasing need for

Myocardial Revascularization: Novel Percutaneous Approaches, Edited by George S. Abela.
ISBN 0-471-36166-6   Copyright © 2002 Wiley-Liss, Inc.

alternative antianginal therapies for an increasing number of patients with advanced coronary artery disease who remain symptomatic despite maximal medical or invasive treatment.

Transmyocardial laser revascularization (TMR) is a new surgical approach for treating angina in patients with end-stage coronary artery disease. During the procedure, channels are lased into the myocardium to potentially enhance regional blood flow to ischemic myocardium. The first randomized clinical trials indicate that TMR is effective in reducing symptoms and increasing exercise time in approximately 75% of patients. To reduce the perioperative mortality and morbidity associated with the surgical approach, the procedure is also performed in the cardiac catheterization laboratory with a percutaneous approach to create channels into the endocardial surface (percutaneous myocardial revascularization, PMR).

The exact mechanisms underlying the clinical success of the procedure are still unclear. Direct perfusion of laser channels from the left ventricle and myocardial neovascularization are the most frequently proposed hypotheses. Other hypotheses include an analgesic effect of denervation, a placebo effect, or a combination of these mechanisms. It is questionable whether tissue changes after TMR and the clinical success of the procedure are specific for the laser. There is increasing evidence that energy sources other than the laser result in comparable acute and chronic pathology. In this chapter, we describe acute and chronic pathology of TMR and new alternative approaches for nonlaser TMR.

10.2. BACKGROUND

The initial objective behind TMR was to create communications between the left ventricular cavity and myocardium to allow oxygenated blood to enter and perfuse ischemic tissue. This concept presupposed that channels created during transmyocardial revascularization remain patent and estab-

lish functional connections shunting arteriaized blood directly from the left ventricular cavity into the myocardium. However, histology shows that channels thrombose within hours of the procedures. Chronically there is scar formation and distinct signs of angiogenesis in the original treatment site (Fleischer et al., 1996; Gassler et al., 1997; Gassler and Stubbe, 1997). Animal experiments and preliminary clinical studies suggest that chronic angiogenesis can augment blood flow to ischemic myocardium (Frazier et al., 1999; Horvath et al., 1995, 1996; Yamamoto et al., 1998; Yanagisawa et al., 1992). Consistent with pathology, acute perfusion studies show no evidence of increased blood flow (Hardy et al., 1990), whereas chronically, regional blood flow is increased in treated areas (Donovan et al., 1997; Frazier et al., 1999; Whittaker et al., 1997; Yamamoto et al., 1998).

The mechanism underlying the beneficial clinical effect of TMR may be multifactorial. Other hypotheses explaining the immediate and chronic angina relief following the procedure include nerve fiber destruction and a possible placebo effect (Benson and McCallie, 1979; Schofield et al., 1999). Preliminary data examining a potential anesthetic effect of TMR resulted in conflicting results (Al-Sheikh et al., 1999; Hirsch et al., 1999; Kwong et al., 1997). One recent trial has addressed the potential placebo effect of TMR with percutaneous Biosence laser system (DIRECT trial). At 6 months follow-up, there was no statistical difference between the laser and the placebo groups regarding total exercise time, angina, quality of life, and myocardial perfusion. This study suggests a placebo affect of laser revascularization and has raised significant concern about using laser TMR and PMR in future. It may also be possible that a combination of different mechanisms act simultaneously or in a temporal sequence. Decreased angina perception by nerve damage and a placebo effect may be responsible for the acute benefits, whereas angiogenesis and placebo effect may reduce ischemic symptoms at the chronic stage.

10.3. FIRST RANDOMIZED CLINICAL TRIALS OF TMR

Initial clinical studies evaluating safety and feasibility of laser TMR and PMR show promising results, with an average improvement of ischemic symptoms in more than two-thirds of all treated patients (Gassler and Stubbe, 1997; Horvath et al., 1996; March, 1999; Oesterle et al., 1998). In 1999, four prospective randomized TMR trials were published, three of them confirming previous data (Frazier et al., 1999; Allen et al., 1998; Burkhoff et al., 1999), whereas Schofield's study performed in the United Kingdom showed limited clinical benefit (Schofield et al., 1999). All trials randomized approximately 200 patients to surgical laser TMR or maximal medical treatment. Study design and clinical end points were comparable in all trials, whereas inclusion and exclusion criteria varied. Schofield's patient cohort excluded unstable patients, and only 27% of all patients presented with CCS class IV angina compared to 70–80% in the US trials. Myocardial perfusion was assessed by thallium single-photon emission computed tomography (SPECT).

All three US trials demonstrated symptomatic improvement of two CCS angina classes in approximately 70% of patients in the TMR group compared with approximately 12% in the medically treated group. In contrast, only 25% of patients randomized to laser TMR in the UK study improved clinically compared with 4% in the medical treatment arm. Although the difference between the groups was statistically significant, the investigators felt that a 25% improvement in the TMR group was in the range of a placebo effect. More blinded clinical trials are needed to clarify the role of a potential placebo effect in TMR in the near future. Only one trial demonstrated improved myocardial perfusion at 3-, 6-, and 12-month follow-up. However, the investigators used a nonstandardized method to evaluate the thallium scans, and perfusion in the control group deteriorated as early as 3 months after randomization (Frazier et al., 1999).

Recently, the first clinical study using a catheter-based percutaneous approach has been published. This technique performed comparably to surgical TMR with a significant improvement of angina in the PMR group compared with medical therapy alone (Lauer et al., 1999). Moreover, periprocedural mortality was only 0.5% compared with 5% in the surgical trials.

There is clear evidence that different laser systems induce different clinical outcomes and they may perform equally well. The first catheter-based PMR trial (Lauer et al., 1999) and Allan's surgical trial (Allen et al., 1999) were performed with a Ho:YAG laser system, whereas the other two positive US trials and the negative UK trial used a CO_2 laser. It has been suggested that the placebo effect of the recent DIRECT trial may be related to the type of laser used or to a device specific outcome. Future studies using other energy systems than the laser have to address this important question.

10.4. IS LASER ENERGY NECESSARY TO CREATE CHANNELS?

Initially, investigators assumed that different laser or energy systems affect procedural outcome. Although there are differences in the acute tissue responses associated with various technical TMR approaches, it is questionable whether they translate into significant differences in long-term clinical outcome.

Fisher and colleagues systematically addressed the question of whether different laser types are associated with specific pathologic features (Fisher et al., 1997). They compared CO_2 channels with Ho:YAG laser channels in normal dog hearts. Within 24 h of TMR, all channels were thrombosed regardless of the laser energy used. During the next 21 days, subsequent organization and neovascularization occurred in both treatment groups. Although the CO_2 laser caused less myocardial damage acutely compared with the Ho:YAG laser, overall histologic features including angiogenesis were indistinguishable at the chronic stage. Autopsies from patients who died at various time points after different types of laser TMR reproduced these findings, including prominent neovascularization (Gassler and Stubbe, 1997). Potent natural stimuli of growth factor expression and growth factor receptors are inflammation and chronic hypoxia. Both are associated with TMR: necrosis and an inflammatory cell reaction acutely and scar formation chronically. The initial injury created by the channel causes leukocytes and macrophages to migrate into treated areas. These cells promote angiogenesis by releasing enzymes, growth factors, and cytokines, which initiate endothelial cell activation. After activation, there is disruption of the vascular basement membrane and increased vascular permeability [mediated, e.g., by vascular endothelial growth factor (VEGF)]. Proteolysis around the parent vessel provides a space for endothelial cells migrating from a preexisting vessel toward the angiogenic stimulus. Proliferating endothelial cells sprout from the parent vessel to form an intravascular lumen and collateral branches. Regeneration of the surrounding extracellular matrix completes the process of neovascularization.

It is very likely that angiogenesis after TMR is not specific for the laser and that other energy sources and injury modalities could stimulate neovascularization in a similar way. Therefore, investigators have explored alternative approaches to create channels.

10.5. RADIO FREQUENCY PMR

An alternative energy technique, which is low in cost and can also elevate tissue temperature quickly, is radio frequency (RF) energy. RF catheter ablation has been used successfully for decades to treat patients with cardiac tachyarrhythmias. Tissue reactions after myocardial RF ablation have been well described (Nath et al., 1994, 1995). On the basis of observation that different laser systems induce a similar chronic angiogenic response, investigations have recently started on RF energy for PMR.

The RF-PMR system (Boston Scintific/ Scimed®) consists of a portable RF energy generator (ArthroCare®, Sunnyvale, CA), a steerable 9 F delivery catheter, and an electrode catheter. The instrumentation is easy to handle and considerably less bulky than typical laser equipment. The steerable catheter system allows access to the endocardial surface of the entire left ventricle including the septum, which cannot be treated during the surgical TMR approach (Fig. 10-1). The electrode catheter has two inner lumens with ports at its tip allowing fluid injections into the channel during the procedure. The injection port of the RF-PMR catheter can also be used for additional drug delivery such as growth factors or gene therapy expressing pharmacologically active proteins to enhance the desired angiogenic effect. After each ablation, contrast agent is applied into the channel to mark treated sites. The contrast infiltrates the tissue, and a radiopaque blush appears on the monitor marking the channel. This provides a map of treatment sites as the procedure progresses, thus minimizing the risk of ventricular perforation by ablating the same myocardial area twice.

On pathology, RF-PMR sites are almost identical to treatment sites after laser TMR (Kantor et al., 1998, 1999a, 1999b), suggesting that the laser may not be a necessary component of the long-term outcome of the procedure. Acutely, numerous regions of myocardial hemorrhage are associated with inflammatory cell infiltration (Fig. 10-2). Chronically, all channels are occluded, and both RF-PMR and laser TMR show distinct signs of angiogenesis at the sites of previous channel creation (Fig. 10-3). These tissue responses are almost identical to what is found after laser TMR in pigs, dogs, and humans (Figs. 10-4 and 10-5). To date, it is clear whether heat is necessary to achieve an intense angiogenic response. Future basic research and clinical studies will give more insight into these aspects.

A common problem in all new proangiogenic therapies is imaging and measuring the efficacy of the intervention, especially in

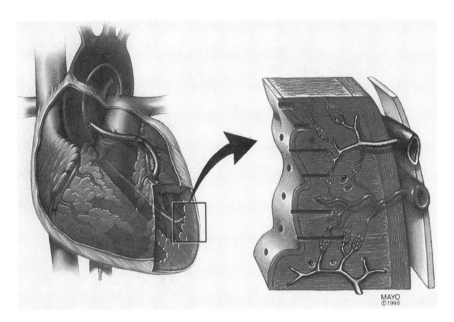

FIGURE 10-1. Percutaneous RF-PMR via standard femoral artery access without general anesthesia. A steerable catheter system and an energy delivery catheter are delivered retrogradely across the aortic valve, allowing access to the endocardium of the entire left ventricular wall (Reprinted with permission from Kantor et al., 1999b).

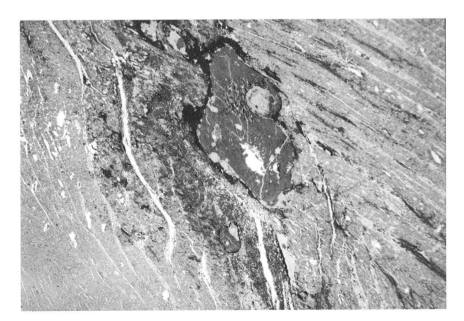

FIGURE 10-2. Histology 4 h after RF PMR. The channel is thrombosed, and there is extensive intramyocardial hemorrhage around the channel site. Hematoxylin and eosin (HE), magnification ×50.

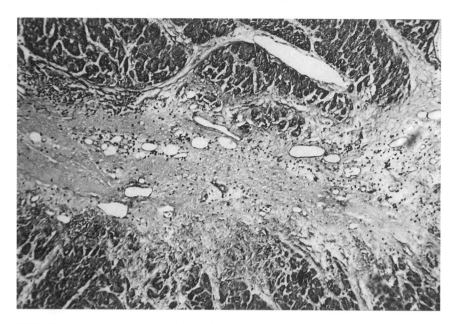

FIGURE 10-3.   Chronic findings 28 days after RF-TMR in normal porcine myocardium. The channels are replaced by highly vascular scar tissue. HE, magnification ×40.

clinical trials. In animal experiments, blood flow can be measured with labeled microspheres. The limited spatial resolution of histology makes it difficult to analyze the complex three-dimensional architectures and the collateralizing connections of the newly formed vascular networks. In addition, attempts to show increased perfusion late after TMR have shown conflicting results. We use a new microscopic imaging modality (Micro-CT) to quantify and visualize complex microvascular structures. This technique allows us to follow the course of arterial blood supply from the epicardial arteries to the area of angiogenesis. After RF-PMR, three-dimensional microscopic imaging demonstrated direct connections among epicardial coronary arteries, intramyocardial vessels, and the newly developed anastomosing capillary network in the RF-PMR-treated regions (Kantor et al., 1998). These data indicate that the angiogenic region after RF-PMR connects to the surrounding myocardial vasculature, thus potentially enhancing local perfusion.

The RF PMR system has recently entered phase I clinical trial in four centers in the United States. Preliminary data on safety and feasibility of the procedure in patients will soon be available.

10.6. FOCUSED ULTRASOUND FOR TRANSMYOCARDIAL REVASCULARIZATION

A new, experimental method to generate TMR channels has very recently been tested by vaporizing myocardium at the focal spot with focused ultrasound (Smith et al., 1998) (see Chapter 12). This new technique has recently been explored in vitro using bovine myocardium and evaluated in vivo in normal dogs. The most important potential for using ultrasound for TMR is its ability to generate channels completely noninvasively.

The desired shape and size of the channel can be modified and is dependent on the ultrasound exposure parameters used: frequency, amplitude, pulse period, duty cycle, focal depth, and exposure time. If pressure amplitudes are high enough the formation of gas bubbles (cavitation) can additionally be used to disintegrate the tissue. Variations in

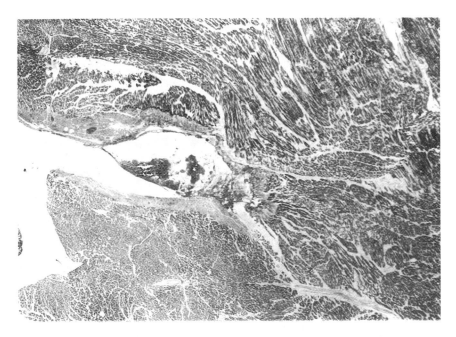

FIGURE 10-4.   Acute effects of TMR in patient who died 1 day after the procedure. The histologic appearance is comparable to RF-PMR in the porcine model including extensive blood-filled spaces in the neighborhood of a thrombosed TMR channel. HE, magnification ×55.

the intensity and exposure time are the main factors manipulated to increase cavity size. Channels are typically 1 mm × 8 mm in size surrounded by a small region of damaged tissue similar to what laser or RF-PMR achieves.

There are three potential advantages of using ultrasound for TMR. First, exposure parameters of ultrasound make channel formation of any shape possible. Second, the ability to focus ultrasound does not require direct contact of the applicator with the cavitation site. Therefore, this technique may allow for a completely noninvasive image-guided procedure from an external ultrasound source. Finally, ultrasound, like all alternative TMR equipment, is considerably less expensive than current laser systems. Future studies must compare acute and chronic histology to laser TMR and assess perfusion before and after treatment in ischemic myocardium. Clinical trials will address safety, feasibility, and efficacy in patients.

10.7. MECHANICAL TMR

In 1965, Sen initiated the concept of mechanical transmyocardial revascularization by creating channels with acupuncture needles. In an ischemic canine model, he demonstrated lower mortality and smaller infarct size in the TMR group compared with nontreated control animals (Sen et al., 1965). White and Hershey described restoration of normal sinus rhythm after transmyocardial acupuncture in a patient with refractory ischemic ventricular fibrillation (Hershey and White, 1969). Histology from their animal data published in 1969 shows a highly vascular scar in the acupunctured myocardium 3 months after the procedure (Fig. 10-6). This histologic appearance is comparable to chronic histologic findings after modern laser TMR, indicating similar tissue responses to these therapeutic approaches.

Considering the significant cost of laser TMR, several investigators have explored mechanical punctures further. The early

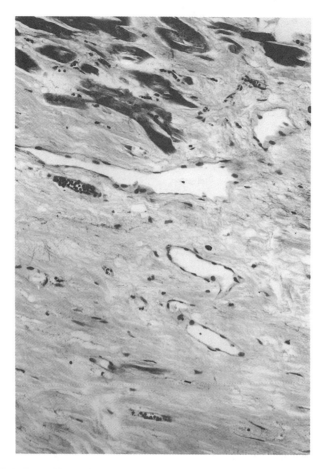

FIGURE 10-5. Chronic findings after laser TMR in a patient who died a year after the procedure. The original treatment site is healed as highly vascular scar tissue comparable to RF-PMR. HE, magnification ×55.

experimental studies available show conflicting results. Mack and co-workers compared channels created by the excimer laser with mechanically induced channels in normal sheep hearts (Mack et al., 1997). At 30 days, they found a combination of partially patent channels and neovascularization around the treatment site. On pathology, 56 of the lased channels were identifiable as partially endothelialized "channel derivatives," whereas all mechanical channels were occluded. Laser-treated myocardium showed a significantly higher angiogenic response than mechanical channels.

Whitaker et al. found no neovascularization at all when comparing laser- and needle-created channels in rats. Needle-created channels showed less fibrosis than laser-made channels. There was no increase in overall capillary density in both treatment arms, although hearts treated with needle-created channels had smaller infarct sizes after coronary artery occlusion than those treated with lased channels. Differences in the study results may be explained by the different models used.

Malekan et al. compared CO_2 laser channels with channels induced by a power drill in an ovine model (Malekan et al., 1998). Both techniques resulted in significant chronic neovascularization regardless of the energy used. Others confirmed these results in ischemic

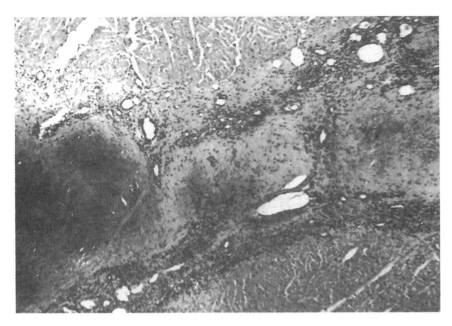

FIGURE 10-6. Mechanical acupuncture TMR in a chronic canine model. Original histology published by White and Hershey in 1969 shows a highly vascular scar in the acupunctured myocardium 3 months after the procedure. This histologic appearance is comparable to chronic histologic findings after modern laser TMR and RF-PMR, indicating similar tissue responses to all therapeutic approaches (Reprinted with permission from Hershey and White, 1969).

rat and porcine models and demonstrated concomitant growth factor expression (VEGF, basic fibroblast growth factor, and transforming growth factor-β) in both models (Chu et al., 1999).

Many different methods to induce myocardial collateralization and different direct revascularization methods have been studied in the past. As early as 1935, Beck et al. sutured pectoral muscle and an internal mammary vessel graft to the pericardium of patients with severe angina to induce collateralization (Beck, 1935). Later, they added inflammatory agents (powdered talc, asbestos, metal) to stimulate additional vessel growth. Inflammation is now well known as a potent stimulus of angiogenesis, with monocytes being a major source of growth factors. Recently, Meerkin and others reworked this concept by implanting metal screws into the myocardium in pigs. Two weeks after surgery, the implants were sur-

rounded by fibrous tissue with prominent vascularization (Meerkin et al., 1998).

Future studies must address functional significance of these newly formed vessels in response to mechanical injury. Clinical trials must confirm whether the potential similarities between laser-induced and mechanical channels shown in animal models translate into clinical benefits in patients.

10.8. CONCLUSIONS AND FUTURE DIRECTIONS

Transmyocardial laser revascularization appears to be successful in treating angina in patients with intractable ischemic symptoms due to end-stage coronary artery disease. This group of patients will expand in the next decade as modern pharmacological and interventional approaches allow them to survive even advanced stages of coronary atherosclerosis disease. If restenosis after angioplasty remains a major clinical problem, this group of patients will expand even further. TMR and PMR have the potential to become widely accepted procedures, especially adjunctive to incomplete bypass surgery or as an adjunct to percutaneous interventions. The mechanisms underlying the clinical benefit of TMR are incompletely understood. There is increasing evidence that chronic angiogenesis is a key factor for the clinical success, which appears to be not confined to the laser. Other approaches show comparable morphologic and pathologic results after application of RF energy, focused ultrasound, and mechanical channel creation. For the high-risk patient cohort currently treated with TMR, the safest and most cost-effective approach should be chosen. In the next few years, data from further animal experiments and randomized clinical trials will become available to provide a better assessment of the efficacy and durability of the clinical benefit of these new revascularization techniques. Recent advances in gene therapy make the consideration of using angiogenic factors in combination with TMR worthwhile to further enhance perfusion. Future studies will determine the maximal extent of clinical improvement that can be expected of laser and nonlaser TMR and of its combination with injected angiogenic substances.

References

Allen KB, Delrossi AJ, Realyvasquez F et al. Transmyocardial revascularization combined with coronary artery bypass grafting versus coronary artery bypass grafting alone: results of a prospective randomized, multi-center trial (abstract). *Circulation* 1998; 98: I-217.

Allen KB, Dowling RD, Fudge TL et al. Comparison of transmyocardial revascularization with medical therapy in patients with refractory angina. *N Engl J Med* 1999; 341: 1029–1036.

Al-Sheikh T, Allen KB, Straka SP et al. Cardiac sympathetic denervation after transmyocardial laser revascularization. *Circulation* 1999; 100: 135–140.

Beck CS. The development of a new blood supply to the heart by operation. *Ann Surg* 1935; 102: 801–813.

Benson H, McCallie DP. Angina pectoris and the placebo effect. *N Engl J Med* 1979; 300: 1424–1429.

Burkhoff D, Schmidt S, Schulman SP et al. Transmyocardial laser revascularization compared with continued medical therapy for treatment of refractory angina pectoris: A prospective randomized trial. *Lancet* 1999; 354: 885–890.

Chu VF, Giaid A, Kuang J et al. Angiogenesis in transmyocardial revascularization: Comparison of laser versus mechanical punctures. *Ann Thorac Surg* 1999; 68: 301–308.

Donovan CL, Landolfo KP, Lowe JE et al. Improvement in inducible ischemia during dobutamine stress echocardiography after transmyocardial laser revascularization in patients with refractory angina pectoris. *J Am Coll Cardiol* 1997; 30: 607–612.

Fisher PE, Kohmoto T, DeRosa CM et al. Histologic analysis of transmyocardial channels: comparison of CO_2 and holmium:YAG lasers. *Ann Thorac Surg* 1997; 64: 466–472.

Fleischer KJ, Goldschmidt-Clermont PJ, Fonger JD et al. One-month histologic response of transmyocardial laser channels with molecular intervention. *Ann Thorac Surg* 1996; 62: 1051–1058.

Frazier OH, March RJ, Horvath KA. Transmyocardial revascularization with a carbon dioxide laser in patients with end-stage coronary artery disease. *N Engl J Med* 1999; 341: 1021–1028.

Gassler N, Stubbe M. Clinical data and histological features of transmyocardial revascularization with CO_2-laser. *Eur J Cardiothorac Surg* 1997; 12: 25–30.

Gassler N, Wintzer HO, Stubbe HM et al. Transmyocardial laser revascularization: Histological features in human nonresponder myocardium. *Circulation* 1997; 95: 371–375.

Hardy RI, James FW, Millard RW et al. Regional myocardial blood flow and cardiac mechanics in dog hearts with CO_2 laser-induced intramyocardial revascularization. *Basic Res Cardiol* 1990; 85: 179–197.

Hershey JE, White M. Transmyocardial puncture revascularization. *Geriatrics* 1969; 12: 101–108.

Hirsch GM, Thompson GW, Arora RC et al. Transmyocardial laser revascularization does not denervate the canine heart. *Ann Thorac Surg* 1999; 68: 460–469.

Horvath KA, Smith WJ, Laurence RG et al. Recovery and viability of an acute myocardial infarct after transmyocardial laser revascularization. *J Am Coll Cardiol* 1995; 25: 258–263.

Horvath KA, Mannting F, Cummings N et al. Transmyocardial laser revascularization: operative techniques and clinical results at two years. *J Thorac Cardiovasc Surg* 1996; 111: 1047–1053.

Kantor B, Kwon H, McKenna C et al. 3-D Micro-CT: a new method for 3-dimensional rendering of myocardial channels and the microcirculation after percutaneous RF myocardial revascularization. *Z Kardiol* 1998; 87 (*Suppl* I): 95.

Kantor B, McKenna C, Ritman E et al. Does channel depth affect chronic outcome after catheter-based myocardial revascularization? A histologic and 3D-microcomputed tomography study (abstract). *J Am Coll Cardiol* 1999a; 33 (*Suppl* IIA): 333A.

Kantor B, McKenna C, Caccitolo J et al. Transmyocardial revascularization: current and future role in the treatment of coronary artery disease. *Mayo Clin Proc* 1999b; 74: 585–592.

Kwong KF, Schuessler RB, Kanellopoulos GK et al. Transmyocardial laser treatment denervates canine myocardium. *J Thorac Cardiovasc Surg* 1997; 114: 883–890.

Lauer B, Junghans U, Stahl F, Kluge R, Oesterle SN, Schuler G. Catheter-based percutaneous myocardial laser revascularization in patients with end-stage coronary artery disease. *J Am Coll Cardiol* 1999; 34: 1663–1670.

Mack CA, Magovern CJ, Hahn RT et al. Channel patency and neovascularization after transmyocardial revascularization using an excimer laser: results and comparisons to nonlased channels. *Circulation* 1997; 96 (*Suppl* II): II-65–II-69.

Malekan R, Narula N, Kelley ST et al. Transmyocardial laser revascularization provides a unique and effective intervention for symptomatic relief and improvement of myocardial perfusion in diffuse cardiac allograft vasculopathy. *Circulation* 1998; 98: II-62–II-66.

March R. Transmyocardial laser revascularization with the CO_2 laser: one year results of a randomized, controlled trial. *Semin Thorac Cardiovasc Surg* 1999; 11: 12–18.

Meerkin D, Pellerin M, Aretz TH et al. Transmyocardial transplants: A novel approach to transmyocardial revascularization. *J Am Coll Cardiol* 1998; 31 (*Suppl* 2): 813–816.

Nath S, Whayne J, Kaul S et al. Effects of RF catheter ablation on regional myocardial blood flow. *Circulation* 1994; 89: 2667–2672.

Nath S, Haines DE. Biophysics and pathology of catheter energy delivery systems. *Prog Cardiovasc Dis* 1995; 37: 185–204.

Oesterle SN, Reifart NJ, Meier B et al. Initial results of laser-based percutaneous myocardial revascularization for angina pectoris. *Am J Cardiol* 1998; 82: 659–662.

Schofield PM, Sharples LD, Caine N et al. Transmyocardial laser revascularization in patients with refractory angina: a randomized control trial. *Lancet* 1999; 353: 519–529.

Sen PK, Udwadia TE, Kinare SG et al. Transmyocardial acupuncture: a new approach to myocardial revascularization. *J Thorac Cardiovasc Surg* 1965; 50: 181–189.

Smith NB, Hynynen K. The feasibility of using focused ultrasound for transmyocardial revascularization. *Ultrasound Med Biol* 1998; 24: 1045–1054.

Whittaker P, Rakusan K, Kloner RA. Transmural channels can protect ischemic tissue: assessment of long-term myocardial response to laser- and needle-made channels. *Circulation* 1997; 93: 143–152.

Yamamoto N, Kohomoto T, Gu A et al. Angiogenesis is enhanced in ischemic canine myocardium by transmyocardial laser revascularization. *J Am Coll Cardiol* 1998; 31: 1426–1433.

Yanagisawa-Miva A, Uchida Y, Nakamura F. Salvage of infarcted myocardium by angiogenic action of basic fibroblast growth factor. *Science* 1992; 257: 1401–1403.

11

Cryoenergy-Induced Neovascularization for Myocardial Reperfusion: A Novel Alternative to Percutaneous Myocardial Revascularization

Richard Gallo, M.D., and Marc Dubuc, M.D.

Department of Medicine
Montreal Heart Institute
Montreal, Quebec, Canada

SUMMARY

With increasing evidence that the use of alternative energy sources to create myocardial channels produces results comparable to those of laser energy, an association between neovascularization and cryoenergy has been demonstrated.

There are many potential advantages of using cryoenergy versus radio frequency energy, including visualization of the catheter tip via echocardiography, more controlled delivery of energy, enhanced adherence to underlying tissue, and the ability to create reversible lesions through temperature variations.

It is believed that the inflammatory environment created by freezing and thawing the myocardial tissue will stimulate an angiogenic or vasculogenic response.

In initial studies of dogs and swine attempting to prove the feasibility of cryoenergy versus PMR, there was greater vascularity overall at treatment sites than in controls after 6 weeks.

Studies have shown that the use of cryoenergy has not been associated with endocardial thrombus or overt device-related safety concerns.

11.1. INTRODUCTION

During the last few years laser myocardial revascularization has emerged as a nonconventional therapeutic option for a number of patients with end-stage coronary artery disease. Although the precise mechanisms of action remain unclear, the notion that new vessel formation or angiogenesis is responsible for the clinical benefits observed remains appealing. However, angiogenesis, as shown in other chapters of the present work, has

Myocardial Revascularization: Novel Percutaneous Approaches, Edited by George S. Abela.
ISBN 0-471-36166-6   Copyright © 2002 Wiley-Liss, Inc.

been demonstrated to occur in response to various stimuli and is not exclusive to laser energy. There is increasing evidence that alternative energy sources such as radio frequency and acupuncture-type mechanically created channels may result in pathologic changes comparable to those observed with laser energy. An association between neovascularization and cryoenergy has been reported (Theodossiadis, 1981). After sealing peripheral retinal tears in retinal detachment surgery by means of cryoapplications, neovascularization stemming from the choroidal circulation appeared. This supports the hypothesis that angiogenesis and/or vasculogenesis may be a nonspecific response to injury.

Our institution, in collaboration with CryoCath Technologies Inc, Canada, has developed a percutaneous catheter system using cryoenergy for the treatment or arrhythmias (Dubuc et al., 1998). This system has been used safely for the treatment supraventricular arrhythmias and atrial flutter in humans (Khairy et al., 1999). Potential advantages of cryoenergy over radio frequency energy in the electrophysiology setting include enhanced adherence to underlying tissue with greater catheter stability, the ability to create reversible lesions before definitive tissue damage through variations in temperature levels, visualization of the catheter tip by echocardiography, more controlled delivery of energy, and histologic evidence of greater homogeneity with sharper demarcations between normal and ablated tissue.

We, therefore, sought to evaluate the potential of this system to deliver cryoenergy to the myocardium and to assess its effects on neovascularization. This chapter describes and discusses the method and novel devices of cryo-percutaneous myocardial revascularization (cryo-PMR). We review the historical beginnings of cryo-PMR, the mechanisms of tissue injury involved with cryoenergy, and the first preclinical results.

11.2. HISTORICAL BEGINNINGS

Cryogenics involves the freezing of a volume of tissue using appropriate techniques and instruments to control the freezing process. The basic features of cryosurgical techniques were established early on as rapid freezing, slow thawing, and repetition of the freeze-thaw cycle (Gage et al., 1998). The modern era of cryosurgery began with the development of automated cryosurgical equipment cooled by liquid nitrogen in the 1930s (Cooper et al., 1963). Since this time cryoenergy is regularly used to treat a variety of pathologies including cutaneous, gynecologic, prostatic, hepatic, ophthalmologic, neurosurgical, and oncologic disorders (Baust et al., 1997).

Cryoenergy has until recently been used in the heart exclusively in the treatment of arrhythmias. Haas and colleagues first described the production of controlled predictable myocardial lesions with cryoenergy in 1948 (Taylor et al., 1951). With the use of CO_2 in the cooling process, the ability of hypothermia to produce a homogeneous, sharply demarcated lesion free of intracardiac thrombosis was demonstrated. Cardiac transmural lesions were created without subsequent rupture or aneurysmal dilation. The absence of such complications and the maintenance of ultrastructural tissue integrity have been attributed to the remarkable resilience of collagen and fibroblasts to hypothermic injury (Gage et al., 1998).

In 1964, Lister reported the first study of cooling applied to specialized cardiac conductive tissue (Lister et al., 1964). A 4-mm "U"-shaped silver tube was sutured to the atrial septum near the His bundle. Passage of a cooling mixture composed of alcohol and CO_2 inhibited atrioventricular (AV) node function at $-10°C$ to $-20°C$. AV node function was altered by progressively decreasing the temperature. Almost immediately after termination of the cooling process, AV conduction returned to its baseline state.

The initial prototype for the current cryo-PMR system was designed by Dr. Peter Freidman in 1993. He first demonstrated the capability of a cryoablation system to produce cryogenic temperatures at the end of a long shaft catheter in the ventricles of sheep. Since this time numerous animal trials have been conducted; although most of these animal trials were carried out in the field of electrophysiology, the results have broad applicability to angiogenesis, specifically those results in the left ventricle. The system initially used for angiogenesis will be the same as the electrophysiology system, and the placement and access are similar (percutaneous endocardial cryoapplications in the left ventricle).

At the time of this printing, over 100 patients have undergone cryoablative therapy for supraventricular tachycardia and atrial flutter.

11.3. MECHANISMS OF TISSUE INJURY BY CRYOAPPLICATION

The rapid and intense freezing of tissue in situ, as done in cryosurgical procedures, results in a localized, sharply demarcated lesion (Gage et al., 1998; Mazur et al., 1970). The nature of the tissue response varies with the intensity of the cryoapplication. Minor cryogenic lesions show varying degrees of inflammatory response, but greater injury will result in tissue destruction. Commonly, the intent of modern cryosurgery is to destroy tissue, such as neoplasms. However, lesser degrees of tissue injury such as that used for our purposes will take advantage of the localized inflammatory response.

The effects of freezing tissue are the result of a number of factors that can be grouped into three major mechanisms, one immediate and the others delayed. The immediate cause of injury is the direct deleterious effect of the freeze-thaw cycle on the cells. A more delayed inflammatory effect accompanied by vascular stasis and microcirculatory failure is observed within 24–48 h of freeze injury. In the final phase of cryoinjury, replacement fibrosis occurs within weeks, forming a well-circumscribed, dense fibrotic lesion (Gage et al., 1998; Mazur et al., 1984).

In the freeze-thaw phase, rapid cooling of cells to subzero temperatures results in ice crystal formation. Crystals are initially produced in the extracellular matrix (Budman et al., 1995) but subsequently form intracellu-

larly as well. The density and size of ice crystals is a function of their proximity to the cryoenergy source, the tissue temperature, and freezing rate. Although the crystals themselves do not seem to disrupt the integrity of the cellular membrane, they compress and deform adjacent nuclei and cytoplasmic components (Whittaker et al., 1984). The earliest changes occur in mitochondria with predominantly central irreversible damage (Gage et al., 1998; Tsvetkov et al., 1985). Subsequent warming, referred to as the "thawing effect," is an integral part of the cryodestructive process (Baust et al., 1997; Gage et al., 1998; Mazur et al., 1984). During the warming cycle, small, high-energy intracellular crystals enlarge and fuse, thereby conglomerating into larger crystals with potentially deleterious effects. To re-establish the osmotic equilibrium disturbed by ice crystal formation, water gradually migrates from within myocardial cells, resulting in an increased intracellular solute concentration. The hyperosmotic state ensuing from this "solution effect" chemically damages cell membranes (Muldrew et al., 1994). Subsequent restoration of the microcirculation to the previously frozen tissue results in edema with exudation of fluid across damaged microvascular endothelial cells and circumscribed ischemic necrosis.

Vascular stasis characterizes the delayed second phase of tissue destruction and occurs within 48 h of thawing (Gage et al., 1998; Giampapa et al., 1981). The initial response to cooling of tissue is vasoconstriction and a decrease in the flow of blood. After freezing, circulation returns, accompanied by vasodilatation. The hyperemic response is usually brief, and increased vascular permeability occurs within a few minutes. Edema develops and progresses over a few hours and days. The endothelial damage induced by freezing results in exudation of proteins, protracted cell permeability, and microthrombus formation (Bowers et al., 1973; Whittaker et al., 1984). The extracellular matrix is now rich in mononuclear cells, lymphocytes, fibroblasts, platelets, and free proteins constituting a highly inflammatory microenvironment. It is precisely this protracted inflammatory environment that we hypothesize will stimulate an angiogenic or vasculogenic response.

11.4. CHARACTERISTICS OF A CRYOLESION

Animal studies have shown that the size of the cryolesion depends on such factors as temperature of the cryoprobe, diameter of the probe in contact with cardiac tissue, exposure time, and number of freeze-thaw cycles (Holman et al., 1983; Hunt et al., 1989; Rodriguez-Santiago et al., 1999). Repeating the freeze-thaw cycle generates lesion dimensions larger than those obtained by a single cryoapplication of longer duration (Cage et al., 1985). Thus, by varying such parameters, early cryosurgical experience demonstrated the ability of cryoenergy to produce predictable, discrete electrophysiologically inert lesions that are sharply delineated from normal cardiac tissue (Dubuc et al., 1999; Markovitz et al., 1988).

Immediately after cryoapplication, the tissue appears normal. There is no destruction of tissue, and the myocardial architecture appears intact (Dubuc et al., 1999; Gage et al., 1998). No macroscopic thrombi have been observed. After a few days cryolesions are visibly more homogeneous, with clearer and smoother demarcations from underlying normal myocardium. At the center of the cryolesion myocardial cells are replaced by collagen and vessel growth. The periphery contains a blend of living and dead myocytes now replaced by fibrous tissue. In addition, there is significant new large conduit vessel (arterioles and muscular arteries) formation observed in a 1- to 2-mm-wide margin of the periphery.

11.5. DEVICE DESCRIPTION

The CryoCath Freezor® (CryoCath Technologies Inc., Canada) system consists of a deflectable 9 F delivery catheter and accompanying console (Fig. 11-1).

The central console houses the electronics and software for controlling and recording the cryo-PMR procedure, stores and controls delivery of liquid refrigerant under high pressure through the injection umbilical to the

AZ-20 CryoCath System

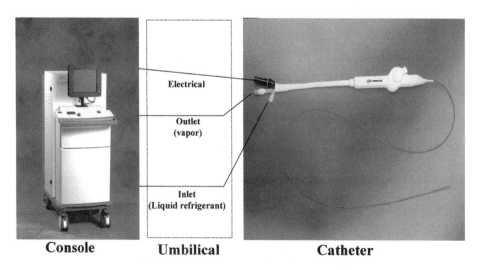

Console   **Umbilical**   **Catheter**

FIGURE 11-1. The CryoCath Freezor system consists of a central console, umbilicals, and a 9 F deflectable catheter (a 7 F catheter is now available).

catheter, recovers the expanded refrigerant vapor from the catheter under vacuum, and recompresses the vapors into a recovery container.

The current 9 F cryocatheter (a 7 F catheter is now available) has a 3 mm wide gold-plated copper-tellurium tip electrode and three proximal platinum electrodes that, in addition to cryoapplication, can also be used for cardiac pacing and intracardiac electrogram recording (Fig. 11-2). The handle of the catheter contains a deflection mechanism that aids in directing the catheter tip to the desired site. The cryocatheter has a hollow shaft with a closed electrode tip. The central console containing freon-derived refrigerant fluid (Gentron® AZ-20) releases the cryogen under pressure. The cooling fluid travels through the inner delivery lumen to the distal electrode, which is maintained under constant vacuum. At the cryocatheter tip, the liquid cooling fluid is boiled. This accelerated liquid-to-gas-phase change results in rapid cooling of the distal catheter tip to temperatures as low as −60°C. Temperature is recorded at the distal tip by an integrated thermocouple device. The gas is then conducted away from the catheter tip via a vacuum return lumen and back to the console where it is collected and restored to its liquid state.

11.6. SAFETY AND FEASIBILITY STUDIES IN ANIMAL MODELS

An initial study attempted to prove the feasibility of cryoenergy as an alternative PMR technique. This first experiment was conducted in 15 healthy mongrel dogs (Khairy et al., 2000).

Under fluoroscopic and electrocardiographic guidance, a standard 9 F cryocatheter was positioned against the left and right ventricular cavities. When the cooling tip of the cryocatheter appeared to be in contact with the endocardium a double freeze-thaw cycle at the lowest attainable temperature was applied for 5 min each. The catheter was then repositioned, and cryoapplications were repeated to a maximum of four per ventricle. Six animals were immediately euthanized for acute pathologic analysis. Chronic histologic

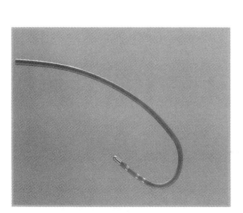
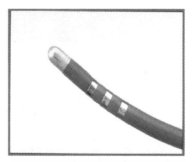
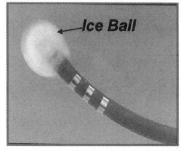

FIGURE 11-2. A close-up view of the 9 F catheter showing catheter deflectability and its gold-plated tip with ice ball.

analysis was performed on nine animals (4 animals were euthanized at 3 weeks and 5 at 6 weeks). There were no device-related procedural complications (Khairy et al., 2000).

Histologic analysis of acute lesions revealed clear demarcations between cryo-injured tissue and normal tissue. Notably, myocardial architecture remained intact. There were no macroscopic endocardial thrombi present. However, intratissue hemorrhage and contraction band necrosis were present (Fig. 11-3). Chronic lesions were also clearly demarcated. At both 3 and 6 weeks, lesions showed well-delineated fibrotic tissue with prominent neovascularization (Fig. 11-4). The average volume for chronic lesions was $55.3 \pm 20.5\,mm^3$, with no significant differences observed between lesions at different locations and at 3 and 6 weeks.

Because this was a feasibility study, the predetermined end point was quantification on vascularity. We limited ourselves to vessel counts in control (distal unaffected) myocardium, in the cryotreated area, and in a 1-mm-wide border zone between cryolesions and uninjured myocardium. Only vessels having at least one layer of smooth muscle cells were accepted. Analysis at both 3 and 6 week sections ($n = 140$) revealed a greater vessel density in the cryotreated area (12.7 ± 5.6 vessels/mm^3) and at the border zones (3.3 ± 1.2 vessels/mm^3) compared with uninjured myocardium (0.6 ± 0.4 vessels/mm^3) ($P < 0.0001$). Blood vessels were more abundant at 3 weeks compared with 6 weeks (14.3 ± 6.3 vs. 11.2 ± 4.6/mm^3; $P = 0.002$; Fig. 11-5). However, vessels were significantly larger at 6 weeks (0.017 ± 0.009 vs. $0.022 \pm 0.015\,mm^3$; $P = 0.04$). Blood vessels at 6 weeks were anatomically more mature, showed signs of branching, and meandered through the cryolesion and its border area (Fig. 11-6) (Khairy et al., 2000).

Preclinical experience with the cryo-PMR system extended to a swine model. This study, performed on 12 nonischemic swine was designed to evaluate the feasibility and safety of the Freezor system in a large animal.

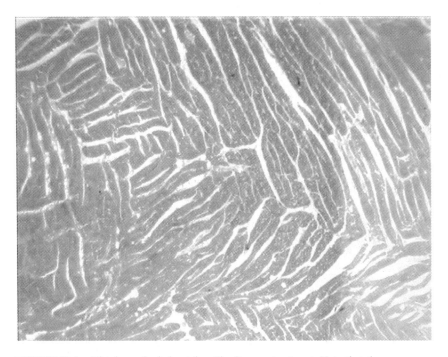

FIGURE 11-3. Histology of a lesion taken 1 h after cryotreatment. Note that the myocardial ultrastructure is not disrupted. There is myocyte edema, but no macroscopic thrombi.

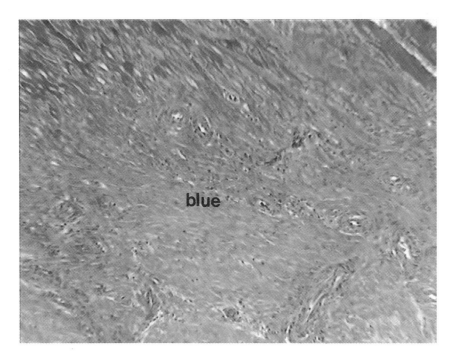

FIGURE 11-4. High-power magnification (×120) of a chronic 6-week lesion in a nonischemic canine model. A well-demarcated fibrotic lesion (blue) has replaced the site of cryoinjury. An abundance of small arterioles (at least 1 layer of smooth muscle cells) is present.

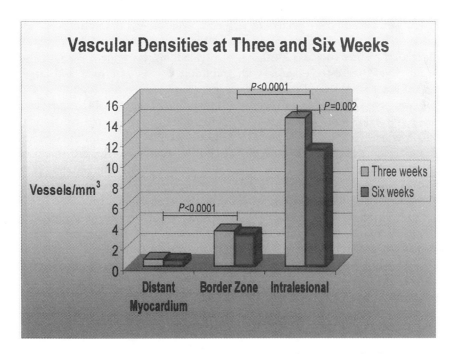

FIGURE 11-5. Comparison of vessel densities in cryo-treated zones, 1-mm border zones, and control myocardium from a nonischemic canine model. Only vessels exhibiting at least 1 smooth muscle cell layer were counted. Vessels appear more numerous at 3 weeks than at 6 weeks. However, morphometric analysis reveals vessels at 6 weeks to be significantly larger than at 3 weeks, suggesting maturation of vessel development.

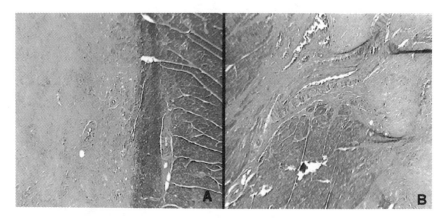

FIGURE 11-6.   (A) A 6-week histologic section taken at the border zone of a cryo-treated zone of myocardium. Numerous mature vessels are visible. (B) Vessels are seen branching and meandering from border area to cryotreated zone.

Multiple (up to 9) cryotreatments in the left ventricle were not associated with increased risk of perforation, serious arrhythmias, or other observable adverse events.

Unlike the experiments performed on the canine model, we attempted to determine a dose-response effect of cryotreatments on neovascularization. Three doses (2-min, 3-min, and 4-min single freeze-thaw cycles) with a minimum of six to eight applications per left ventricle were performed. No correlation between dose, cryolesion size, or neovascularization was observed.

Finally, we evaluated the compatibility of the simultaneous use of the CryoCath system with an electromagnetic ventricular navigation system. The Endocardial Solutions, Inc (ESI) EnSite™ 3000 electromagnetic mapping system was used successfully and permitted adequate placement of the cryocatheter. The ESI EnSite™ system consists of a 9 F over-the-wire electrode recording catheter with a 64-electrode array. This system is commercially available for the recording and mapping electrical potentials from the left ventricle or right atrium. Vascular access was obtained through the left femoral artery. The mapping catheter was advanced under fluoroscopic guidance into the left ventricle. The cryocatheter was inserted via the right femoral artery retro-

gradely through the aortic valve. A three-dimensional electromagnetic map of the left ventricle was obtained before proceeding with the cryotreatments (Fig. 11-7). In most cases, the mapping and cryotreatments could be completed in less than 30 min.

Visual assessment of histology specimens revealed impressive neovascularization. Large conduit vessels, arterioles and larger muscular arteries were abundant (Figs. 11-8 and 11-9). The density of both arterioles and large muscular vessels increased significantly in border zones and within the cryolesion (Fig. 11-10). Morphometric assessment of cryoinjury sites suggests that cryoenergy stimulates large new vessel formation, as seen by growth and penetration of arterioles and muscular arteries from the border zones to the treatment area. Overall, there was greater vascularity at treatment sites than in controls after 6 weeks. The increased vessel density is consistent with other modalities of transmyocardial revascularization. Before pathologic sectioning the coronary arteries were injected with a barium solution. The presence of barium in these new vessels suggests a connection with epicardial coronary arteries, continued patency, and functionality. Regardless of their size, whether these new vessels perfuse myocardium remains undetermined at this time and can probably be best studied

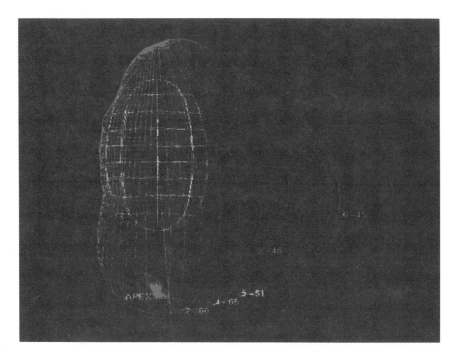

FIGURE 11-7. A 3-dimensional electromagnetic map of a pig left ventricle, obtained with the cryocatheter and the EnSite 3000™ mapping system from EndoCardial Solutions. Cryo-treated sites are clearly marked and separated. The green line indicates in real time the position of the cryocatheter relative to the reference multielectrode catheter.

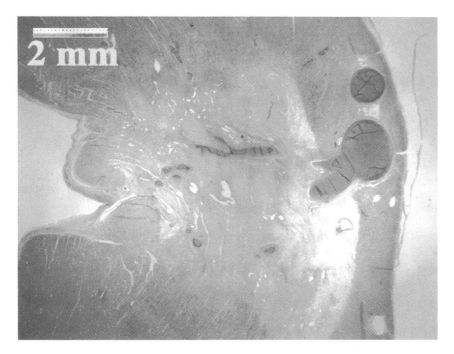

FIGURE 11-8. A trichrome/elastin histology section taken at 6 weeks from a nonischemic porcine model. The cryo-treated zone appears in blue. Abundant large muscular arteries and arterioles are present. After perfusion fixation, coronary arteries were injected with a barium solution. Barium-filled muscular arteries are easily identified in this picture. The presence of barium in these conduit vessels strongly suggests patency and connections with epicardial vessels.

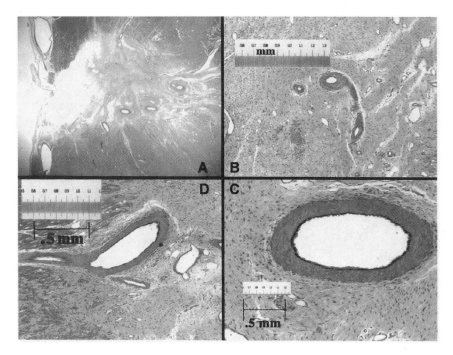

FIGURE 11-9. Further examples of muscular arteries present 6 weeks after cryotreatment in nonischemic porcine myocardium. Muscular arteries were identified by the presence of both smooth muscle cells and elastin-positive immunohistochemical stains. The presence of large muscular arteries contrasts with the relatively immature single-cell vessels observed with lasers. However, regardless of the size observed, the physiologic significance of these vessels remains to be determined.

by performing perfusion studies in a chronic ischemic model.

11.7. THE CRYO-PMR ADVANTAGE

11.7.1. Safety

Any heat-based source, such as lasers, will cause the formation of myocardial channels. Indeed, many physicians still falsely believe that the creation of a physical hole in the myocardium is a necessary precursor to the initiation of an inflammatory response. A significant risk of creating holes with heat in the myocardium is the thromboembolic complications from the charring as well as tamponade caused by perforations. Myocardial architecture is not disrupted with cryoenergy, thus significantly reducing the risk of myocardial perforation. Indeed, extensive preclinical and human experience in the electrophysiol-

ogy field has repeatedly demonstrated the safety of cryoenergy.

11.7.2. Efficacy

Data obtained during the examination of double 5-min freeze-thaw cycles in healthy canine myocardium and single 2-min freeze-thaw cycles in porcine myocardium indicate vasculogenesis superior to that seen with laser-based systems. One should always be cautious when comparing experimental data to previously published data because of differences in methodology, experimental models, and measurement methods. Nevertheless, an ad hoc comparison of the above animal experiments shows a vascular density of approximately 3000 vessels/cm^2 at 6 weeks as compared to one study using a Ho-YAG laser (Yamamoto et al., 1998) that showed

Arteriolar Density

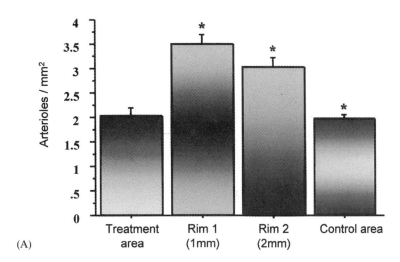

(A)

Density of Muscular Arteries

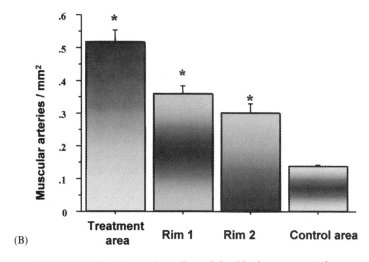

(B)

FIGURE 11-10. Comparison of vessel densities between control areas and cryo-treated, and 1-mm and 2-mm border zones. There is an increased arteriolar density in the border zones of cryo-treated areas (A). There are significantly more muscular arteries in both the border areas and cryo-treated sections (B).

approximately 150 vessels/cm^2 at 8 weeks. This represents a 20-fold difference in vessel density. A similar comparative difference between cryoenergy and lasers is seen with another study (Malekan et al., 1998). That study shows vessel densities on the order of 2.1 vessels per ×40 high-power field (HPF) with laser, whereas our results show densities of approximately 50 vessels per ×40 HPF. This again represents a more than 20-fold difference between observations from cryoenergy and lasers.

Similarly, whereas laser-generated vessels are relatively immature with single cell layer walls, cryogenerated vessels tend to be larger conduit vessels with one or more smooth muscle layers and an external elastic lamina (Fig. 11-8).

11.7.3. Navigation

Intuitively, the capability to guide and position a revascularization catheter at the targeted area with increased precision has its advantages. At this moment, the only available system combining PMR and an electromagnetic mapping system is the biosense NOGA/DMR system. As we have shown in our preclinical studies the CryoCath Freezor system is compatible with the ESI EnSite 3000™ system (Fig. 11-7). Furthermore, because of their separate platforms, the CryoCath Freezor system can be used independently. This offers the physician the flexibility of using or not using a mapping system, as desired.

11.7.4. Speed

A typical laser hole is approximately 1 mm in diameter; its accompanying acoustic shock can affect a border zone anywhere from 1 to 4 mm around. Cryo-PMR on the other hand creates a continuous, well-demarcated border zone of about 4 mm in diameter. Because area is proportional to the square of diameter a rough estimate is that cryo-PMR can cover the same area as laser with about one-quarter ($4 mm^2$ vs. $16 mm^2$ per application) the number of applications. As an example, a typical 25-laser hole procedure could be replaced with 5 or 6 cryoapplications. This will yield significantly improved procedure times. Preclinical work in the porcine model has consistently demonstrated complete procedure times in the range of 25–30 min (including electromagnetic mapping and 6–8 cryoapplications).

11.8. CONCLUSIONS

Significant angiogenesis/vasculogenesis appears to be induced by cryoenergy application to the myocardium of healthy dogs and swine. The present study suggests that arterioles grow from the border zone and then pen-

etrate the lesion core, where they mature into muscular arteries. In contrast to the immature single cell layer vessels often observed with lasers, the present observations are striking. At 6 weeks, the presence of barium within these vessels suggests their continued patency, and their size suggests functionality.

In accordance with previous animal and human studies, the delivery of cryoenergy was not associated with the presence of endocardial thrombus. No device-related safety concerns were raised.

If elected by the operator, the CryoCath Freezor system can he used safely and effectively with an electromagnetic mapping system, allowing for increased positioning of the cryocatheter.

However, as with other available energy sources, the functional and physiologic significance of these new vessels remains to be determined.

11.9. FUTURE DIRECTIONS

Given the relative inexperience with this new percutaneous system compared with laser or even radio frequency energy, its use is limited by obstacles that all new technologies face. With the aid of further animal experiments and clinical studies, optimal procedural settings regarding duration of the freeze-thaw cycle, temperature setting, and size of the catheter tip are in the process of refinement. Given the proven safety record of this technology for the treatment of supraventricular arrhythmias, we have designed a phase I safety trial involving 20 patients with end-stage coronary artery disease. Trial completion is planned for the fall of 2000. At the time of printing, we have enrolled 19 patients in this Phase I Trial. Results, including device, safety and efficacy will be available in the fall of 2001.

References

Baust J, Cage A, Ma H et al. Minimally invasive cryosurgery-technological advances. *Cryobiology* 1997; 34: 373–384.

Bowers W, Hubbard R, Daum R et al. Ultrastructural studies or muscle cells and vascular endothelium immediately after freeze-thaw injury. *Cryobiology* 1973; 10: 9–21.

Budman H, Shitzer A, Dayan J. Analysis of the inverse problem of freezing and thawing of a binary solution during cryosurgical processes. *J Biomed Eng* 1995; 117: 193–202.

Cage A, Guest K, Montes M et al. Effect of varying freezing and thawing rates in experimental cryosurgery. *Cryobiology* 1985; 22: 175–182.

Cooper I. Cryogenic surgery: a new method of destruction or extirpation of benign or malignant tissue. *N Engl J Med* 1963; 268: 743–749.

Dubuc M, Talajic M, Roy D et al. Feasibility of cardiac cryoablation using a transvenous steerable electrode catheter. *J Interv Card Electrophysiol* 1998; 2: 285–292.

Dubuc M, Roy D, Thibauk B et al. Transvenous catheter ice mapping and cryoablation of the atrioventricular node in dogs. *Pacing Clin Electrophysiol* 1999: 1488–1498.

Gage A, Baust J. Mechanisms of tissue injury in cryosurgery. *Cryobiology* 1998; 37: 171–186.

Giampapa V, Oh C, Aufses A. The vascular effect of cold injury. *Cryobiology* 1981; 8: 49–54.

Holman W, Ikeshita M, Douglas J et al. Cardiac cryosurgery: effects of myocardial temperature on cryolesion size. *Surgery* 1983; 93: 268–272.

Hunt C, Chard R, Johnson D et al. Comparison of early and late dimensions and arrhythmogenicity of cryolesions in the normothermic canine heart. *J Thorac Cardiovasc Surg* 1989; 97: 313–318.

Khairy P, Rodriguez-Santiago A, Talajic M et al. Catheter cryo-ablation in man: early clinical experience(abstract). *Can J Cardiol* 1999; 15: 173D.

Khairy P, Dubuc M, Gallo R. Percutaneous cryoinjury induces neovascularization: a novel approach to myocardial revascularization(abstract). *J Am Coll Cardiol* 2000; 35: 5A.

Lister J, Hoffman B. Reversible cold block of the specialized conduction tissues of the anaesthetized dog. *Science* 1964; 145: 723–725.

Malekan R, Reynolds C, Narula N et al. Angiogenesis in transmyocardial laser revascularization: a nonspecific response to injury. *Circulation* 1998; 98: II-62–II-66.

Markovitz L, Frame L, Josephson M et al. Cardiac cryolesions: factors affecting their size and a means of monitoring their formation. *Ann Thorac Surg* 1988; 46: 531–535.

Mazur P. Cryobiology: the freezing of biological systems. *Science* 1970; 68: 939–949.

Mazur P. Freezing of living cells: mechanisms and implications. *Am J Physiol* 1984; 143: C125–C142.

Muldrew K, McGann L. The osmotic rupture hypothesis of intracellular freezing injury. *Biophys J* 1994; 66: 532–541.

Rodriguez-Santiago A, Dubuc M, Talajic M et al. Percutaneous catheter cryoablation in dogs: chronic lesion characterization(abstract). *Can J Cardiol* 1999; 15: 102D.

Taylor C, Davis C, Vawter G et al. Controlled myocardial injury produced by a hypothermal method. *Circulation* 1951; 3: 239.

Theodossiadis G. Choroidal neovascularization after cryoapplication. *Opthalmologie* 1981; 215: 203–208.

Tsvetkov T, Tsonev L, Meranzov N et al. Functional changes in mitochondrial properties as a result of their membrane cryodestruction. II. Influence of freezing and thawing on ATP complex activity of intact liver mitochondria. *Cryobiology* 1985; 22: 111–118.

Whittaker D. Mechanisms of tissue destruction following cryosurgery. *Ann R Coll Surg Engl* 1984; 66: 313–318.

Yamamoto N, Kohmoto T, Gu A et al. Angiogenesis is enhanced in ischemic canine myocardium by transmyocardial laser revascularization. *J Am Coll Cardiol* 1998; 31: 1426–1433.

12

Ultrasonic Surgery: Mechanism of Action and Implications for Transmyocardial Revascularization

Rudolf Verdaasdonk, Ph.D., Henk Cobelens, B.Sc.,
Christiaan van Swol, Ph.D., Matthijs Grimbergen, B.Sc.,
Paul F. Gründeman, Ph.D.

Department of Clinical Engineering and Physics and Heart-Lung Institute
University Medical Center
Utrecht, The Netherlands

and

Stephen Fry, Ph.D.

CardioCavitational Systems, Inc.
Hanalei, Hawaii

SUMMARY

It is hypothesized that tissues can be ruptured, fragmented, and vaporized by inducing cavitation effects via ultrasound.

Ultrasonically induced effects can be delivered to the tissue by various devices, including extracorporeal application, transcutaneous application, percutaneous catheter-based device, and an intraoperative device.

The intraoperative surgical ultrasonic myocardial revascularization device is a handheld piece that is user friendly and requires only a short learning curve to operate the system.

In vivo myocardial revascularization with ultrasonic needle has been tested in animals and found to produce channels comparable with those created by a laser.

Ultrasonic myocardial revascularization can be more cost-effective than laser, as well as having the additional benefits of not requiring the training, safety precautions, calibration, and maintenance necessary with PMR/TMR laser systems.

Myocardial Revascularization: Novel Percutaneous Approaches, Edited by George S. Abela.
ISBN 0-471-36166-6   Copyright © 2002 Wiley-Liss, Inc.

12.1. INTRODUCTION

Ultrasound equipment has been used in the cardiovascular field for many years for diagnostic purposes (Roelandt, 1998). Cutaneous transducers enable high-resolution real-time imaging of the heart, providing information on such functional parameters as wall motion and valve condition (Mulvagh et al., 2000; Plein, 2000). To obtain better image quality, transesophageal transducers are used to provide cardiac images without requiring the ultrasonic energy to pass through the lungs and ribs. Also, catheter-based devices (intravascular ultrasound, or IVUS) have been developed to obtain cross-sectional images of arterial walls to determine the degree of stenosis and calcification in atherosclerotic patients (Berry et al., 2000; Di Mario et al., 2000). The typical frequencies of the cutaneous devices are 500 kHz to 4 MHz, whereas the IVUS systems utilize higher frequencies, in the range of 30–50 MHz (Quinn et al., 2000).

The energy densities used for diagnostics are assumed to be below damage threshold. However, at higher frequencies and power densities, temporal or permanent damage might be induced because of either local heating of tissue or mechanical damage (American Institute of Ultrasound, 2000). Density waves within the tissue can induce the formation of small bubbles. At a low-density front, water can start boiling, forming a low-pressure vapor bubble. This bubble formation is called cavitation (Miller, 1998). The collapse of these bubbles can be very forceful mechanically on a small scale, inducing localized tissue damage. The damage can include DNA deformation, cell membrane leaking and rupture, cell matrix disruption, and secondary damage due to free radical formation (Barnett et al., 1997, 2000; Suhr et al., 1991).

Several medical procedures have been developed based on the mechanical tissue-modifying effects of ultrasonic cavitation. One of the most widely known therapies is kidney stone lithotripsy, in which a short burst of high-energy ultrasound is focused

from a source outside the body to a target stone within the kidney (Kupeli et al., 1998). Because of the high energy densities obtained locally near the stone, cavitation effects and stresses within the stone break the stone to pieces. For cardiovascular applications, high local energy densities can be used for thrombolysis and decalcification of heart valves (Rosenschein et al., 2000).

Besides transcutaneous focusing, ultrasonic energy can also be transported into the body by rigid devices that induce effects at the distal tip of the device. These devices consist of a hand piece with a tapered tip a catheter with a metal wire along which the energy is transported, or a transducer at the tip of the device. Cavitation effects are induced at the tip of these devices, resulting in tissue disruption. They are mostly applied in neurosurgery and liver surgery for selective resection of soft and more dense tissues in favor of elastic tissues like blood vessels. This enables the removal of tumors with minimal loss of blood, because the vasculature remains intact while the surrounding tissue is removed (Brotchi et al., 1992). There are several systems on the market based on this principle, each with similar characteristics. One of the pioneering systems in this type of surgery is called the cavitron ultrasonic surgical aspirator, or CUSA (Bond et al., 1996; Fasulo et al., 1992). These devices are used in the cardiovascular field for valve decalcification. The harmonic knife is a system in which ultrasound is applied in combination with electrosurgery, taking advantage of both systems, for example, for harvesting arteries for bypass surgery.

In this chapter, the mechanism of action of the various ultrasonic devices is discussed in view of their potential application to transmyocardial revascularization. Some ultrasonic or cavitational systems have already been developed and tested. One device in particular is discussed because it has already been tested and proven in vivo. The use of ultrasound is compared with laser systems in terms of its mechanism, effectiveness, and cost.

12.2. PHYSICAL MECHANISMS OF INTERACTION OF ULTRASOUND WITH BIOLOGICAL TISSUES

12.2.1. Definition of Ultrasonic Phenomena

First, some definitions are given, because the terminology of physical phenomena related to ultrasound is often ambiguous.

12.2.1.1. Ultrasound
Ultrasound describes the sound of a frequency greater than 20,000 Hz, which is above the audible frequencies for humans.

12.2.1.2. Ultrasound Wave
An ultrasound wave is a sound wave consisting of a series of slight density variations moving longitudinally through a medium. The density varies gradually like a sinusoidal wave around normal density or pressure. These density waves typically travel at the speed of sound, which is specific to each medium. For gases the speed is around 300 m/s, for liquids/tissue around 1,500 m/s, and for solids 5,000 m/s. The corresponding wavelength of, for example, 1-MHz ultrasound in tissue is 1.5 mm.

12.2.1.3. Cavitation
Cavitation is the formation of vapor bubbles, caused by sudden reductions in pressure in a liquid, making it boil. Cavitation typically occurs at the trailing edge of ship propellers and in liquids subject to ultrasonic waves of high power density. The cavitation bubbles condense at higher pressure, resulting in a forceful implosion. These implosions can induce mechanical damage. The deterioration of ship propellers is a typical example of this effect. The mechanism of action of ultrasonic cleaning is also based on imploding cavitation bubbles dissolving dirt on surfaces.

12.2.1.4. Shock Wave
A shock wave is an explosion or implosion that can produce an expanding wave of a large amplitude across which density, temperature, and pressure change abruptly. This shock wave causes local stresses and a nonlinear response in the medium, which may result in permanent deformation. A shock wave can travel at speeds higher then the speed of sound.

12.2.2. Basic Mechanisms: Thermal

During motion of a wave through a medium the local variation in density causes friction between the molecules, resulting in absorption of the acoustic energy and transformation to thermal energy (Clarke et al., 1997). The magnitude of absorption depends on the properties of the tissue. Body liquids have a typically low absorption, whereas bone has a high absorption. Similar to light-tissue interactions, the local temperature rise depends on the absorption coefficient, the energy density (W/cm^2), and the cooling rate due to diffusion and perfusion.

12.2.3. Basic Mechanism: Nonthermal

12.2.3.1. Pressure Waves
Ultrasonic waves are accompanied by negative and positive pressures in the fluid and the surrounding tissue. At higher intensities (amplitudes) of the waves, the pressure change along the wave front induces stress and torque in the tissue structure, potentially rupturing the cell matrix of tissues (Barnett et al., 1997).

12.2.3.2. Microcavitation Bubbles
At higher amplitude and frequencies, the pressure change becomes so abrupt that at the lower-pressure end of the wave, the liquid goes into the vapor phase, resulting in small gas bubbles (Miller et al., 1996, 1998). The original size of each bubble will determine its lifetime. Smaller bubbles will resolve or implode instantly, whereas bigger bubbles can expand and compress in a cyclic way induced and sustained by the ultrasonic energy. Because of their behavior, these bubbles are referred to as "ultrasonic microcavitations" and are believed to contribute to the ultrasonic surgery mechanism. The size of the

bubbles is on the order of micrometers. However, in an ultrasonic field, the bubbles may expand up to 100 times and become stable because of mechanical resonance.

Because of their spherical shape, the bubbles will eventually implode toward a central point. The momentum of the surrounding liquid that is accelerated to the center is enormous. The forces associated with the "collision" of the fluid in the center can induce extremely high pressures and temperatures and can generate high-intensity shock waves traveling at supersonic speed from the center. Under these circumstances, free radicals such as hydroxyl (OH) and hydrogen (H) can be formed, inducing biochemical reactions (Suhr et al., 1991).

Ultrasonic cavitation is expected to occur above energy densities of $1,500\,W/cm^2$ and peak positive pressure and peak negative pressure exceeding $5\,MPa$. Cavitation phenomena occur especially at abrupt local changes in densities, such as boundaries between different types of tissue, and at boundaries of tissue and liquid or air. Because of this, bone surfaces and lung tissue are at risk of fractures or hemorrhage when subjected to intense ultrasonic energy (Delius et al., 1990, 1995).

12.2.3.3. Macrocavitation Bubbles

Another form of cavitation is induced by a fast-moving object in a liquid environment. In front of this moving object liquid is compressed, whereas at the back of the object a hole is left behind. The liquid is too slow to fill the gap that is left behind after the object has passed through. In aerodynamics, this principle is used to generate the force to lift the wing of an airplane. The gap behind a fast-moving object through a liquid environment creates a near-vacuum, inducing the liquid to vaporize at ambient temperatures. Consequently, the low pressure in the gap sucks liquid in, and the momentum of the incoming liquid focused toward a center can create a shock wave at the "collision" of the liquid in the center (Verdaasdonk et al., 1995). A well-known example of this phenomenon are the cavitation bubbles generated by ships' propellers that wear down their

metal surface. Cavitation is also notorious in submarine warfare, because the noise associated with the microbubble implosion can give away the position of the submarine.

12.2.3.4. Focused Ultrasonic Cavitation

With focused ultrasound, the extreme power densities at the focal point create nonlinear effects, with very high temperatures and pressures locally inducing shock waves and exploding vapor bubbles (Hill et al., 1995; ter Haar, 1995). After cooling down during expansion, these bubbles implode, which can again be associated with a shock wave.

12.2.3.5. Acoustic Streaming

Another phenomenon associated with imploding cavitation bubbles is microstreaming. Locally, the liquid is accelerated to tremendous speed, forming microstreams. Parallel to a surface, the fast-moving fluid induces shear stress on tissue surfaces and can easily damage superficial cell layers (Laborde et al., 2000). A cavitation bubble near a tissue surface implodes in a particular way, forming a microjet that is directed perpendicular to the surface. This fast-moving jet can easily perforate the tissue surface.

12.3. POTENTIAL TRANSMYOCARDIAL REVASCULARIZATION ULTRASOUND MODALITIES

With the above background, we now consider the different interactions of ultrasound that can be useful for transmyocardial revascularization. By inducing cavitation effects, tissues can be ruptured, fragmented, and vaporized. The thermal effects and shock waves may also induce the release of particular cellular factors. Also, the biochemical effects associated with the formation of free radicals might have potential beneficial effects in transmyocardial revascularization and angiogenesis. Ultrasonically induced effects can be delivered to the tissue by various devices that are described below. They can be distinguished primarily by the method of application.

12.3.1. Extracorporeal Application

In principle, the most "ideal" method of treatment would be totally noninvasive—without any surgery—as performed using an extracorporeal device. An extracorporeal shock wave lithotripsy (ESWL) system is commonly used for breaking up kidney or ureteral stones (Kupeli et al., 1998). The system generally utilizes a spark device and a reflector to create a focused shock wave that penetrates tissue and impinges at great amplitude on the stone to be fractured by a combined shock wave and cavitation effect. In the original ESWL systems, the patient was positioned in a water bath that provided the boundary-matching for the focused ultrasound wave to penetrate the body with minimal distortion. Smaller, and more focused systems, that can be positioned directly adjacent to the body using a gel pad rather than the water bath, are available for lithotripsy and are currently being developed in Europe for the treatment of joints.

A similar system potentially could be used to focus ultrasound on a particular spot in the myocardium to induce shock waves and cavitation effects, resulting in tissue defects or channels similar to laser transmyocardial revascularization lesions (Smith et al., 1998).

An important aspect of this system is that the shock waves are transmitted and focused only through tissue, water, or some other solid/liquid medium. Air spaces between the skin and the myocardium will preclude delivery of shock waves. In addition, shock waves travel differently in harder tissues, such as bone, and could be defocused by traveling through the ribs (Delius et al., 1995). Some implementations of the system would utilize a fluid-filled balloon, inserted by a needle, between the ribs, inflated, and utilized to transmit the shock waves to the myocardium. The shock waves are applied to the balloon using minimally invasive or entirely noninvasive methods, relying on the density uniformity provided by the fluid to conduct the shock wave energy to a localized region within the heart tissue.

As with laser transmyocardial revascularization systems, it may be desirable to synchronize the shock wave with the heartbeat, to occur at a specified phase (e.g., T wave) of the beat. Synchronization might not be required with the use of sufficiently small amplitude shock waves. The amplitude of the shock wave delivered to the myocardium can be varied over a wide range; this may allow cumulative doses of shock waves sufficient to induce angiogenesis while further minimizing damaging myocardial tissue effects of the treatment (Dalecki et al., 1997).

12.3.2. Transcutaneous Application

A transcutaneous application of shock waves could be achieved using a combination lithotripsy probe/balloon system. The system could comprise a needle and cannula-tipped balloon that can be inserted through the skin at a point between the ribs into the cavity beneath the chest wall and overlying the heart. A fluid injector is connected to the balloon, allowing it to be inflated with saline to fill any intervening space (for transmission of shock waves and/or to displace tissue such as lung) and contact the surface of the heart. A shock wave (acoustic) generator is used to generate shock waves through, or at the tip of, the lithotripsy probe, which travel through the fluid-filled balloon and into the myocardial tissue. The fluid provides a uniform medium for transmission of the acoustic energy, allowing precise focus and direction of the shock wave to induce repeatable cavitation events, producing small fissures that are created by the cavitation bubbles. In this case, channels may not need to be "drilled" into the heart muscle, minimizing trauma to the tissue while still creating conditions that might stimulate increased expression of angiogenic growth factors. The fluid in the balloon also stabilizes the myocardium, reducing variations that can occur because of movement of the heart as it beats, because the balloon remains in contact with the surface of the heart throughout the procedure. Visualization of the target area can be achieved using known methods including an integrated shock wave generating/transmitting endoscope or a separate optical or video-based viewing endoscope.

12.3.3. Percutaneous Catheter-Based Device

Similar to the catheter-based laser angioplasty devices, ultrasound energy can be delivered via a catheter that is positioned on the endocardial surface of the ventricles of the heart. The acoustic energy can be transported along a rigid wire incorporated in the catheter, or the ultrasound transducer can be positioned on the distal tip of the catheter near or directly in contact with the myocardium. The tip of the catheter may also include a fluid-filled balloon as described above to couple the shock wave directly to the myocardium. In one design, a pulsed laser is coupled to an optical fiber which extends coaxially through the flexible catheter. The laser light is absorbed in a metal cap at the tip of the catheter, converting it into acoustic energy. This can induce a rapid tip motion to create a highly localized cavitation effect, or it can induce an explosive vapor bubble associated with shock waves and cavitation effects.

In another design, the laser fiber itself acts as the rigid wire along which ultrasonic waves are transported to the catheter tip. The motion of the tip induces cavitation bubbles. In this design continuous wave (CW) laser energy can be combined with the acoustic energy for independent control of the thermal and cavitational components of the treatment (Tschepe et al., 1994).

12.3.4. Intraoperative Device

For intraoperative surgical application, a handheld ultrasound device, similar to the CUSA systems, but utilizing a much smaller tip that produces 1-mm channels in myocardium during a coronary artery bypass graft (CABG) procedure is used. The ultrasound transducer can be incorporated in a hand piece, which transmits ultrasonic waves through a tapered metal needle. At the 1-mm-diameter tip of the needle, cavitation bubbles are formed, enabling the penetration of tissue

and creating a small channel. This device has been prototyped and tested at the University Medical Center, Utrecht, The Netherlands and is being developed by CardioCavitational Systems, Inc. This device, discussed in detail below, has been demonstrated to produce channels that are essentially identical, in terms of myocardial histology, to laser-produced transmyocardial revascularization channels.

12.4. DESCRIPTION OF INTRAOPERATIVE ULTRASONIC TRANSMYOCARDIAL REVASCULARIZATION DEVICE

12.4.1. System Description

The intraoperative surgical transmyocardial revascularization system consists of a hand piece connected to a console that provides the electronic signals and controls as well as an integrated irrigation system (Fig. 12-1, 12-2).

The signal from the console powers a piezoelectric or ferromagnetic transducer in the hand piece. The transducer generates density waves with a typical frequency between 24 and 35 kHz (Verdaasdonk et al., 1998a). These waves are passed through a titanium needle that tapers gradually in a precisely determined curve to a long, thin, 1-mm-diameter tip. Because of its shape, the original longitudinal vibration amplitude of around 10 μm is amplified to 350-μm expansion and contraction at the needle tip. The titanium needle is enveloped by a plastic sheath through which saline is flushed, which acts as a lubricant and cools the needle. The irrigation system can be adjusted to provide flow rates that provide a range of thermal versus cavitational effects. The titanium tip incorporates specialized materials technology and design characteristics to provide the amplitude and frequency of motion required, without being damaged. However, extended repeated use can erode the tip. Initially, the hand piece has been designed for open surgical applications, but it can be modified for endoscopic procedures, including potential use with robotic cardiac surgery systems.

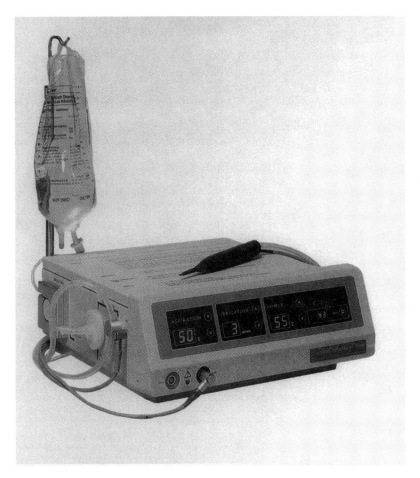

FIGURE 12-1.   Surgical ultrasonic transmyocardial revascularization system with hand piece and irrigation console.

12.4.2. Clinical Application

The surgical ultrasonic transmyocardial revascularization system is user friendly, and surgeons and operating room nurses will require only a short learning curve to operate the system. The system is activated in a preset menu by a key turn. The sterile hand piece and tip are connected to the console and irrigation system. The needle tip is placed on the myocardial surface and, while activated, pushed gently into the tissue, creating a hole. The surgeon can determine the moment of perforation into the ventricle by tactile feedback. The needle can be retracted with or without activation. Similar to laser-created channels, blood spills out of the hole for several minutes before the epicardial surface is sealed off by a clot. The tissue penetration is a continuous process that takes several seconds, and ECG triggering is optional. Although the small needle tip could be mechanically forced into the tissue without activation, there is a clear difference in resistance. The penetration mechanism is explained further below.

12.4.3. Mechanism of Action

12.4.3.1. Cavitation Bubbles

The mechanism of action of the ultrasonic (US) needle is mainly ascribed to macrocavitation bubbles. These cavitation bubbles are formed in a fluidlike environment (water, blood, organic tissue). To characterize and understand the working mechanism of the

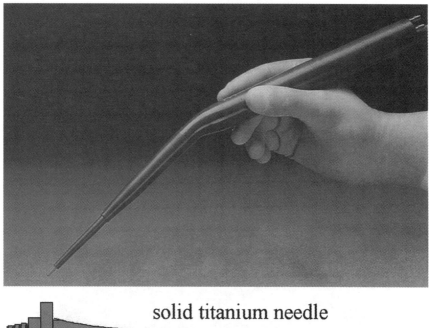

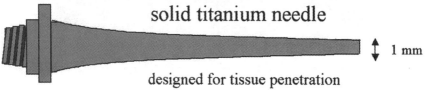

solid titanium needle

↕ 1 mm

designed for tissue penetration

FIGURE 12-2.   Ultrasonic hand piece (top) and schematic of solid titanium needle (bottom).

US needle, high-speed visualization techniques were employed (Verdaasdonk et al., 1995, 1998b). The US needle was placed in a water bath, and close-up high-speed photographs were taken at 5-μs intervals during the 40-μs motion cycle of the tip (Figs. 12-3 and 12-4). Using Schlieren techniques (Verdaasdonk, 1995), very high contrast images are obtained enabling the visualization of shock waves (Figs. 12-4 to 12-6).

The needle motion in the liquid can be considered best as a cosine function. In the first half-period the needle protrudes, whereas in the second half-period the needle retracts. The frames in Figures 12-3 and 12-4 show the sequence of a cavitation bubble formation and collapse during the retraction period of the needle.

During tip retraction, the cylindrical tip moves at maximum speed of about 20 m/s through a liquid environment. The fluid has difficulty filling the gap that is left behind (frames A–D). This hole is near vacuum. Because of the extreme underpressure, the surrounding fluid is sucked inward from all directions at the same time (frames D–F). The acceleration of the fluid is tremendous. During this process, fragments or layers of soft tissue near the cavitation bubble are separated from the underlying tissue. The moment the hole is filled, there will be collapse of fluid near the center of the original gap.

Because this process is usually not symmetric, so-called jet streams are formed, focusing the momentum of the accelerated fluid at particular positions preferentially at the surface of tissue. The mechanism described can be selective for tissue structure. Soft tissue is easily fragmented. Hard tissue does not give way and therefore amplifies the jet streams focused on the tissue surface that

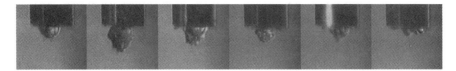

FIGURE 12-3. Expanding and imploding cavitation bubble sequence at the tip of the US needle in a liquid environment (A–F).

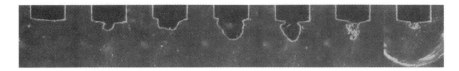

FIGURE 12-4. High-contrast images of cavitation bubble sequence at the tip of the US needle in a liquid environment with a shock wave visible in the last frame (A–G).

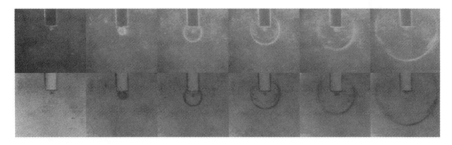

FIGURE 12-5. Sequence of expanding shock wave in liquid ("normal" Schlieren, top; inverse image, bottom).

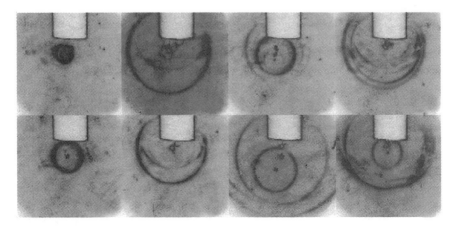

FIGURE 12-6. Close-up view of multiple shock waves under needle tip (inverse Schlieren image).

fragment it locally. Elastic tissue can partly follow the "low"-speed part of the expansion and implosions and deform without breaking, and so it stays intact. The extremely high forces during the collapse can also induce shock waves as described in the next section.

12.4.3.2. Shock Waves

Figure 12-5 shows the sequence of a shock wave as it "grows" after the collapse of one cavitation bubble in a liquid environment. The implosion takes place about $200\,\mu m$ underneath the needle surface. As the shock wave grows, one can see that it rebounds from the surface of the titanium needle tip. Because the shock wave moves at speeds over $1,500\,m/s$, the total sequence in Figure 12-5 is only a few microseconds long.

The multiple shock waves in Figure 12-6 reveal that the cavitation bubble implosion is not symmetric, resulting in multiple foci of implosion. The original cavitation bubble breaks up in fragments during the implosion process. The presence of cavitation bubbles and shock waves has also been confirmed in a transparent polyacrylamide gel with and without a biological tissue boundary.

12.4.3.3. Mechanical Cutting and Breaking

In addition to the cavitation effects, "ordinary" mechanical effects are also present. When the titanium tip is in direct contact with the tissue, it will push against the tissue with extreme forces. The relatively sharp rim (90°) of the tip can cut easily into the soft tissue, and biological hard tissue, which does not deform at all because of the bubble implosions in this case, is no competition for a metal like titanium. The metal tip will pound on the tissue surface, shattering it to small pieces.

12.4.3.4. Thermal Effects

During vibration, the tip will move at high speed through the fluid and tissue. Tissue in contact with the front and side surface of the needle will not follow the motion. Because of friction and mechanical resistance, energy is dissipated, heating the tissue in the regions of contact. The temperature rise can be considerable, because of the high-speed motion and the friction. In the design of the tip, friction is accounted for by using the irrigation fluid from the plastic protective sheath passing over the needle as a lubricant and cooling medium.

The presence and extent of thermal effects was visualized using a special optical method based on color Schlieren imaging techniques (Verdaasdonk, 1995). Temperature increases in an transparent model tissue are visualized as colors of the rainbow, where red represents the highest temperature. Figure 12-7 shows the temperature effects around the tip during penetration into tissue. The temperature rise is highest at the tip because of energy dissipation of the cavitation bubbles and friction. During tissue penetration a "thermal tail" is left behind while the tissue is cooling down. The extent of thermal effects depends on the needle penetration speed. The upper panel in Figure 12-7 shows the thermal effects while penetrating at $0.3\,mm/s$ and the lower panel at $1.8\,mm/s$. The thermal effects are also dependent on the power applied. By activating the tip sequentially, as one would do during ECG triggering, the thermal effects would decrease because of sufficient cooling between the activations.

12.4.4. In Vivo Transmyocardial Revascularization Experiments with Ultrasonic Needle

The US transmyocardial revascularization needle was investigated in a pig model in comparison to laser modalities. The animals underwent surgery according to standard protocols approved for animal experiments. After thoracotomy, the heart was locally immobilized using the "octopus" stabilization techniques for off-pump bypass surgery (developed in Utrecht and distributed by Medtronic). Between the "tentacles" of the "octopus," holes were drilled while close-up images were recorded with a video system (Fig. 12-8). During tissue penetration, the ECG was recorded to identify any potential

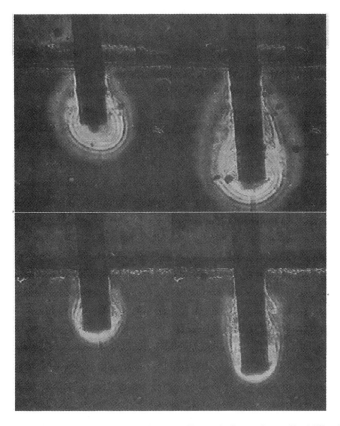

FIGURE 12-7.   Visualization of thermal effects of ultrasonic needle drilling in transparent gel at 0.3 mm/s (top) and at 1.8 mm/s (bottom).

arrhythmias. The animal was euthanized after 1 h, and the myocardium containing the channels was taken out and fixated for histologic examination.

Figure 12-9 shows the myocardium with H&E staining in normal light (top) and polarized light (bottom). Along the channel wall, small fissures can be appreciated, and the zone of thermal injury can be seen up to 500 μm from the channel in polarized light. These channels are comparable to the channels created with the 308-nm excimer laser.

At higher magnification, in a cross-sectional view of the bottom of the channel, a mass of totally pulverized tissue can be appreciated in Figure 12-10. Individual cells can no longer be discriminated, although cell nuclei are present in the pulp material. This clearly shows how effectively the tissue is "ground" to pieces by the forces of the cavi-

tation bubbles. Also, the zone of thermal damage can be well distinguished because of the loss of polarization of the muscle fibers.

12.4.5. Comparison of Ultrasonic Transmyocardial Revascularization Needle to Laser Transmyocardial Revascularization

Figure 12-11 shows a schematic of the characteristics of channels created by lasers obtained in another study comparing the different laser modalities (Verdaasdonk et al., 1998b) and the US needle device. The shape and size of the US needle channels resemble those of the channels obtained with the excimer laser most. The in vivo experiments, however, showed a thermally damaged zone extending approximately 500 μm from the channel wall. This is more comparable to the

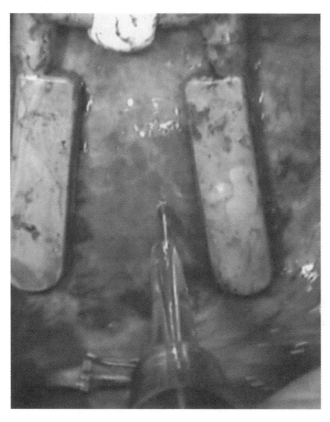

FIGURE 12-8.   US needle penetrating into the myocardium of locally immobilized pig heart.

thermal damage induced by the holmium laser. As illustrated in Figure 12-7, the thermal effects are related to various parameters such as penetration speed. It is not known to what extent the thermal and mechanical damage contributes to the formation of capillaries in the myocardium.

12.4.6. Advantages of Handheld Ultrasonic Transmyocardial Revascularization System Compared with Laser Systems

12.4.6.1. User Friendly
The surgical transmyocardial revascularization system is similar to conventional electrosurgical units (ESUs), in terms of size and controls. Many surgeons are already familiar with cavitational surgical ultrasonic aspiration (CUSA). Much less warm-up is required,

and bulky articulated arms or fragile silica fibers are not needed.

12.4.6.2. No Requirements for Safety in the Operating Room
Laser systems—especially of the high-peak-power laser transmyocardial revascularization systems—generally require the hospital to have a safety committee, hazard lights that illuminate over the operating room doors when the laser is in use, wearing of safety goggles by surgeons and staff in the operating room, and biomedical personnel who can keep the system maintained.

12.4.6.3. Easy Application
The surgical procedure is simple technically. Just as the laser is aimed at a grid of locations for the channels, the surgical US transmyocardial revascularization system is used

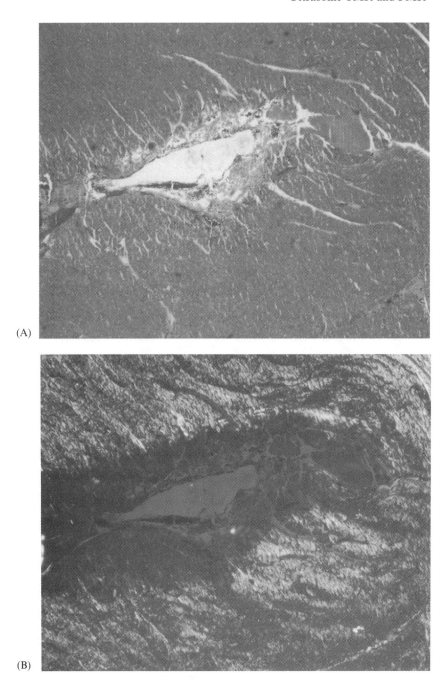

(A)

(B)

FIGURE 12-9.   H&E-stained histologic sample of channel created with US needle in porcine myocardium, using regular transmission microscopy (A, top), and polarized light (B, bottom).

to make channels directly, with tactile feedback. This is more like the way surgeons typically operate and what they are comfortable with.

12.4.6.4. Reliable

The output of surgical US transmyocardial revascularization system is reliable and calibrated, whereas the output of medical lasers

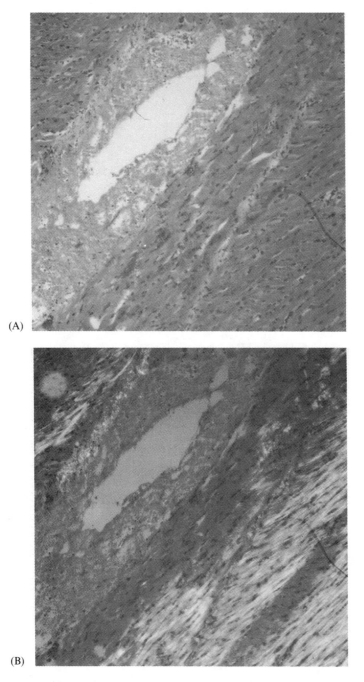

(A)

(B)

FIGURE 12-10. Cross section of channel through porcine myocardium, using regular transmission microscopy (A, top), and polarized light (B, bottom).

may vary depending on laser fluctuations, and the output to tissue depends on transmission of the delivery system (including misalignment of an articulated arm or mismatched input to an optical fiber in a catheter-based system). Therefore, laser procedures are typically preceded by calibrated measurements of the output of the delivery system, which will not be required using the US transmyocardial revascularization system.

Exc CO_2 Holm   US

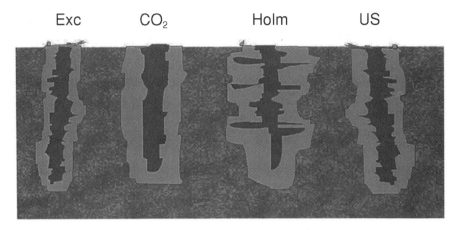

FIGURE 12-11.   Channel characteristics (fissures and thermal damage zone) of excimer (EXC), CO_2, and holmium (Holm) lasers and ultrasound (US) needle-drilled channels.

12.4.6.5. The Equipment Is Less Expensive

The US transmyocardial revascularization surgical system is expected to be only 1/5 or even 1/10 of the price of a typical laser transmyocardial revascularization system. Such reduced system costs would be advantageous for the acceptance of transmyocardial revascularization technology by clinicians as well as hospital administrators and insurance companies.

12.4.6.6. Low Maintenance and Service Costs

Gas lasers (such as CO_2 and excimer) require periodic replenishing of their gas supply—either by adding bottles of gas or by refilling a sealed laser. Solid-state lasers have flashlamps to be replaced, and the optics of all of these high-peak-power laser systems must periodically be cleaned or replaced. In contrast, the maintenance for the surgical US transmyocardial revascularization system is expected to be minimal compared with laser systems because it does not have consumable components.

12.5. DISCUSSION AND CONCLUSIONS

Although the precise mechanism of transmyocardial revascularization has still not been elucidated, published data have indicated that several pulsed laser systems have the capability to improve patient symptoms. Both CO_2 and Ho-YAG lasers have been FDA approved, and more than 11,000 patients have now been treated using these systems. Other transmyocardial revascularization laser systems, including excimer, are also being developed.

At the same time, it appears that continuous wave (CW) lasers do not create the same transmyocardial revascularization results. The original needle technique used by Sen (Sen et al., 1965) also does not work, and the literature on other mechanical devices—although mixed—also tends to show lack of an angiogenic response. Therefore, the injury required for transmyocardial revascularization appears to be rather specific, and it appears unlikely that general, nonspecific myocardial trauma or injury will create the conditions required for angiogenesis.

Transmyocardial revascularization may be a result of one or more of the possible laser-tissue interactions, which include illuminating tissue, initiating a photochemical reaction, heating tissue, fragmenting the tissue by cavitation, and passing shock waves through the tissue (Verdaasdonk, 2000).

It seems quite unlikely that merely illuminating the myocardium will result in angiogenesis. Although photobiological responses do occur, these are mainly at the cellular level. Because several different laser wavelengths have been used for transmyocardial revascularization, the effect cannot be dependent on absorption of light by a single chromophore. Also, because of the long wavelength of most transmyocardial revascularization lasers, there is not expected to be any photochemical reaction involved.

Although some investigators are attempting transmyocardial revascularization with a thermal source (e.g., radio frequency transmyocardial revascularization), there is little evidence that heat alone can be responsible for the clinically observed transmyocardial revascularization results. Heat has been delivered to the myocardium in many types of cardiac surgeries (such as valve replacement)—using conventional electrosurgical devices—without evidence of reduced postoperative or longer-term angina. Also, if heat alone were responsible for the effects seen in transmyocardial revascularization, then CW lasers would have shown better results.

The only effects that are obtained in tissue only through pulsed—not CW—lasers include cavitation and shock waves. Cavitation occurs when tissue is rapidly heated, raising the temperature locally to well above the boiling point of water, resulting in bubble formation and collapse, similar to what we have observed using the ultrasonic system. Shock waves can emanate from the bubble collapse and can travel several millimeters into the tissue.

Whether there are baroreceptors that feel the pressure waves caused by the pulsed lasers and subsequently cause release of growth factors, or there are other—still to be determined—effects of the cavitation and shock waves, it is very clear that expensive laser systems are not the most efficient or cost-effective way to deliver cavitational energy.

The present research has aimed to provide tissue effects similar to those of the transmyocardial revascularization laser systems, utilizing relatively simple and conventional surgical ultrasound equipment and specialized delivery systems. The solid titanium needle described in this chapter is one such device. On the basis of the experiments performed to date, the tissue effects of the ultrasonic transmyocardial revascularization system appear to be extremely similar to those provided by laser transmyocardial revascularization systems. Human studies are required to demonstrate and confirm the clinical effect of the ultrasonic transmyocardial revascularization system, and such studies are currently being designed.

Ultrasonic transmyocardial revascularization can be implemented in a variety of ways, including surgical and minimally invasive handheld probes, robotic surgical probes, catheter-based ultrasonic delivery systems, and potentially extracorporeal systems, with suitable delivery devices. These systems can be very cost-effective compared with laser transmyocardial revascularization systems and do not require the training, safety precautions, calibration, and maintenance necessary with the laser transmyocardial revascularization systems.

By providing a simpler and much more cost-effective approach to transmyocardial revascularization, transmyocardial revascularization may be adopted more rapidly, and become available in centers throughout the world to improve the treatment of patients with coronary artery disease.

References

American Institute of Ultrasound. Selected papers on bioeffects of ultrasound in tissue. *J Ultrasound Med* 2000; 19: 1–168.

Barnett SB, Rott HD, Ter Haar GR et al. The sensitivity of biological tissue to ultrasound. *Ultrasound Med Biol* 1997; 23: 805–812.

Barnett SB, Ter Haar GR, Ziskin MC et al. International recommendations and guidelines for the safe use of diagnostic ultrasound in medicine. *Ultrasound Med Biol* 2000; 26: 355–366.

Berry E, Kelly S, Hutton J et al. Intravascular ultrasound-guided interventions in coronary artery disease: a systematic literature review, with decision-analytic modelling of outcomes and cost-effectiveness. *Health Technol Assess* 2000; 4: 1–117.

Bond LJ, Cimino WW. Physics of ultrasonic surgery using tissue fragmentation. *Ultrasonics* 1996; 34: 579–585.

Brotchi J, Noterman J, Baleriaux D. Surgery of intramedullary spinal cord tumours. *Acta Neurochir Wien* 1992; 116: 176–178.

Clarke RL, ter Haar GR. Temperature rise recorded during lesion formation by high-intensity focused ultrasound. *Ultrasound Med Biol* 1997; 23: 299–306.

Dalecki D, Raeman CH, Child SZ et al. Effects of pulsed ultrasound on the frog heart: III. The radiation force mechanism. *Ultrasound Med Biol* 1997; 23: 275–285.

Delius M, Denk R, Berding C et al. Biological effects of shock waves: cavitation by shock waves in piglet liver. *Ultrasound Med Biol* 1990; 16: 467–472.

Delius M, Draenert K, Al Diek Y et al. Biological effects of shock waves: in vivo effect of high energy pulses on rabbit bone. *Ultrasound Med Biol* 1995; 21: 1219–1225.

Di Mario C, Gorge G, Peters R et al. Clinical application and image interpretation in intracoronary ultrasound. Study Group on Intracoronary Imaging of the Working Group of Coronary Circulation and of the Subgroup on Intravascular Ultrasound of the Working Group of Echocardiography of the European Society of Cardiology. *Eur Heart J* 1998; 19: 207–229.

Fasulo F, Giori A, Fissi S et al. Cavitron ultrasonic surgical aspirator (CUSA) in liver resection. *Int Surg* 1992; 77: 64–66.

Hill CR., ter Haar GR. Review article: high intensity focused ultrasound—potential for cancer treatment. *Br J Radiol* 1995; 68: 1296–1303.

Kupeli B, Biri H, Isen K et al. Treatment of ureteral stones: comparison of extracorporeal shock wave lithotripsy and endourologic alternatives. *Eur Urol* 1998; 34: 474–479.

Laborde JL, Hita A, Caltagirone JP et al. Fluid dynamics phenomena induced by power ultrasounds. *Ultrasonics* 2000; 38: 297–300.

Miller MW, Miller DL, Brayman AA. A review of in vitro bioeffects of inertial ultrasonic cavitation from a mechanistic perspective. *Ultrasound Med Biol* 1996; 22: 1131–1154.

Miller DL. Frequency relationships for ultrasonic activation of free microbubbles, encapsulated microbubbles, and gas-filled micropores. *J Acoust Soc Am* 1998; 104: 2498–2505.

Mulvagh SL, DeMaria AN, Feinstein SB et al. Contrast echocardiography: current and future applications. *J Am Soc Echocardiogr* 2000; 13: 331–342.

Plein S, Williams GJ. Developments in cardiac ultrasound. *Hosp Med* 2000; 61: 240–245.

Quinn RR, Pflugfelder PW, Kostuk WJ et al. Intracoronary ultrasound imaging: methods and clinical applications. *Can J Cardiol* 2000; 16: 911–917.

Roelandt JR. Three-dimensional echocardiography: the future today. *Acta Cardiol* 1998; 53: 323–336.

Rosenschein U, Furman V, Kerner E et al. Ultrasound imaging-guided noninvasive ultrasound thrombolysis: preclinical results. *Circulation* 2000; 102: 238–245.

Sen PK, Udwadia TE, Kinare SG. Transmyocardial acupuncture: a new approach to myocardial revascularization. *J Thorac Cardiovasc Surg* 1965; 50: 189.

Smith NB, Hynynen K. The feasibility of using focused ultrasound for transmyocardial revascularization. *Ultrasound Med Biol* 1998; 24: 1045–1054.

Suhr D, Brummer F, Hulser DF. Cavitation-generated free radicals during shock wave exposure: investigations with cell-free solutions and suspended cells. *Ultrasound Med Biol* 1991; 17: 761–768.

Ter Haar G. Ultrasound focal beam surgery. *Ultrasound Med Biol* 1995; 21: 1089–1100.

Tschepe J, Desinger K, Helfmann J et al. Transmission of laser radiation and acoustic waves via optical fibers for surgical therapy. In: *Optical Fibers in Medicine IX, SPIE Proceedings*. 1994. Bellingham, WA.

Verdaasdonk RM. Imaging laser induced thermal fields and effects. In: *Laser-Tissue Interaction VI, SPIE Proceedings* 1995 (ed. S. L. Jacques); 2391: 165–175. Bellingham, WA.

Verdaasdonk RM, Sachinopoulou A, Grundeman PF et al. Working mechanism of pulsed CO_2, holmium and excimer laser systems in view of trans-myocardial revascularization (transmyocardial revascularization): in vivo implications. In: *TMLR Management of Coronary Artery Diseases* (ed. Klein M, Schulte HD, Gams E), 1998a; 143–151. Springer-Verlag, Berlin.

Verdaasdonk RM, Swol CFP, Grimbergen MCM. High-speed and thermal imaging of the mechanism of action of the cavitational ultrasonic surgical aspirator (CUSA). *SPIE Proceedings* 1998b; 3249: 72–84. Bellingham, WA.

Verdaasdonk RM. Transmyocardial revascularization: the magic of drilling holes in the heart. *Critical Reviews* 2000; 75: 99–135, SPIE Bellingham.

Color Plates

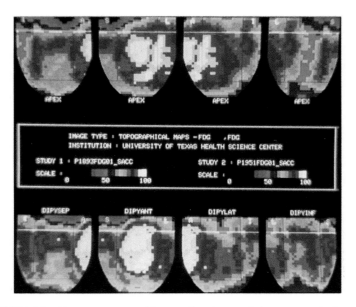

FIGURE 6-3. Computer-processed images of positron emission tomography from patient with inferior wall ischemia before and after TMR. The images after TMR show reduction of ischemia. Areas of ischemia are depicted in green and perfused areas in orange and red (Courtesy of O.H. Frazier, Texas Heart Institute, Texas Heart Institute Journal.)

Biosense DMR

An Electromechanical Mapping and Guidance System for Direct Myocardial Revascularization

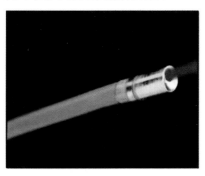

Laser catheter

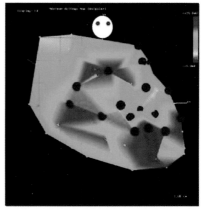

Noga Map

FIGURE 8-6. DMR laser catheter system (left) and the Noga™ navigation (right) used in the DIRECT Trial (Courtesy of Cordis, J&J, Miami, FL.)

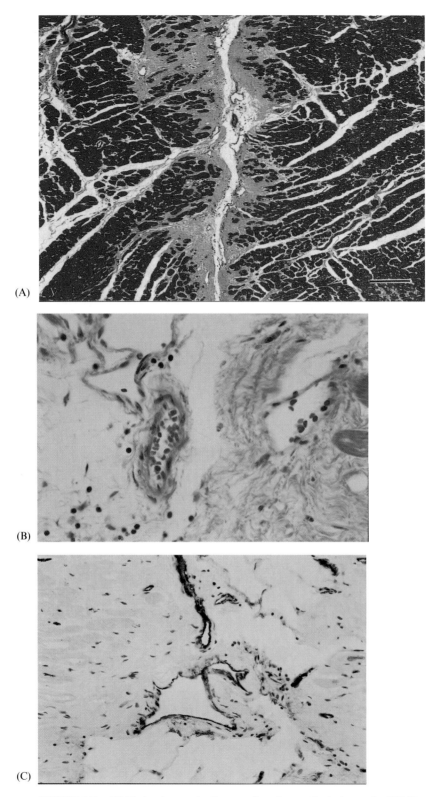

FIGURE 6-5. (A) Photomicrograph of myocardium from patient who received TMR 7 months before heart transplantation for progressive ischemia and failure despite early relief from symptoms for 6 months. (B) Photomicrograph of high-power magnification showing neoblood vessels containing red blood cells. (C) Factor VII antibody stain demonstrates endothelial lined vessels adjacent to channel remnant. For full caption, see page 89.

Color Plates

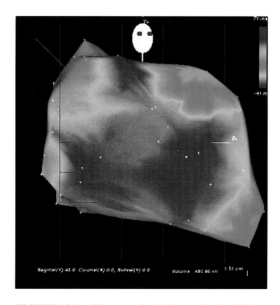

FIGURE 13-1. Electromechanical map, in the right anterior oblique projection, showing the activation sequence of the left ventricle. The dark shade indicates the earliest activation, and the lighter shade indicates the latest activation.

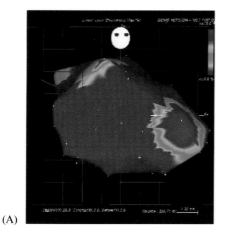

(A)

FIGURE 13-4. Data obtained before percutaneous catheter intervention. (A) Electromechanical map. For full caption, see page 190.

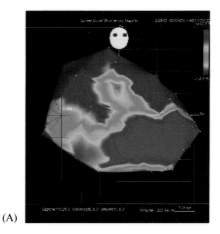

(A)

FIGURE 13-5. (A) Electromechanical map obtained after percutaneous catheter intervention (PCI). For full caption, see page 192.

Color Plates

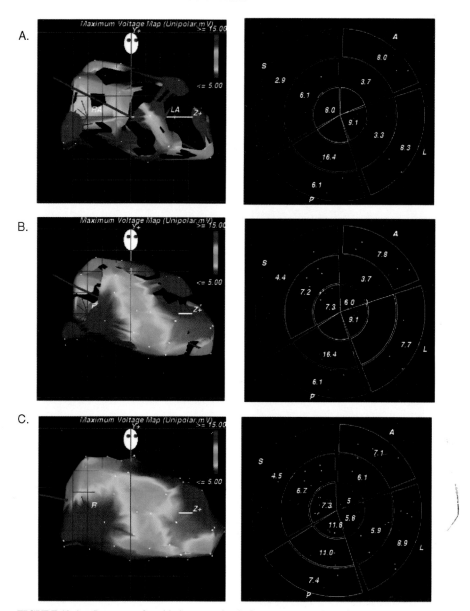

FIGURE 13-6. Sequence of rapid electromechanical map construction: (A) Reference map with 19 data points. (B) Regional map of the septal area with 28 data points. (C) Complete map with 65 data points.

13

Left Ventricular Electromechanical Mapping As a Diagnostic Method

Emerson C. Perin, M.D., F.A.C.C.

New Interventional Cardiovascular Technology
Texas Heart Institute
Baylor College of Medicine and University of Texas Health Science Center
Houston, Texas

Guilherne V. Silva, M.D.

Cardiology Research Fellow
Texas Heart Institute/Baylor College of Medicine
Houston, Texas

and

Rogério Sarmento-Leite, M.D., Ph.D

Cardiology Research Fellow
Texas Heart Institute/Baylor College of Medicine/CAPES-Brazil
From the Department of Adult Cardiology
Texas Heart Institute/St. Luke's Episcopal Hospital and Baylor
College of Medicine
Houston, Texas

SUMMARY

Electromechanical mapping (EMM) is a new process that produces three-dimensional representations of left ventricular electrical and mechanical function in real time.

The EMM method was first described in 1997 by Gepstein et al., and its accuracy and reproducibility were confirmed in a pig model. By directly assessing the myocardial voltage, the different states of perfusion can ultimately be defined. In this way, EMM of the left ventricle offers a unique perspective on myocardial function and viability.

Myocardial Revascularization: Novel Percutaneous Approaches, Edited by George S. Abela.
ISBN 0-471-36166-6   Copyright © 2002 Wiley-Liss, Inc.

Initial studies have shown a clear difference in voltage values when areas of infarcted myocardium have been compared with viable myocardium, indicating that EMM can accurately distinguish between normal and infarcted tissue.

The local linear shortening (LLS) function of the EMM system has been found to be a valuable tool for assessing mechanical function because it has a proven capacity for differentiating various states of perfusion and of myocardial mechanical function.

There are pitfalls associated with EMM, most commonly poor map quality. The authors are working to develop a "mapping excellence program" in which mapping criteria are established and categorized.

The diagnostic value of EMM in assessing myocardial viability, perfusion, and function is very important, and prospective randomized trials can help further validate this technique.

13.1. INTRODUCTION

Electromechanical mapping (EMM) (NOGA; Biosense-Webster, Diamond Bar, CA) is an innovative technology that produces three-dimensional (3D) representations of left ventricular electrical and mechanical function in real time. Chapter 7 describes the EMM system in detail. Briefly, EMM utilizes ultra-low magnetic fields that are generated by a triangular location pad positioned beneath the patient. These fields help determine the location and orientation of a magnetic location sensor just proximal to the deflectable tip of a 7F mapping catheter. The catheter also incorporates electrodes to measure endocardial electrical signals.

To construct the electromechanical map, a series of location and voltage points are acquired at multiple locations on the LV endocardial surface, gated for the conventional electrocardiogram. Data points are obtained only when the catheter tip is in stable contact with the endocardium. Computer algorithms later use all the data points to recreate the LV electrical and mechanical maps. The resultant 3D map can be spatially manipulated in real time on a computer workstation (Silicon Graphics, Mountain View, CA).

The potential for navigation and direct delivery of myocardial therapy (e.g., laser revascularization, gene therapy) offered by the EMM system is widely appreciated (Kornowski and Leon, 1998). Underlying the blueprint for navigation, however, is a myriad of colors that represent a wealth of electrical and mechanical data concerning the function of the left ventricle (LV). The interpretation of these data is currently being explored, but they are already rendering invaluable diagnostic information.

The electrical data obtained by the system are expressed in terms of unipolar or bipolar voltage. Unipolar voltage (UniV) is more commonly utilized in clinical practice, despite the fact that bipolar voltage (BiV) has better spatial and time resolution. This difference is mainly caused by the consistency of the electrical signals obtained, because UniV is not sensitive to catheter orientation. The analysis of the electrical data is mainly utilized to assess myocardial viability (identify areas of healthy or previously infarcted myocardial tissue). Mechanical function is assessed by determining the spatial motion of the catheter tip, which represents the contractile state of the underlying myocardium. This variable is expressed by a numerical value obtained through an algorithm called linear local shortening (LLS). Interpretation of EMM involves the combined analysis of both electrical and LLS data. A further step, which integrates these functions, involves the concept of myocardial discordance (Perin et al., 2000b), which defines an area of the LV with ischemic dysfunction.

13.2. BASIC MAP INTERPRETATION

13.2.1. Hemodynamic Measurements and Map Accuracy

Gepstein et al. were the first to describe the EMM method and to confirm its accuracy and reproducibility in a pig model (Gepstein et al., 1997a). Subsequently, the same authors described the method's accuracy in measuring LV volumes (Gepstein et al., 1997b). The system was found to be highly accurate for simple phantoms (mean ± standard deviation, 2.3 ± 1.1%), LV casts (9.6 ± 1.3%), and a dynamic test jig (Gepstein et al., 1997a). In measuring the LV end-systolic volume (ESV), end-diastolic volume (EDV), and ejection fraction (EF) in 12 swine, Fuchs et al. (1999) encountered minimal intraobserver and inter-observer variability (EF, 6.5 ± 1.9% and 7.1 ± 2.0%; stroke volume, 4.5 ± 1.0% and 11.3 ± 2.4%, respectively).

LV volumes obtained with EMM are usually underestimated compared with those obtained with echocardiography and angiography. This discrepancy is a consequence of (1) the difficulty encountered by EMM operators in reaching all areas of the endocardium with the catheter tip and (2) the geometric constraints involved in reproducing the LV cavity from a limited number of endocardial points. In our experience with 29 patients who underwent both LV angiography and EMM (Sarmento-Leite et al., 2000), the correlation index between these two methods was $r^2 = 0.66$ for EF, $r^2 = 0.74$ for EDV, and $r^2 = 0.88$ for ESV ($P = 0.001$). A coefficient of $16.6 + (1.03 \times \text{EMM EF})$ was defined as a correction index for calculating LVEF from EMM EF.

In EMM, EDV and ESV can be used to assess the completeness of mapping. The angiographic or echocardiographic volumes are used as gold standards, and EDVs and ESVs that range between 75% and 100% of these gold standards are associated with complete maps.

13.2.2. Map Data Representation

Electromechanical map data may be represented in qualitative or quantitative form. Both types of representations can exhibit electrical-activation-sequence, UniV and BiV, and LLS data. A 3D, color-coded shell representing the LV endocardial surface provides a qualitative view of all LV segments (Fig. 13-1) and can be manipulated and viewed in any axis. This type of representation is useful for

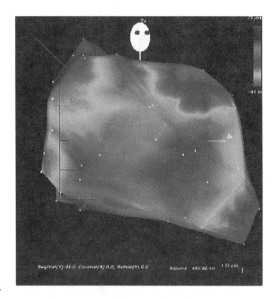

FIGURE 13-1. Electromechanical map, in the right anterior oblique projection, showing the activation sequence of the left ventricle. The dark shade indicates the earliest activation, and the lighter shade indicates the latest activation.(See color plates.)

a global understanding of the distribution of the different parameters that the system can exhibit. This is especially true of the activation sequence map, which (notwithstanding its electrophysiologic merits) is particularly useful for ascertaining uniform rhythm during map acquisition. This uniformity is essential to assure the integrity of the acquired data. The global representation gives the operator the relative certainty of having a map free of premature beats (which would dramatically alter its appearance).

The cylindrical polar reference coordinate, or bull's eye, map representation is the quantitative representation in which values are assigned to each segment. The mean value of the data points in each segment is displayed. Along its long axis, the LV is divided into three parts: apex, mid-zone, and base. The bull's eye is commonly divided into 9 or 12 segments (Fig. 13-2), much in the same manner as SPECT findings are represented. The apical, mid-zone, and base respectively represent 20%, 40%, and 40% of the LV. Because the EMM bull's eye is centered on the apex, the acquisition of a true LV apical point

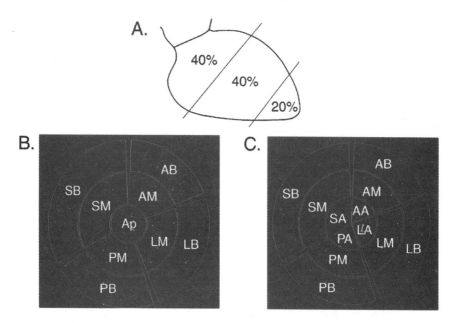

FIGURE 13-2.   Segmental distribution of the bull's eye. (A) The left ventricle, in the
right anterior oblique projection, is divided into 3 regions (apical, mid-zone, and
basal), whose respective sizes are shown as percentages. (B) Nine-segment bull's eye
distribution. (C) Twelve-segment bull's eye distribution. AA = anteroapical; AB =
anterior-basal; AM = anterior-mid; Ap = apex; LA = lateral-apical; LB = lateral-basal;
LM = lateral-mid; PA = posteroapical; PB = posterior-basal; PM = posterior-mid; SA =
septal-apical; SB = septal-basal; SM = septal-mid.

cannot be overemphasized as a critical part of
the mapping procedure.

13.2.3. Electrical Data (Unipolar and Bipolar Voltage) and Myocardial Viability

Defining the presence, extent, and nature of
dysfunctional myocardial tissue remains a
cornerstone of diagnostic cardiology. Electromechanical mapping of the LV offers a
unique perspective on myocardial function
and viability. By directly assessing the myocardial voltage, one can ultimately define the
different states of perfusion.

Early work was performed in animal
models to determine whether EMM could
accurately distinguish chronically infarcted
areas of myocardium from healthy areas.
Gepstein et al. mapped the LV in 11 dogs with
chronic infarctions (4 weeks after ligation of
the left anterior descending artery) and in
6 control dogs (Gepstein et al., 1998). The

average bipolar amplitude was significantly
lower in the infarcted zone (2.3 ± 0.2 mV; $P <
0.01$) than (1) in the same region in control
animals (10.3 ± 1.3 mV) and (2) in the noninfarcted regions (4.0 ± 0.7 to 10.2 ± 1.5 mV; $P
< 0.01$) in the infarcted group. In addition, the
electrical maps could accurately delineate
both the location and extent of the infarct, as
demonstrated by the maps' high correlation
with pathologic studies (Pearson's correlation
coefficient $= 0.90$) and precise identification of
the infarct border.

Further data delineating differences between infarcted and normal tissue were presented by Kornowski et al., who analyzed
both animal and patient subsets (Kornowski
et al., 1998a). Measurements of LV endocardial UniV and BiV were obtained from dogs
at baseline ($n = 12$), at 24h ($n = 6$), and at
3 weeks ($n = 6$) after occlusion of the left
anterior descending coronary artery. Also, 12
patients with a previous myocardial infarc-

tion (MI) and 12 control patients underwent LV endocardial mapping to assess electromechanical function in infarcted versus healthy myocardial regions. In the canine model, a significant decrease in voltage potentials was noted in the MI zone at 24 h (UniV, 42.8 ± 9.6 to 29.1 ± 12.2 mV; $P = 0.007$; BiV, 11.6 ± 2.3 to 4.9 ± 1.2 mV; $P < 0.0001$) and at 3 weeks (UniV, 41.0 ± 8.9 to 13.9 ± 3.9 mV; $P < 0.0001$; BiV, 11.2 ± 2.8 to 2.4 ± 0.4 mV; $P < 0.0001$). No change in voltage was noted in areas remote from the MI zone. In patients with a previous MI, the average voltage was 7.2 ± 2.7 mV (UniV)/1.4 ± 0.7 mV (BiV) in the MI zones, 17.8 ± 4.6 mV (UniV)/4.5 ± 1.1 mV (BiV) in healthy areas remote from the MI zones, and 19.7 ± 4.4 mV (UniV)/5.8 ± 1.0 mV (BiV) in control patients without a previous MI ($P < 0.001$ for MI values vs. remote zones or control patients).

In a pivotal study, Kornowski et al. correlated the results of SPECT with those of EMM (Kornowski et al., 1998b). The different perfusional states were correlated with the voltage values in 18 patients (mean age 58 ± 12 years); all patients had symptomatic chronic angina, with reversible and/or fixed myocardial perfusion defects on SPECT studies using (201)Tl at rest and 99 m Tc-sestamibi after adenosine stress testing. The average UniV potentials (14.0 ± 2.0 mV) were highest when measured in myocardial segments with normal perfusion ($n = 56$) and were lowest (7.5 ± 3.4 mV and $3.4 \pm 3.4\%$) when measured in myocardial segments with fixed perfusion defects ($n = 20$) ($P < 0.0001$). Myocardial segments with reversible perfusion defects ($n = 66$) had intermediate UniV amplitudes (12.0 ± 2.8 mV; $P = 0.048$ vs. normal segments and $P = 0.005$ vs. fixed segments). These initial studies showed a clear difference in voltage values when areas of infarcted myocardium were compared with viable myocardium. According to these studies, the absolute UniV that can be used to distinguish viable myocardium from scar tissue ranges from 7.2 to 7.5 mV.

We compared EMM findings with the results of magnetic resonance imaging (MRI), using a delayed hyperenhancement technique that has been shown to accurately detect myocardial scar tissue (Kim et al., 1999a, 1999b; Ramani et al., 1998; Rehwald et al., 1999). In 15 patients who underwent both EMM and cardiac MRI, bull's eye representations comprising a total of 275 myocardial segments were obtained with both methods. On the basis of MRI assessment 64 segments were considered to have transmural or subendocardial scar tissue, and 211 segments were deemed healthy tissue. Electromechanical mapping was able to distinguish normal tissue from subendocardial scar and transmural scar. Using a threshold of 6.9 mV, EMM identified normal versus transmural scar segments with an accuracy of 94%, for a sensitivity of 93% and a specificity of 88% (Perin et al., 2001). Electromechanical voltage maps allow the interventional cardiologist to assess myocardial viability online, directly, in the catheterization laboratory, based on UniV values. This important feature of EMM is used when targeting treatment zones for direct laser myocardial revascularization (Kornowski et al., 1999a; Kornowski et al., 1999b) and gene transfer therapy (Vale et al., 1999; Vale et al., 2000).

13.2.4. Mechanical Data (Linear Local Shortening)

Electromechanical mapping introduces cardiologists to a new concept of myocardial mechanical function. The methods that are traditionally used to assess the contractile function of the myocardium focus on a specific plane (echocardiography, MRI) or projection (angiography). In contrast, the LLS function (Fig. 13-3) of the EMM system places the focus on the movement of a data point. The system automatically calculates the LLS of a data point by means of an algorithm that compares the distance between a given data point and its neighbors during systole and diastole. The shortening of the distance between points in endsystole and enddiastole, as well as the change in LV volume, is taken into account in the LLS algorithm. Furthermore, the influence of points that are too close or too distant and of points

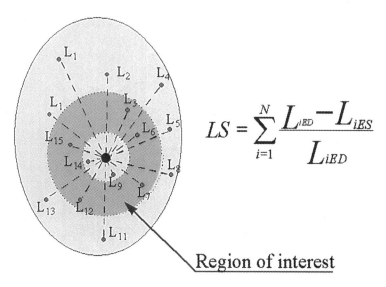

$$LS = \sum_{i=1}^{N} \frac{L_{iED} - L_{iES}}{L_{iED}}$$

Region of interest

FIGURE 13-3.   Formula for calculating linear local shortening. Data points outside the region of interest (too close or too far from the target) are not computed in the analysis. ED = end diastole; ES = end systole.

that present in clusters is eliminated by a weighting algorithm. Finally, all the LLS data points in a particular segment are displayed as a mean value for that segment in the bull's eye.

Linear local shortening has been proven to be an accurate tool for identifying and differentiating between infarcted and healthy myocardium. Early canine studies (Gepstein et al., 1998) showed that, compared with healthy areas, infarcted areas had significantly lower LLS values. In humans, the initial work of Kornowski et al. in 12 patients with previous myocardial infarction showed that the mean LLS in the infarcted segments was ≤8%, as opposed to ≥12% in the healthy myocardium (Kornowski et al., 1998a). Also, compared with SPECT findings (Kornowski et al., 1998b), the LLS values reflected the degree of myocardial perfusion (normal, reversible, and fixed perfusion defects). The normally perfused myocardium had an LLS value of $12.5 \pm 2.8\%$; the values for reversible and fixed perfusion defects were $10.3 \pm 3.7\%$ and $3.4 \pm 3.4\%$, respectively. When those values were compared overall by means of analysis of variance (ANOVA), the differ-

ences reached significance ($P < 0.0001$). Normal and reversible values also differed significantly from fixed values ($P < 0.0001$ and $P < 0.001$, respectively). However, the difference between normal and reversible values was not significant ($P = 0.067$). This finding was likely due to the fact that a rest/stress method for detecting ischemia (SPECT) was being compared to a rest-only method (EMM). It is reasonable to postulate that, if used during EMM, a stress modality such as dobutamine testing or atrial pacing could yield LLS values more closely associated with a reversible perfusion state, that is, diagnostic of myocardial ischemia. This would enable the cardiologist to evaluate the patient for the presence of myocardial ischemia (and simultaneously for myocardial viability) in the setting of angiographic studies, online, in the cardiac catheterization laboratory. Stress modalities for use during EMM are currently being investigated.

Linear local shortening has also been compared with other methods of assessing mechanical function. We compared LV angiography and EMM with respect to EF and regional wall motion (Sarmento-Leite et al., 2000). Electromechanical maps were acquired in 29 patients after biplane LV angiography. Visual assessment by two blinded readers defined LV contractility in 145 myocardial segments as akinetic/dyskinetic, hypokinetic, or normokinetic. These findings were correlated with the corresponding EMM LLS values. The angiographic EF, EDV, and ESV were calculated by means of the area-length method and were compared to the EMM EF, EDV, and ESV. Table 13-1 shows the segmental wall motion, as indicated by LLS, in the three groups. A discriminant analysis model was applied, and the cut-off values for wall motion comparison were found to be LLS ≥ 12% for normokinetic segments, 6–12% for hypokinetic segments, and ≤6% for akinetic/dyskinetic segments.

In comparing EMM with echocardiography, Lessick et al. (2000) showed that LLS values were concordant with echocardiographic scores 73% of the time. The ability to differentiate normal from abnormal segments, as defined by receiver-operating characteristic (ROC) graphs combining sensitivity and specificity, was 0.75.

In conclusion, the LLS function of the EMM system is a valuable tool for assessing mechanical function. It has a proven capacity for differentiating various states of perfusion and of myocardial mechanical function. An LLS value of >12% generally reflects a normally contractile segment (normokinetic), and a value of <6% reflects a severely impaired segment (akinetic or dyskinetic) (Kornowski et al., 1998a, 1998b). The range of values that reflect stress-induced ischemia remains to be defined.

13.3. ADVANCED MAP INTERPRETATION

13.3.1. Integration of Electrical and Mechanical Data

The EMM workstation displays a UniV and an LLS bull's eye side by side. The integration of both electrical and mechanical data yields a distinctive manner of analyzing LV function. Four principal conditions can be considered:

1. Normal LLS (≥12%) and preserved UniV (≥6.9 mV) indicate viable and normally contractile myocardium.
2. Compromised LLS (<12%) and preserved UniV (≥6.9 mV) generally indicate hibernating or profoundly ischemic segments or simply resting ischemia. Viability is suggested by the preserved UniV. Mechanical impairment within an area of preserved electrical activity indicates electromechanical dissociation or discordance.
3. Preserved LLS (≥12%) and compromised UniV (<6.9 mV) indicate reverse discordance or preserved mechanical function in an area with little electrical activity. The presence of mechanical function, even in the absence of normal electrical activity, suggests some degree of viability. These findings may represent areas of subendocardial or patchy infarction.
4. Severely impaired LLS (<6%) and compromised UniV (<6.9 mV) indicate nonviable, or infarcted, myocardium.

Although important diagnostic information can be obtained with EMM, as explained above, the system is most often used in clinical practice to settle questions related to myocardial viability. To illustrate the utility of this modality in the clinical setting, Figure 13-4 shows the UniV and LLS bull's eye representation of an electromechanical map of the LV in a 60-year-old man with known coronary artery disease. Two weeks before hospital admission, the patient had presented with recurrent angina (Canadian class III) and new-onset dyspnea after sustaining a non-Q-wave MI. He had previously undergone

TABLE 13-1. **Segmental Wall Motion, as Indicated by Linear Local Shortening (Mean ± Standard Deviation)**

Patient Group*	Linear Local Shortening (%)
Akinetic/Dyskinetic	3.2 ± 3.1
Hypokinetic	8.3 ± 5.2
Normokinetic	13.9 ± 5.6

* All intergroup comparisons were significant.

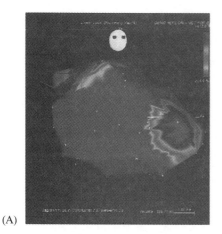

(A)

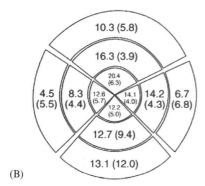

(B)

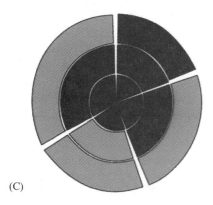

(C)

FIGURE 13-4. Data obtained before percutaneous catheter intervention. (A) Electromechanical map. (B) Bull's eye distribution of values denoting voltage (numbers outside parentheses) and linear local shortening (numbers within parentheses) in each segment. (C) Bull's eye highlighting 8 segments with electromechanical discordance (black areas). (See detail in color plates.)

triple-vessel coronary artery bypass grafting. Coronary angiography revealed a severe stenosis (90%) of the left main coronary artery (LMCA), which supplied a large first septal and a large diagonal branch. The left anterior descending artery was occluded at the diagonal branch and was supplied by a patent left internal mammary artery. The circumflex artery was occluded at the LMCA. The saphenous vein graft to the right coronary artery was widely patent, as was the first marginal branch. The EF was severely reduced (20%), and global hypokinesis was evident. On angiography, the LMCA was the only flow-limiting lesion present. As Figure 13-4 shows, 8 of the 12 segments in the bull's eye representation had preserved UniV values (>7.5mV) and severely reduced LLS values (<6%). Those segments were interpreted as being discordant (viable with profound resting ischemia), thus justifying an interventional procedure to restore the blood supply in the culprit artery.

13.4. INTERPRETIVE PITFALLS

To interpret an electromechanical map of the LV, one must be familiar with the EMM system and with aspects of map acquisition and display. The data can be easily misinterpreted, for example, if the map is incomplete but the interpreter does not realize it or if an apical point is misplaced.

The most common underlying pitfall is poor map quality. The most critical aspects of map quality are data point quality (which may be poor for points acquired during ventricular ectopy or ST elevation, reflecting excessive pressure of the catheter against the endocardium) and map completeness (all LV areas should be represented adequately). A common mistake is to inadequately map areas around the mitral and aortic valves (fibrous annuli) that constitute an important part of the LV base. This area is significant in terms of the volume that it represents and that it reflects on the overall distribution of points on the bull's eye.

In analyzing electromechanical maps from 32 patients without a previous history of MI, the authors found that $14 \pm 11\%$ of the LV area had a very low UniV ($<7.5\,mV$) in the anterior and septal basal areas. In specifically analyzing the septum and anterior basal areas, one should keep in mind that, physiologically, the perivalvular areas have low LLS and UniV values. This is clearly a limitation of the EMM method, and the operator should be careful when diagnosing conditions in the basal regions.

To improve mapping techniques and establish uniform criteria for assessing map quality, the authors have worked with Biosense-Webster (Diamond Bar, CA) to develop a "mapping excellence program," in which mapping criteria have been established and categorized. Tables 13-2 and 13-3, respectively, describe ideal and acceptable mapping standards.

13.5. FUTURE PERSPECTIVES

13.5.1. Pre- and Postinterventional Electromechanical Mapping

One important advantage of EMM over other diagnostic methods is its ability to

TABLE 13-2. Ideal   Electromechanical   Mapping Criteria

The volume of the map is $\pm 15\%$ of the corresponding fluoroscopic image or echocardiographic volume.

With respect to visual morphology, the map matches the size and shape of the corresponding fluoroscopic images.

The map has at least 65 acquired data points, including at least 3 points per segment (12-segment bull's eye).

TABLE 13-3. Acceptable Electromechanical Mapping Criteria

The volume of the map is $\pm 25\%$ of the corresponding fluoroscopic image or echocardiographic volume.

With respect to visual morphology, the map matches the size and shape of the corresponding fluoroscopic images.

The map has at least 45 acquired data points, including at least 3 points per segment, no more than 1 segment having only a single point (12-segment bull's eye).

assess myocardial function online in the catheterization laboratory. Using this feature of the system, we assessed the immediate electromechanical effects of percutaneous catheter intervention (PCI) on myocardial function (Perin et al., 2000d, 2001). Electromechanical mapping was performed in 48 patients before and after successful elective PCI. Five patients who had two consecutive maps without an intervening PCI in the same clinical setting were regarded as the control group. The maps were analyzed with a histographic tool that allowed us to select LV areas of interest that had a particular electromechanical characteristic (e.g., LLS $>12.5\%$) and, therefore, to quantify the exact percentage that this area represented in comparison with the entire LV. In each map, we quantified the percentages of the LV with normal ($>12.5\%$) LLS and with a severely impaired ($<7.5\,mV$) UniV. Variations in those values were compared with the results observed in the control group. The patients were then rated as better, worse, or unaltered in terms of the LLS and UniV changes, and an ANOVA was performed. Of the 48 patients who underwent a PCI, 38 patients had a stent implantation and 10 patients had a rotational atherectomy. The UniV did not differ significantly between the control group and the PCI group. However, the intergroup LLS differed significantly ($P = 0.002$), evidently changing immediately after PCI. Therefore, EMM affords a unique viewpoint on the functional assessment of PCI and may reflect previously undetected acute changes in mechanical and electrical function.

To further illustrate the usefulness of pre- and postinterventional EMM, Figure 13-5 shows the postinterventional map from the case described above, under *Integration of Electrical and Mechanical Data*. The patient was subjected to rotablation of the LMCA. In the postinterventional map, the regions that originally had discordant electromechanical values either were improved or remained unaltered, reflecting the benefits of increased blood flow and confirming the accuracy of the preinterventional EMM data (Fig. 13-4) regarding myocardial viability.

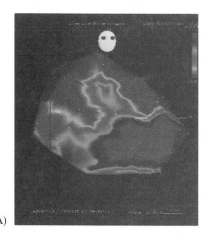

(A)

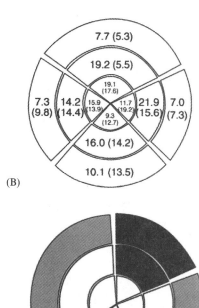

(B)

(C)

In the postprocedural assessment of myocardial function EMM remains an experimental tool, but it may eventually play a diagnostic role in the hands of the interventional cardiologist.

13.5.2. Stress Electromechanical Mapping

EMM is presently performed in the resting state and, even so, has shown good correlation with SPECT perfusion imaging in identifying reversible versus nonreversible defects according to UniV values. We have postulated that a stress model of EMM would allow more precise identification of myocardial viability and also allow the system to identify the presence myocardial ischemia. In the assessment of viability, there would be less overlap in the range of electrical values corresponding to the different myocardial states. The presence of ischemic myocardial segments would be signaled by stress-induced mechanical changes. Stress EMM was successfully accomplished with atrial pacing in a group of 22 patients. A stress response associated with atrial pacing at 85% of the maximal predicted heart rate consistently showed a generalized decrease in LLS values and an increase in UniV values. Comparison with SPECT imaging preliminarily suggests that stress EMM may become a useful tool in the diagnosis of myocardial ischemia. Furthermore, in the "no-option" patient undergoing targeted direct myocardial therapies stress EMM may prove especially useful by accurately identifying viable and nonviable myocardium, even in areas considered by SPECT to benonreversibly ischemic (unpublished data).

13.6. RAPID ELECTROMECHANICAL MAPPING

In our experience and that of others (Kornowski and Leon, 1999; Lessick et al., 2000), one of the major limitations of EMM is the time involved in obtaining a complete map and the difficulty of mapping the entire LV because of ectopy in specific segments. To solve this problem, we have devised a method by which maps can be constructed rapidly so

FIGURE 13-5. (A) Electromechanical map obtained after percutaneous catheter intervention (PCI). (B) Bull's eye distribution of values denoting voltage (numbers outside parentheses) and linear local shortening (numbers within parentheses) in each segment. (C) Bull's eye distribution obtained after PCI. Six of the previously discordant segments are no longer discordant (white areas), but 2 segments (black areas) remain discordant. (See detail in color plates.)

as to focus on a region of interest without compromising the accuracy of the electrical, mechanical, and anatomic information present in a standard map (Perin et al., 2000c). In 10 patients, we performed EMM in three stages (Fig. 13-6): (1) A reference map that represented most of the myocardial segments was acquired to serve as framework for further datapoint acquisition. (2) Data point acquisition was continued so as to create a "regional" map that focused on a particular region of interest (apical, mid-zone, and basal segments in the anterior, lateral, inferior, or septal regions). (3) Data point acquisition was continued until the map was completed according to an "ideal map" standard. The reference maps consisted of 18 ± 3 data points that represented 10 ± 2 segments of the 12-

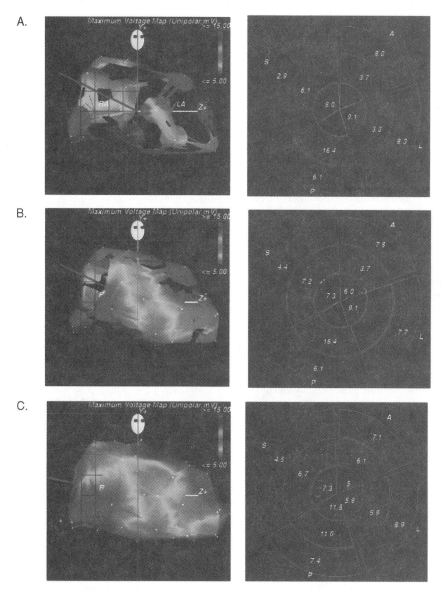

FIGURE 13-6. Sequence of rapid electromechanical map construction: (A) Reference map with 19 data points. (B) Regional map of the septal area with 28 data points. (C) Complete map with 65 data points. (See color plates.)

segment bull's eye. The regional and complete maps consisted of 34 ± 7 and 58 ± 11 points, respectively, with mean acquisition times of $21:32$ and $40:51$. The correlation between regional and complete maps for both the EDV and ESV was 0.99 ($P < 0.0001$). For all segments, the LLS and UniV values had a correlation of 0.94 and 0.96, respectively ($P < 0.0001$).

Electromechanical mapping according to the above-described technique reduced the mapping time by 48%; when we compared the region of interest in the regional map with that in the complete map with respect to anatomic and EM data, the correlation was excellent. Therefore, this new approach permits accurate therapeutic delivery while reducing the mapping time.

13.7. CONCLUSION

Electromechanical mapping of the LV is able to assess hemodynamic measurements, distinguish electrical states of the myocardium (infarcted vs. noninfarcted areas), determine myocardial viability, distinguish different mechanical states, and correlate with different functional states (myocardial perfusion). By integrating mechanical and electrical data, EMM introduces the concept of myocardial discordance. Mapping can be done online, in the cardiac catheterization laboratory and can precisely guide the delivery of direct treatments such as laser myocardial revascularization and growth factor therapy. Although it is an ideal platform for therapeutic delivery, EMM remains an experimental tool for the interventional cardiologist. Nevertheless, its diagnostic value in the assessment of myocardial viability, perfusion, and function cannot be overemphasized. Prospective randomized trials are needed to further validate this unique technique and to define its utility in day-to-day practice.

References

Fuchs S, Kornowski R, Shiran A et al. Electromechanical characterization of myocardial hibernation in a pig model. *Coron Artery Dis* 1999; 10: 195–198.

Gepstein L, Hayam G, Ben-Haim SA. A novel method for nonfluoroscopic catheter-based electroanatomical mapping of the heart: In vitro and in vivo accuracy results. *Circulation* 1997a; 95: 1611–1622.

Gepstein L, Hayam G, Shpun S et al. Hemodynamic evaluation of the heart with a nonfluoroscopic electromechanical mapping technique. *Circulation* 1997b; 96: 3672–3680.

Gepstein L, Goldin A, Lessick J et al. Electromechanical characterization of chronic myocardial infarction in the canine coronary occlusion model. *Circulation* 1998; 98: 2055–2064.

Kim RJ, Fieno DS, Parrish TB et al. Relationship of MRI delayed contrast enhancement to irreversible injury, infarct age, and contractile function. *Circulation* 1999a; 100: 1992–2002.

Kim RJ, Rafael A, Chen EL et al. Contrast-enhanced MRI predicts wall motion improvement after coronary revascularization (abstract). *Circulation* 1999b; 100: I797–I798.

Kornowski R, Hong MK, Gepstein L et al. Preliminary animal and clinical experiences using an electromechanical endocardial mapping procedure to distinguish infarcts from healthy myocardium. *Circulation* 1998a; 98: 1116–1124.

Kornowski R, Hong MK, Leon MB. Comparison between left ventricular electromechanical mapping and radionuclide perfusion imaging for detection of myocardial viability. *Circulation* 1998b; 98: 1837–1841.

Kornowski R, Leon MB. Left ventricular electromechanical mapping: current understanding and diagnostic potential. *Cathet Cardiovasc Interv* 1999; 48: 421–429.

Kornowski R, Fuchs S, Tio FO et al. Evaluation of the acute and chronic safety of the Biosense injection catheter system in porcine hearts. *Cathet Cardiovasc Interv* 1999a; 48: 447–453.

Kornowski R, Moses J, Baim D et al. Percutaneous direct myocardial revascularization guided by Biosense left ventricular mapping in patients with refractory coronary ischemia (abstract). *J Am Coll Cardiol* 1999b; 33: 354A.

Lessick J, Smeets JLRM, Reisner SA et al. Electromechanical mapping of regional left ventricular function in humans: comparison with echocardiography. *Cathet Cardiovasc Interv* 2000; 50: 10–18.

Perin EC, Howell M, Sarmento-Leite R et al. Comparison between left ventricular electromechanical mapping and cardiac magnetic resonance imaging for detection of myocardial scar (abstract). *Am J Cardiol* 2000a; 86(Suppl 8A): 108i–109i(Abst. TCT-284).

Perin E, Silva GS, Sarmento-Leite R. Left ventricular electromechanical mapping: A case study of functional assessment in coronary intervention. *Tex Heart Inst J* 2000b; 27: 314–315.

Perin EC, Silva GV, Sarmento-Leite R et al. Rapid NOGA: a new technique for navigation and accurate delivery of direct myocardial therapy (abstract). *Am J Cardiol* 2000c; 86(Suppl 8A): 108i–109i(Abst. TCT-282).

Perin EC, Silva GV, Vaughn W et al. NOGA: a window to the microvasculature? Immediate mechanical changes following PCI (abstract). *Circulation* 2000d; 102: II-815.

Perin EC, Silva G, Sarmento-Leite R et al. Predicting hemodynamic data and presence of scar tissue from electromechanical mapping: Correlation with cardiac magnetic resonance imaging (abstract). *J Am Coll Cardiol* 2001; 34: 441A.

Ramani K, Judd RM, Holly TA et al. Contrast magnetic resonance imaging in the assessment of myocardial viability in patients with stable coronary artery disease and left ventricular dysfunction. *Circulation* 1998; 98: 2687–2694.

Rehwald WG, Fieno DS, Chen EL et al. Relationship of regional Gd-DTPA concentrations to myocardial elec-trolytes following reversible and irreversible ischemic injury (abstract). *Circulation* 1999; 100: I797.

Sarmento-Leite R, Silva GV, Vaughn WK et al. Predicting LV ejection fraction from electromechanical mapping: correlation with angiographic parameters (abstract). *Am J Cardiol* 2000; 86(Suppl 8A): 108i(Abst. TCT-284).

Vale PR, Losordo DW, Tkebuchava T et al. Catheter-based myocardial gene transfer utilizing nonfluoro-scopic electromechanical left ventricular mapping. *J Am Coll Cardiol* 1999; 34: 246–254.

Vale PR, Losordo DW, Milliken CE et al. Left ventricu-lar electromechanical mapping to assess efficacy of phVEGF$_{165}$ gene transfer for therapeutic angiogenesis in chronic myocardial ischemia. *Circulation* 2000; 102: 965–974.

14

Percutaneous Gene Therapy for Myocardial Angiogenesis

Steven W. Werns, M.D.

Division of Cardiology
University of Michigan Medical School
Ann Arbor, Michigan

SUMMARY

Acidic fibroblast growth factor (aFGF) and basic fibroblast growth factor (bFGF) are monomeric polypeptides that induce endothelial and smooth muscle cell proliferation in vitro and angiogenesis in vivo.

A porcine model demonstrated that epicardial placement of microspheres loaded with bFGF resulted in improved collateral blood flow and regional left ventricular function.

There have been many experimental studies that have demonstrated that vascular endothelial growth factor (VEGF) is capable of stimulating angiogenesis in vivo, however some studies have suggested that an unregulated expression of VEGF in the myocardium could have adverse effects.

Problems with gene therapy for myocardial angiogenesis include hypotension (with both bFGF and VEGF) as well as the possibility of promoting plaque rupture, proliferative retinopathy, and oncogenic effects.

Several new strategies are under investigation for the delivery of gene therapy, including transplantation of transfected heart cells

and the combination of transmyocardial revascularization with an excimer laser and adenovirus-mediated gene transfer of growth factors.

14.1. EXPRESSION OF ANGIOGENESIS FACTORS IN ISCHEMIC AND INFARCTED MYOCARDIUM

Both experimental and clinical studies have demonstrated that angiogenesis factors are expressed in myocardium after ischemia or infarction. Vascular endothelial growth factor (VEGF) is a homodimeric glycoprotein that is a specific growth factor for vascular endothelial cells in vitro (Leung et al., 1989). Experimental studies have demonstrated the rapid induction of VEGF mRNA in hypoxic rat myocytes in vitro and ischemic or infarcted rat myocardium in vivo (Hashimoto et al., 1994; Li et al., 1996). Also, receptors for VEGF are upregulated by endothelial cells that have been exposed to medium conditioned by hypoxic myoblasts in vitro (Brogi et al., 1996) and by viable myocardium adjacent to infarcted myocardium in vivo (Li et al., 1996).

Myocardial Revascularization: Novel Percutaneous Approaches, Edited by George S. Abela.
ISBN 0-471-36166-6 Copyright © 2002 Wiley-Liss, Inc.

Several studies have demonstrated that expression of VEGF is increased after myocardial infarction in humans. Lee et al. (2000c) investigated the expression of VEGF and hypoxia-inducible factor 1 (HIF-1), a transcriptional activator of VEGF, in ventricular biopsy specimens obtained from patients undergoing coronary artery bypass surgery. VEGF or HIF-1 mRNA was not detectable in specimens obtained from normal ventricular tissue. HIF-1 mRNA was detected in myocardial specimens with pathologic evidence of either acute ischemia or early infarction (<24 h before surgery). VEGF mRNA was detected in specimens with evidence of either acute ischemia or evolving infarction (24–120 h before surgery). Also, the serum concentration of VEGF increased after acute myocardial infarction (Hojo et al., 2000; Kranz et al., 2000).

14.2. EXPERIMENTAL STUDIES OF ANGIOGENESIS FACTORS

Several angiogenesis factors have been studied in multiple species and models of acute and chronic ischemia and infarction of skeletal muscle and myocardium, utilizing a variety of delivery techniques and experimental end points to demonstrate diverse results (Table 14-1).

14.2.1. Fibroblast Growth Factor

The fibroblast growth factor family consists of at least nine structurally related polypep-

TABLE 14-1 Angiogenic Growth Factors

aFGF	Acidic fibroblastic growth factor
Angiopoietin	
bFGF	Basic fibroblast growth factor
HB-EGF	Heparin-binding epidermal growth factor
HGF	Hepatocyte growth factor
IGF	Insulinlike growth factor
PlGF	Placental growth factor
PDGF	Platelet-derived growth factor
TGF-β	Transforming growth factor-β
VEGF	Vascular endothelial growth factor

tides. Acidic fibroblast growth factor (aFGF or FGF-1) and basic fibroblast growth factor (bFGF or FGF-2) are monomeric polypeptides that induce endothelial and smooth muscle cell proliferation in vitro and angiogenesis in vivo. A daily intracoronary infusion of bFGF for 1 month increased collateral blood flow to ischemic myocardium in a canine model of chronic coronary artery occlusion (Unger et al., 1994). Six months after treatment with the same regimen for 1 week, however, collateral perfusion of chronically ischemic myocardium was similar among dogs treated with bFGF or saline (Shou et al., 1997). Using a porcine model of chronic myocardial ischemia, Lopez et al. (1997a) demonstrated that epicardial placement of microspheres loaded with bFGF resulted in improved collateral blood flow and regional left ventricular function.

aFGF is an endothelial cell mitogen that has been shown to stimulate angiogenesis in vivo. Using a porcine model of chronic myocardial ischemia, Lopez et al. (1998a) demonstrated that perivascular delivery of aFGF in the form of a sustained-release polymer resulted in improved collateral blood flow and regional left ventricular function. Tabata et al. (1997) utilized a rabbit ischemic hind limb model to investigate the angiogenic effects of intra-arterial gene transfer. A plasmid encoding aFGF along with a signal sequence that permitted protein secretion increased the formation of angiographically visible collaterals and improved perfusion of the ischemic skeletal muscle (Tabata et al., 1997). Intramyocardial injection of an adenovirus vector containing the cDNA for recombinant, secreted aFGF induced neovascularization of nonischemic rabbit myocardium and reduced the size of the risk region after coronary artery occlusion (Safi et al., 1999).

Giordano et al. (1996) studied the effects of recombinant adenovirus expressing human FGF-5 on blood flow and contractile function of ischemic myocardium in pigs subjected to chronic coronary artery stenosis. Intracoronary injection of the adenovirus vector resulted in messenger RNA and protein expression of the transferred gene within the heart. Microscopic analysis demonstrated increased capillary density, and regional perfusion and contractile function were improved 2 weeks after gene transfer.

14.2.2. Vascular Endothelial Growth Factor

14.2.2.1. Models of Limb Ischemia

Numerous experimental studies have demonstrated that VEGF is capable of stimulating angiogenesis in vivo. Initial studies were performed using a model of rabbit unilateral hind limb ischemia created by ipsilateral excision of the femoral artery (Takeshita et al., 1994a, 1994b). A single intra-arterial bolus of the 165-amino acid isoform of recombinant human VEGF to the ipsilateral internal iliac artery of the ischemic hind limb produced angiographically visible collaterals and improved calf blood pressure (Takeshita et al., 1994b). Daily intramuscular injection of VEGF for 10 days increased collateral formation and improved limb perfusion in the same model (Takeshita et al., 1994a). A single bolus of intravenous VEGF also increased collateral blood flow to the ischemic rabbit hind limb (Bauters et al., 1995). The combined administration of both VEGF and bFGF stimulated greater development of the collateral circulation compared with administration of either growth factor alone (Asahara et al., 1995).

Subsequently, the same laboratory studied the effect of intramuscular injection of naked plasmid DNA encoding for VEGF (Tsurumi et al., 1996). Human VEGF mRNA was demonstrated by reverse transcriptase-polymerase chain reaction (RT-PCR) from day 3 to day 14 after gene transfection in the ischemic hind limb muscle, but not in the contralateral limb or other organs. Thirty days after transfection, increased collaterals were visible by angiography and improved blood flow was measurable by both an intra-arterial Doppler wire and colored microspheres.

Gowdak et al. (2000) reported the effects of adenovirus-mediated gene transfer of $VEGF_{121}$ on tissue perfusion of the rabbit hind limb. The vector was administered by intramuscular injection 4 weeks before removal of the femoral artery in the injected limb. Compared with animals that were transfected with a control vector, the animals transfected with VEGF exhibited greater blood flow measured by radioactive microspheres, more collaterals visible by angiography, and improved bioenergetic reserve measured by ^{31}P-NMR spectroscopy (Gowdak et al., 2000). The results imply that reduced resting blood flow is not a prerequisite for successful induction of collaterals by administration of $VEGF_{121}$.

14.2.2.2. Models of Myocardial Ischemia

Several studies of VEGF have used canine or porcine models of chronic myocardial ischemia that entail placement of a constrictor on the left circumflex coronary artery (Banai et al., 1994; Harada et al., 1996; Lazarous et al., 1999; Lopez et al., 1998b). Banai et al. (1994) studied the effect of VEGF on collateral blood flow in dogs subjected to gradual occlusion of a coronary artery by a constricting device. Beginning 10 days after placement of the device, VEGF was infused distal to the occlusion via an intracoronary catheter. After treatment with VEGF for 28 days there was a 40% increase in collateral blood flow to the ischemic zone (Banai et al., 1994). In another study, pigs received an intracoronary bolus of VEGF or saline 3 weeks after placement of a coronary constrictor (Lopez et al., 1998b). Three weeks after the injections there was increased myocardial blood flow and improved regional ventricular function in the VEGF-treated pigs compared with controls (Lopez et al., 1998b). Both intracoronary and intramyocardial injections of an adenovirus vector coding for $VEGF_{121}$ improved the development of coronary collaterals and regional myocardial perfusion in the ischemic territory of the porcine heart (Lee et al., 2000a; Mack et al., 1998).

Plasmid DNA expressing VEGF has been injected into the border zone of myocardial infarcts in rats 1 month after coronary artery occlusion (Schwarz et al., 2000). Thirty days after the injections angioma-like formations of new blood vessels were observed protruding from the surface of the hearts. The same plasmid DNA was administered to the popliteal artery of a patient with limb ischemia, and three spider angiomas developed on the foot and ankle 1 week later (Isner et al., 1996). Recently, Lee et al. (2000b) reported that myocardial implantation of murine myoblasts expressing the murine VEGF gene caused formation of intramural vascular tumors resembling hemangiomas and a high mortality rate among the mice, suggesting that unregulated expression of VEGF in myocardium could have adverse effects.

14.2.3. Hepatocyte Growth Factor

Hepatocyte growth factor (HGF) is a potent mitogen for endothelial cells that may have therapeutic potential. Somewhat conflicting results have been reported regarding the expression of HGF within ischemic myocardium. Ono et al. (1997) reported that there was increased expression of both HGF and its receptor within ischemic rat myocardium between 3 hours and 5 days after coronary artery occlusion followed by reperfusion. Aoki et al. (2000), however, reported that HGF was significantly decreased 2 weeks after myocardial infarction. HGF and VEGF demonstrated equipotent effects on proliferation and migration of endothelial cells in vitro (Van Belle et al., 1998). The combination of these factors exerted an additive effect on proliferation and a synergistic effect on migration of endothelial cells (Van Belle et al., 1998). Addition of HGF to cultured human smooth muscle cells caused induction of VEGF mRNA and protein (Van Belle et al., 1998). In the rabbit hind limb ischemia model, it was demonstrated that combined administration of HGF and VEGF stimulated greater collateral artery development than administration of either factor alone (Van Belle et al., 1998). Transfection of infarcted rat myocardium with HGF vector induced formation of new blood vessels (Aoki et al., 2000).

14.3. CLINICAL STUDIES OF MYOCARDIAL EFFECTS OF ANGIOGENESIS FACTORS

14.3.1. Fibroblast Growth Factor

Schumacher et al. (1998) reported the results of a randomized trial of human aFGF treatment in 20 patients undergoing coronary artery bypass surgery (CABG). A solution of aFGF was injected into the myocardium distal to the anastomosis of the left internal mammary artery (IMA) graft to the left anterior descending coronary artery. A control group received injections of heat-denatured aFGF. The IMA bypass grafts were imaged selectively 12 weeks after surgery, revealing an accumulation of radiographic contrast medium at the sites of aFGF injection.

Laham et al. (1999c) conducted a randomized, double-blind, placebo-controlled trial of human recombinant bFGF in 24 patients undergoing CABG. Sustained-release heparin-alginate microcapsules containing bFGF were implanted in ischemic and viable but ungraftable myocardial territories. Stress nuclear perfusion imaging was performed before hospital discharge and 3 months after CABG. The size of the perfusion defect, expressed as a percentage of the left ventricle, increased in the placebo group (20.7–23.3%; $n = 8$; $P = 0.06$), and decreased in the patients treated with 100 µg of bFGF (19.2–9.1%; $n = 8$; $P = 0.01$). There was no significant change in the patients who were treated with 10 µg of bFGF.

Udelson et al. (2000) reported a preliminary, uncontrolled, dose-escalation study of intracoronary ($n = 45$) or intravenous ($n = 14$) bFGF in patients with angina and inducible ischemia who were suboptimal candidates for CABG or angioplasty. The 37 patients who had at least one segment with a resting thallium-201 perfusion abnormality of mild to moderate severity exhibited an improvement in resting perfusion 1, 2, and 6 months after therapy. Among the entire group of 59 patients, the baseline thallium studies demonstrated inducible ischemia in 51 patients, and there was a sustained reduction of the extent and severity of inducible ischemia after treatment with bFGF. Segments with fixed defects at baseline, however, remained unchanged throughout the study.

14.3.2. Vascular Endothelial Growth Factor

Several preliminary studies of intramyocardial injection of VEGF cDNA have been reported (Losordo et al., 1998; Symes et al., 1999; Vale et al., 2000a). In a study of 20 patients with severe exertional angina and "inoperable" coronary artery disease, naked plasmid DNA encoding VEGF (phVEGF$_{165}$) was injected into ischemic myocardium via a minithoracotomy (Symes et al., 1999). Two months after treatment, myocardial perfusion was improved as measured by SPECT-sestamibi perfusion imaging and angiographic assessment of coronary collaterals. Left ventricular electromechanical mapping performed before and 60 days after treatment of 13 patients provided evidence of improved local myocardial shortening within the treated regions (Vale et al., 2000a).

Rosengart et al. (1999a, 1999b) reported the results of a phase I trial of intramyocardial administration of an adenovirus vector expressing VEGF$_{121}$ cDNA. The adenovirus vector was injected into an ischemic area of myocardium that could not be bypassed in 15 patients undergoing concomitant CABG. The myocardial injections were delivered via a minithoracotomy as sole therapy in six additional patients. Coronary angiograms performed 30 days after vector administration demonstrated improvement in collateral circulation in both groups of patients and no evidence of hemangiomas or other pathology. Resting and stress (adenosine) Tc-99m-sestamibi studies were performed before and 1 month after treatment. Among the patients who underwent gene therapy only, four of the six showed an improvement in the proportion of myocardium that showed reversible stress-induced ischemia. Although the results demonstrate the feasibility of the technique, it is difficult to assess the clinical benefits of the treatment because most of the patients underwent CABG and there was no control group.

Hendel et al. (2000) reported the results of a phase I study of intracoronary infusion of recombinant human VEGF in patients with severe coronary artery disease (CAD) who were not optimal candidates for angioplasty or CABG. Fourteen patients underwent SPECT perfusion imaging before and 30 and 60 days after administration of VEGF. Ten of the fourteen patients demonstrated improvement of resting perfusion, including five of the six patients who received the higher dose of VEGF. For the entire group there was no change in the stress perfusion score, but five of the six patients in the high-dose group exhibited improvement in stress perfusion.

A double-blind, placebo-controlled trial of recombinant human VEGF in patients with CAD, known as the VIVA (VEGF to improve left ventricular function and angiogenesis) trial, has been published in abstract form (Henry et al., 2000). One hundred seventy-eight patients were randomized to three treatment groups and received two 10-min intracoronary infusions (17 or 50 ng/kg/min VEGF or placebo) on day 0, followed by three 4-h intravenous infusions (17 or 50 ng/kg/min VEGF or placebo) on days 3, 6, and 9. After 60 days, all three groups exhibited significant improvement in exercise time, Canadian angina class, and quality of life, with no differences between the groups. Between 120 days and 1 year after treatment, the severity of angina increased in all groups, with only a trend for sustained improvement in the patients treated with VEGF.

14.4. FUTURE ISSUES

The side effects of angiogenesis therapies remain relatively unknown. Hypotension caused by release of nitric oxide is a well-documented side effect of intravascular infusions of both bFGF (Unger et al., 2000) and VEGF (Lopez et al., 1997b). FGF-1 has been shown to induce angiogenesis in vasa vasorum, a process that may promote plaque rupture and resulting acute coronary syndromes (Nabel et al., 1993). Additional theoretical adverse effects are proliferative retinopathy and oncogenic effects.

An expert panel recently published a summary of the issues and problems that are involved in the development of angiogenesis as a therapy for CAD (Simons et al., 2000). One problem is the possibility that many medications used to treat CAD, such as aspirin and angiotensin-converting enzyme inhibitors (Simons et al., 2000), and some risk factors for CAD, such as hypercholesterolemia (Van Belle et al., 1997) and advanced age (Rivard et al., 1999), may inhibit angiogenesis. A second problem is the limitations of various trial end points that are used to assess the efficacy of therapy, such as exercise tolerance, quality of life indicators, myocardial perfusion imaging, left ventricular mechanical mapping (Vale et al., 2000a), and angiographic grading of coronary collaterals. Gibson et al. (1999) published a detailed description of angiographic methods that may be useful to assess human coronary angiogenesis.

Kornowski et al. (2000a) reviewed an additional issue in therapeutic angiogenesis, the limitations of various delivery strategies. Several routes of delivery have been utilized in experimental animals, including direct myocardial injection, epicardial (Sellke et al., 1998) or intrapericardial administration (Laham et al., 1999a, 2000), and intracoronary and intravenous infusion (Laham et al., 1999b). Deposition of bFGF in chronically ischemic myocardium in experimental pigs was three- to fourfold greater 1 hour after intracoronary infusion compared with intravenous infusion (Laham et al., 1999b). Recent experimental studies demonstrated that albumin-coated microbubbles markedly augmented expression of an adenoviral transgene within rat myocardium exposed to transthoracic ultrasound during intravenous infusion of the bubbles (Shohet et al., 2000). Both the intracoronary and intravenous routes of administration are associated with the potential for hypotension and other side effects caused by systemic exposure to growth factors.

Direct intramyocardial injection may provide better retention and less systemic recirculation than intravenous or intracoronary delivery, but intramyocardial delivery requires an invasive procedure. Intramyocardial administration may be accomplished at the time of conventional CABG via a

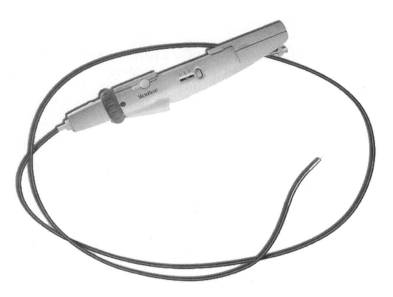

FIGURE 14-1. SteeraJet™ is a fully steerable 7 F catheter-based system for procedures performed in the cardiac catheterization laboratory. It is intended to allow easy access to all treatment regions with single-person operation of the steering and injection controls. (Courtesy of MicroHeart, Mountainview, CA.)

minithoracotomy or, most recently, via percutaneous endocardial injections guided by electromechanical left ventricular mapping (Kornowski et al., 2000b; Vale et al., 1999a, 1999b; 2000b). A catheter produced by Micro-Heart is an example of a catheter delivery approach. It utilizes a mechanism to determine the position of the catheter tip relative to

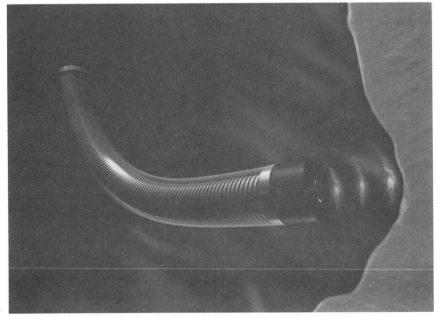

(A)

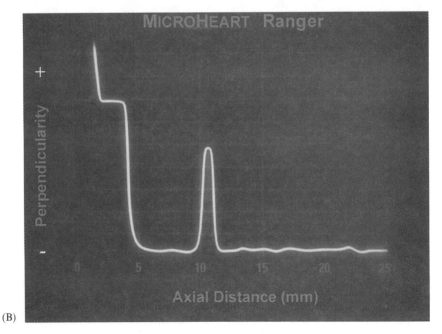

(B)

FIGURE 14-2. (A) Flexible catheter tip with ultrasonic sounding system to confirm contact with the ventricular wall. (B) An alternative catheter uses the MicroHeart Ranger system to detect the distance from the catheter tip to the ventricular wall. (Courtesy of MicroHeart, Mountainview, CA.)

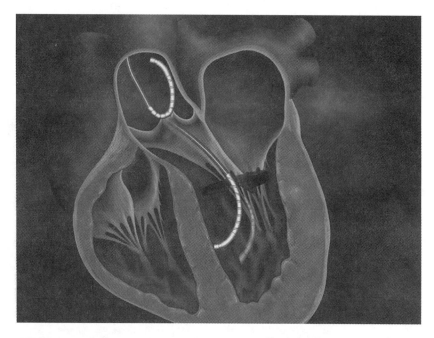

FIGURE 14-3. Catheter system with a radiopaque tip is intended for easy visualization under fluoroscopy. It achieves a tight-radius bend to prolapse across the aortic valve to access the left ventricular wall. (Courtesy of MicroHeart, Mountainview, CA.)

the ventricular wall, and either an ultrasound system or a ranging system mounted in a flexible-tipped catheter to extend the injection needle a preset distance into the myocardium to avoid perforation (Figs. 14-1 to 14-5).

Another delivery strategy that requires a thoracotomy is the epicardial implantation of sustained-release heparin-alginate microcapsules containing bFGF (Laham et al., 1999c).

Numerous issues remain unresolved with respect to the relative merits of protein versus gene therapy (Simons et al., 2000). The putative advantages of protein therapy include limited temporal exposure to the angiogenic factor and the absence of potential immunologic or other reactions to viral vectors. The disadvantages include the short serum half-life that may require repeated administration and/or increased short-term systemic exposure during intravascular infusion. The proposed advantages of gene therapy are sustained production of angiogenic factor after a single administration and

the potential for local delivery. Local gene delivery, however, does not guarantee that the protein product will be confined to the target tissue, because secreted factors such as VEGF may be released into the systemic circulation. The mean time to peak plasma concentration of VEGF after direct intramyocardial injections was 12 days, and the plasma concentration increased from a baseline of 25 pg/ml to a median peak concentration of 78 pg/ml (Freedman et al., 2000). Experimental studies in pigs demonstrated that previous immunization with adenoviral vectors carrying no transgene abrogated transgene expression and was associated with local myocardial necrosis after intracoronary infusion of the adenoviral vector (Szelid et al., 2000). High titers of neutralizing antibody to adenovirus (1:2000) were found in 10 of 26 patients referred for CABG (Szelid et al., 2000). Other theoretical disadvantages of gene therapy are related to the risks of exposure to viral vectors: inflammatory reactions, viral persistence, and in vivo recombination. Leukopenia, thrombocy-

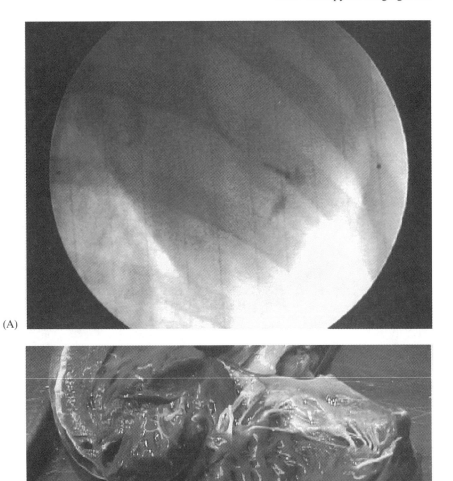

(A)

(B)

FIGURE 14-4. (A) Intraoperative fluoroscopic view of the SteeraJet as used in a porcine model. (B) At autopsy, the sites of successful injection are confirmed with blue dye at the apex and base of the left ventricle. (Courtesy of MicroHeart, Mountainview, CA.)

topenia, and increased liver enzymes were observed after administration of VEGF adenovirus during coronary or peripheral artery angioplasty (Yla-Herttuala et al., 2000). One death has been reported after administration of adenovirus vector to the liver (Hollon, 2000).

New delivery strategies under investigation include transplantation of transfected heart cells to accomplish gene transfer (Yau

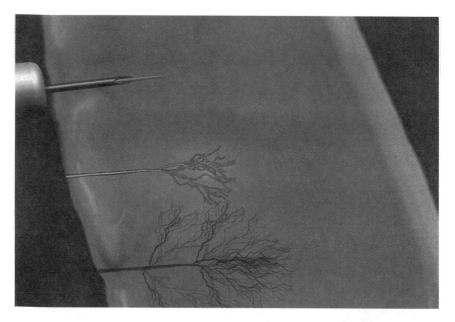

FIGURE 14-5. Using the catheter system above (Figure 14-4), a needle is advanced to a fixed limit that provides midmyocardial delivery while seeking to minimize the risk of perforation. (Courtesy of MicroHeart, Mountainview, CA.)

et al., 2000) and the combination of transmyocardial revascularization with an excimer laser and adenovirus-mediated gene transfer of growth factors (Hamawy et al., 2000).

14.5. CONCLUSION

The functional significance of naturally occurring coronary collateral vessels varies. Patients may experience angina and exercise-induced ischemia despite angiographic visualization of excellent coronary collaterals (Kolibash et al., 1982). Kolibash et al. (1982) analyzed 91 patients with stable coronary artery disease who had 101 totally occluded coronary arteries associated with angiographically visible collateral vessels. Among the 43 cases with normal resting perfusion in the distribution of the occluded artery, 29 had normal perfusion during exercise. Thus 72 of the 101 collateralized myocardial regions had abnormal perfusion at rest and/or during exercise. Di Carli et al. (1994) studied 42 patients with 78 completely occluded coronary arteries that supplied myocardium with severely abnormal wall motion (dyskinesia, akinesia, or severe hypokinesia). Angiographic collateral vessels were graded as absent in 14 cases, minimal in 27 cases, and well developed in 37 cases. There was no correlation between the collateral grade and the severity of perfusion deficit assessed by positron emission tomography. These studies imply that sophisticated techniques will be required to assess myocardial perfusion and function in patients who are enrolled in coronary angiogenesis trials.

References

Aoki M, Morishita R, Taniyama Y et al. Angiogenesis induced by hepatocyte growth factor in non-infarcted and infarcted myocardium: up-regulation of essential transcription factor for angiogenesis, ets. *Gene Therapy* 2000; 7: 417–427.

Asahara T, Bauters C, Zheng LP et al. Synergistic effect of vascular endothelial growth factor and basic fibroblast growth factor on angiogenesis in vivo. *Circulation* 1995; 92 (*Suppl* II): II-365–II-371.

Banai S, Jaklitsch MT, Shou M et al. Angiogenic-induced enhancement of collateral blood flow to ischemic myocardium by vascular endothelial growth factor in dogs. *Circulation* 1994; 89: 2183–2189.

Bauters C, Asahara T, Zheng LP et al. Site-specific therapeutic angiogenesis after systemic administration of vascular endothelial growth factor. *J Vasc Surg* 1995; 21: 314–325.

Brogi E, Schatteman G, Wu T et al. Hypoxia-induced paracrine regulation of vascular endothelial growth factor receptor expression. *J Clin Invest* 1996; 97: 469–476.

DiCarli M, Sherman T, Khanna S et al. Myocardial viability in asynergic regions subtended by occluded coronary arteries: relation to the status of collateral flow in patients with chronic coronary artery disease. *J Am Coll Cardiol* 1994; 23: 860–868.

Freedman B, Vale PR, Kalka C et al. Plasma VEGF levels after intramyocardial and intramuscular VEGF gene transfer in patients with coronary artery and peripheral artery disease(abstract). *Circulation* 2000; 102 (*Suppl* II): II-10.

Gibson CM, Ryan K, Sparano A, Moynihan JL, Rizzo M, Kelley M, Marble SJ, Laham R, Simons M, McClusky TR, Dodge JT. Angiographic methods to assess human coronary angiogenesis. *Am Heart J* 1999; 137: 169–179.

Giordano FJ, Ping P, McKirnan MD, Nozaki S, DeMaria AN, Dillmann WH. Mathieu-Costello O and Hammond HK. Intracoronary gene transfer of fibroblast growth factor-5 increases blood flow and contractile function in an ischemic region of the heart. *Nat Med* 1996; 2: 534–539.

Gowdak LHW, Poliakova L, Wang X et al. Adenovirus-mediated VEGF$_{121}$ gene transfer stimulates angiogenesis in normoperfused skeletal muscle and preserves tissue perfusion after induction of ischemia. *Circulation* 2000; 102: 565–571.

Hamawy A, Samy SA, Leotta E et al. Coadministration of adenovirus encoding for VEGF$_{121}$ and transmyocardial revascularization with an excimer laser increase survival in a double ameroid model of severe myocardial ischemia (abstract). *Circulation* 2000; 102 (*Suppl* II): II-10.

Harada K, Friedman M, Lopez JJ et al. Vascular endothelial growth factor administration in chronic myocardial ischemia. *Am J Physiol* 1996; 270: H1791–H1802.

Hashimoto E, Ogita T, Nakaoka T et al. Rapid induction of vascular endothelial growth factor expression by transient ischemia in rat heart. *Am J Physiol* 1994; 267: H1948–H1954.

Hendel RC, Henry TD, Rocha-Singh K et al. Effect of intracoronary recombinant human vascular endothelial growth factor on myocardial perfusion. Evidence for a dose-dependent effect. *Circulation* 2000; 101: 118–121.

Henry TD, McKendall GR, Azrin MA et al. VIVA trial: one year follow up (abstract). *Circulation* 2000; 102 (*Suppl* II): II-309.

Hojo Y, Ikeda U, Zhu Y et al. Expression of vascular endothelial growth factor in patients with acute myocardial infarction. *J Am Coll Cardiol* 2000; 35: 968–973.

Hollon T. Researchers and regulators reflect on first gene therapy death. *Nat Med* 2000; 6: 6.

Isner JM, Pieczek A, Schainfeld R et al. Clinical evidence of angiogenesis after arterial gene transfer of phVEGF$_{165}$ in patient with ischaemic limb. *Lancet* 1996; 348: 370–374.

Kolibash AJ, Bush CA, Wepsic RA et al. Coronary collateral vessels: spectrum of physiologic capabilities with respect to providing rest and stress myocardial perfusion, maintenance of left ventricular function and protection against infarction. *Am J Cardiol* 1982; 50: 230–238.

Kornowski R, Fuchs S, Leon MB et al. Delivery strategies to achieve therapeutic myocardial angiogenesis. *Circulation* 2000a; 101: 454–458.

Kornowski R, Leon MB, Fuchs S et al. Electromagnetic guidance for catheter-based transendocardial injection: a platform for intramyocardial angiogenesis therapy. *J Am Coll Cardiol* 2000b; 35: 1031–1039.

Kranz A, Rau C, Kochs M et al. Elevation of vascular endothelial growth factor-A serum levels following acute myocardial infarction. Evidence for its origin and functional significance. *J Mol Cell Cardiol* 2000; 32: 65–72.

Laham RJ, Hung D, Simons M. Therapeutic myocardial angiogenesis using percutaneous intrapericardial drug delivery. *Clin Cardiol* 1999a; 22 (*Suppl* I): I-6–I-9.

Laham RJ, Rezaee M, Post M et al. Intracoronary and intravenous administration of basic fibroblast growth factor: myocardial and tissue distribution. *Drug Metab Dispos* 1999b; 27: 821–826.

Laham RJ, Selke FW, Edelman ER et al. Local perivascular delivery of basic fibroblast growth factor in patients undergoing coronary bypass surgery. Results of a phase I randomized, double-blind, placebo-controlled trial. *Circulation* 1999c; 100: 1865–1871.

Laham RJ, Rezaee M, Post J et al. Intrapericardial delivery of fibroblast growth factor-2 induces neovascularization in a porcine model of chronic myocardial ischemia. *J Pharmacol Exp Ther* 2000; 292: 795–802.

Lazarous DF, Shou M, Stiber JA et al. Adenoviral-mediated gene transfer induces sustained pericardial VEGF expression in dogs: effect on myocardial angiogenesis. *Cardiovasc Res* 1999; 44: 294–302.

Lee LY, Patel SR, Hackett NR et al. Focal angiogen therapy using intramyocardial delivery of an adenovirus vector coding for vascular endothelial growth factor 121. *Ann Thorac Surg* 2000a; 69: 14–24.

Lee RJ, Springer ML, Blanco-Bose WE et al. VEGF gene delivery to myocardium. Deleterious effects of unregulated expression. *Circulation* 2000b; 102: 898–901.

Lee SH, Wolf PL, Escudero R et al. Early expression of angiogenesis factors in acute myocardial ischemia and infarction. *N Engl J Med* 2000c; 342: 626–633.

Leung DW, Cachianes G, Kuang WJ et al. Vascular endothelial growth factor as a secreted angiogenic mitogen. *Science* 1989; 246: 1306–1309.

Li J, Brown LF, Hibbert MG et al. VEGF, flk-1, and flt-1 expression in a rat myocardial infarction model of angiogenesis. *Am J Physiol* 1996; 270: H1083–H1811.

Lopez JJ, Edelman ER, Stamler A et al. Basic fibroblast growth factor in a porcine model of chronic myocardial ischemia: a comparison of angiographic, echocardiographic and coronary flow parameters. *J Pharmacol Exp Ther* 1997a; 282: 385–390.

Lopez JJ, Laham RJ, Carrozza JP et al. Hemodynamic effects of intracoronary VEGF delivery: evidence of tachyphylaxis and NO dependence of response. *Am J Physiol* 1997b; 273: H1317–H1323.

Lopez JJ, Edelman ER, Stamler A et al. Angiogenic potential of perivascularly delivered aFGF in a porcine model of chronic myocardial ischemia. *Am J Physiol* 1998a; 274: H930–H936.

Lopez JJ, Laham RJ, Stamler A et al. VEGF administration in chronic myocardial ischemia in pigs. *Cardiovasc Res* 1998b; 40: 272–281.

Losordo DW, Vale PR, Symes JF et al. Gene therapy for myocardial angiogenesis. Initial clinical results with direct myocardial injection of phVEGF$_{165}$ as sole therapy for myocardial ischemia. *Circulation* 1998; 98: 2800–2804.

Mack CA, Patel SR, Schwarz EA. Biologic bypass with the use of a adenovirus-mediated gene transfer of the complementary deoxyribonucleic acid for vascular endothelial growth factor 121 improves myocardial perfusion and function in the ischemic porcine heart. *J Thorac Cardiovasc Surg* 1998; 115: 168–177.

Nabel EG, Zang ZY, Plautz G et al. Recombinant fibroblast growth factor-1 promotes intimal hyperplasia and angiogenesis in arteries in vivo. *Nature* 1993; 362: 844–846.

Ono K, Matsumori A, Shioi T et al. Enhanced expression of hepatocyte growth factor/c-Met by myocardial ischemia and reperfusion in a rat model. *Circulation* 1997; 95: 2552–2558.

Rivard A, Fabre JE, Silver M et al. Age-dependent impairment of angiogenesis. *Circulation* 1999; 99: 111–120.

Rosengart TK, Lee LY, Patel SR et al. Six-month assessment of a phase I trial of angiogenic gene therapy for the treatment of coronary artery disease using direct intramyocardial administration of an adenovirus vector expressing the VEGF121 cDNA. *Ann Surg* 1999a; 230: 466–472.

Rosengart TK, Lee LY, Patel SR et al. Angiogenesis gene therapy. Phase I assessment of direct intramyocardial administration of an adenovirus vector expressing VEGF121 cDNA to individuals with clinically significant severe coronary artery disease. *Circulation* 1999b; 100: 468–474.

Safi J, DiPaula AF, Riccioni T et al. Adenovirus-mediated acidic fibroblast growth factor gene transfer induces angiogenesis in the nonischemic rabbit heart. *Microvasc Res* 1999; 58: 238–249.

Schumacher B, Pecher P, von Specht BU et al. Induction of neoangiogenesis in ischemic myocardium by human growth factors. First clinical results of a new treatment of coronary heart disease. *Circulation* 1998; 97: 645–650.

Schwarz EG, Speakman MT, Patterson M et al. Evaluation of the effects of intramyocardial injection of DNA expressing vascular endothelial growth factor (VEGF) in a myocardial infarction model in the rat-angiogenesis and angioma formation. *J Am Coll Cardiol* 2000; 35: 1323–1330.

Sellke FW, Laham RJ, Edelman ER et al. Therapeutic angiogenesis with basic fibroblast growth factor: technique and early results. *Ann Thorac Surg* 1998; 65: 1540–1544.

Shohet RV, Chen S, Zhou YT et al. Echocardiographic destruction of albumin microbubbles directs gene delivery to the myocardium. *Circulation* 2000; 101: 2554–2556.

Shou M, Thirumurti V, Rajanayagam MAS et al. Effect of basic fibroblast growth factor on myocardial angiogenesis in dogs with mature collateral vessels. *J Am Coll Cardiol* 1997; 29: 1102–1106.

Simons M, Bonow RO, Chronos NA et al. Clinical trials in coronary angiogenesis: issues, problems, consensus. An expert panel summary. *Circulation* 2000; 102: E-73–E-86.

Symes JF, Losordo DW, Vale PR et al. Gene therapy with vascular endothelial growth factor for inoperable coronary artery disease. *Ann Thorac Surg* 1999; 68: 830–837.

Szelid Z, Sinnaeve P, Gillijns H et al. Anti-adenoviral immune response following intracoronary gene transfer: implications for cardiac gene therapy (abstract). *Circulation* 2000; 102 (*Suppl* II): II-10.

Tabata H, Silver M, Isner JM. Arterial gene transfer of acidic fibroblast growth factor for therapeutic angiogenesis in vivo: critical role of secretion signal in use of naked DNA. *Cardiovasc Res* 1997; 35: 470–479.

Takeshita S, Pu LQ, Stein LW et al. Intramuscular administration of vascular endothelial growth factor induces dose-dependent collateral artery augmentation in a rabbit model of chronic limb ischemia. *Circulation* 1994a; 90 (Part II): II-223–II-234.

Takeshita S, Zheng LP, Brogi E. Therapeutic angiogenesis: a single intra-arterial bolus of vascular endothelial growth factor augments revascularization in a rabbit ischemic hind limb model. *J Clin Invest* 1994b; 93: 662–670.

Tsurumi Y, Takeshita S, Chen D et al. Direct intramuscular gene transfer of naked DNA encoding vascular endothelial growth factor augments collateral development and tissue perfusion. *Circulation* 1996; 94: 3281–3290.

Udelson JE, Dilsizian V, Laham RJ et al. Therapeutic angiogenesis with recombinant fibroblast growth factor-2 improves stress and rest myocardial perfusion abnormalities in patients with severe symptomatic chronic coronary artery disease. *Circulation* 2000; 102: 1605–1610.

Unger EG, Banai S, Shou M et al. Basic fibroblast growth factor enhances myocardial collateral flow in a canine model. *Am J Physiol* 1994; 266: H1588–H1595.

Unger EF, Goncalves L, Epstein SE et al. Effects of a single intracoronary injection of basic fibroblast

growth factor in stable angina pectoris. *Am J Cardiol* 2000; 85: 1414–1419.

Vale PR, Losordo DW, Milliken CE et al. Percutaneous myocardial gene transfer of ph VEGF-2. *Circulation* 1999a; 100: 2462–2463.

Vale PR, Losordo DW, Tkebuchava T et al. Catheter-based myocardial gene transfer utilizing nonfluoroscopic electromechanical left ventricular mapping. *J Am Coll Cardiol* 1999b; 34: 246–254.

Vale PR, Losordo DW, Milliken CE et al. Left ventricular electromechanical mapping to assess efficacy of ph VEGF165 gene transfer for therapeutic angiogenesis in chronic myocardial ischemia. *Circulation* 2000a; 102: 965–974.

Vale PR, Losordo DW, Milliken CE et al. Randomized, placebo-controlled clinical study of percutaneous catheter-based left ventricular endocardial gene transfer of VEGF-2 for myocardial angiogenesis in patients with chronic myocardial ischemia (abstract). *Circulation* 2000b; 102 (*Suppl* II): II-563.

Van Belle E, Rivard A, Chen D et al. Hypercholesterolemia attenuates angiogenesis but does not preclude augmentation by angiogenic cytokines. *Circulation* 1997; 96: 2667–2674.

Van Belle E, Witzenbichler B, Chen D et al. Potentiated angiogenic effect of scatter factor/hepatocyte growth factor via induction of vascular endothelial growth factor. *Circulation* 1998; 97: 381–390.

Yau TM, Sarjeant J, Fung K et al. Enhanced myocardial angiogenesis by gene transfer using transplanted cells (abstract). *Circulation* 2000; 102 (*Suppl* II): II-682.

Yla-Herttuala S, Laitinen M, Virtanen AI et al. Safety of VEGF gene therapy with adenovirus and plasmid/liposome vectors in coronary and peripheral vascular disease patients (abstract). *Circulation* 2000; 102 (*Suppl* II): II-10.

15

Myocardial Angiogenesis: Clinical Trial Results

Timothy D. Henry, M.D., and Charlene R. Boisjolie, R.N.

Cardiology Division, Department of Medicine
Hennepin County Medical Center
Minneapolis, Minnesota

SUMMARY

Therapeutic angiogenesis is the use of angiogenic growth factors to enhance the natural process of collateral vessel development in ischemic tissue in an attempt to increase proangiogenic signals to alter the balance to favor new blood vessel growth and vascular remodeling.

Initial clinical trials of therapeutic angiogenesis have been encouraging in regard to both safety and efficacy; however, the number of patients enrolled in placebo-controlled trials remains small.

The VIVA Trial (Vascular Endothelial Growth Factor in Ischemia for Vascular Angiogenesis) was the first large, double-blind, placebo-controlled trial with VEGF, enrolling 178 patients. While there was no significant difference at day 60 due to a prominent placebo effect, at day 120 the high dose VEGF patients had significant improvement in angina and a trend toward improvement in exercise time.

The FIRST trial (FGF-2 initiating revascularization support trial) is the largest double-blind, placebo-controlled trial, enrolling 337 patients with FGF-2. Three month results of the FIRST trial indicate improvements in angina as well as trends toward improvement in exercise time.

Although initial clinical trials offer promising signs of efficacy, many questions remain including the relative safety and efficacy of protein versus gene therapy, optimal dose, dosing schedule, and route of administration.

15.1. BACKGROUND

As the population ages and mortality rates for coronary artery disease decline, an increasing number of patients are left with severe myocardial ischemia not amenable to standard revascularization techniques. For example, in a consecutive series of 500 patients undergoing coronary angiography at the Cleveland Clinic (Mukherjee et al., 1999), 12% had severe coronary artery disease and were not optimal candidates for coronary artery bypass grafting or percutaneous coronary interventions. The most common reasons were poor distal targets (75%); chronic total occlusion (64%), and degenerated vein graft (24%). In addition to increased morbidity and mortality, these "no-option" patients have significant limitations in their

Myocardial Revascularization: Novel Percutaneous Approaches, Edited by George S. Abela.
ISBN 0-471-36166-6 Copyright © 2002 Wiley-Liss, Inc.

quality of life. This increasingly common clinical dilemma has stimulated intense interest in and excitement for novel approaches to myocardial revascularization.

Therapeutic angiogenesis is the use of angiogenic growth factors, or the genes that encode for these growth factors, to enhance the natural process of collateral vessel development in ischemic tissue (Henry, 1999; Ylä-Herttuala and Martin, 2000). Angiogenesis is a complex process modulated by the balance between proangiogenic factors and inhibitors of angiogenesis (Giordano, 1999; Iruela-Arispe and Dvorak, 1997; Isner and Asahara, 1999). Therapeutic angiogenesis is an attempt to increase proangiogenic signals to alter the balance to favor new blood vessel growth and vascular remodeling. An increasing number of angiogenic growth factors have been identified (Table 15-1), but the majority of preclinical and clinical studies are with members of the vascular endothelial growth factor (VEGF) and fibroblast growth factor (FGF) family of proteins. Successful myocardial angiogenesis has been demonstrated with VEGF and FGF using both proteins and genes via a number of delivery techniques. These preclinical trials have prepared the way for an increasing number of clinical trials (Table 15-2). We review the results of these initial clinical trials and address the significant challenges ahead in the attempt to provide an alternative method of myocardial revascularization.

15.1.1. Vascular Endothelial Growth Factor

VEGF is a naturally occurring angiogenic protein that exists in seven isoforms (121, 145, 148, 165, 183, 189, and 206 amino acids) that vary in permeability and heparin binding capabilities (Ferrara, 1999; Ferrara and Davis-Smyth, 1997; Henry and Abraham, 2000; Neufeld et al., 1999). Besides VEGF, referred to as VEGF-1 or VEGF-A, there are a number of VEGF-related proteins including VEGF-B, VEGF-C (commonly called VEGF-2), VEGF-D, placental growth factor, and VEGF-E. Physiologic effects of VEGF include enhanced vascular permeability, nitric oxide-induced vasodilatation, as well as potent endothelial cell proliferation, migration, and differentiation. Although VEGF is relatively specific for endothelial cells, it

TABLE 15-1.   Angiogenic Growth Factors

Angiogenin
Angiopoietin
Fibroblast growth factors (FGF)
    FGF-1 (acidic FGF), FGF-2 (basic FGF), FGF-3,
    FGF-4, FGF-5 (to FGF-20)
Granulocyte colony stimulating factor
Hepatocyte growth factor (scatter factor)
Hypoxia-inducible factor-1α (HIF-1α)
Insulin-like growth factor (IGF)
Interleukin-8
Leptin
Placental growth factor
Platelet-derived growth factor (PDGF)
Proliferin
Thyroxine
Transforming growth factor ($-\alpha$ and $-\beta$)
Tumor necrosis factor-α
Vascular endothelial growth factor (VEGF)
    VEGF A (VEGF-1) (Isoforms$_{121,143,148,165,189,206}$),
    VEGF B, VEGF C (VEGF-2), VEGF D

TABLE 15-2.   Summary of Myocardial Angiogenesis Clinical Trials

	VEGF	Route	FGF	Route
Gene Rx:	VEGF$_{165}$	IM	Ad-FGF-4	IC
	VEGF-2	IM		
	Ad-VEGF$_{121}$	IM		
	Ad-VEGF$_{165}$ local IC			
Protein Rx:	RhVEGF$_{165}$	IC, IV	FGF-1	IM
			FGF-2	IC, IV, IM

IM = intramyocardial; IC= intracoronary; IV= intravenous.

appears there may also be an effect on smooth muscle cells, with cell migration and production of matrix metalloproteinases. It is now clear that VEGF plays a dominant role not only in the natural development of the vascular system during embryogenesis but with angiogenic responses to physiologic and pathologic stresses in the adult as well. The critical role of VEGF in physiologic angiogenesis and the upregulation of its receptors in response to ischemia have generated significant interest in the use of VEGF for therapeutic angiogenesis. At this time, there is clinical experience with VEGF isoforms 165 and 121 as well as VEGF-2.

15.1.2. Fibroblast Growth Factor

FGF is a family of more than 20 proteins that are also potent angiogenic cytokines. Like VEGF, they bind to heparan sulfates (heparin-like molecules) on the surface of endothelial and smooth muscle cells. This binding helps to facilitate attachment to their high-affinity receptors. Although FGF is an endothelial cell mitogen, it is not specific to endothelial cells, with receptors on fibroblast, neuronal, and vascular smooth muscle cells. FGF also stimulates endothelial production of proteases, such as plasminogen activator and matrix metalloproteinases that can digest extracellular matrix, an important step in the angiogenic process (Ware and Simons, 1997). Like VEGF, FGF produces nitric oxide-mediated vasodilatation. However, unlike VEGF, FGF is not associated with vascular permeability. In addition, FGF enhances endothelium-dependent relaxation of collateral-perfused coronary microcirculation. (Selke et al., 1994). Stimuli for the secretion of FGFs are not well understood, although cellular injury such as takes place during ischemia or hemodynamic stress plays important roles. FGF-1, FGF-2, and FGF-4 have been used in clinical trials as discussed below.

15.2. CLINICAL TRIALS OF THERAPEUTIC ANGIOGENESIS

Initial clinical VEGF trials have been performed with intracoronary and intravenous recombinant $VEGF_{165}$ protein and gene therapy using intramyocardial injections of naked plasmid DNA encoding for $VEGF_{165}$ and VEGF-2. In addition, an adenoviral vector encoding for $VEGF_{121}$ has been given both as an adjunct to coronary artery bypass graft (CABG) and alone with intramyocardial injections (Table 15-3). Initial trials with FGF include intravenous and intracoronary FGF-2 protein and intracoronary administration of an adenovirus encoding FGF-4. Also, FGF-2 protein administered via sustained-release heparin-alginate microcapsules and intramyocardial injection of FGF-1 have been utilized in patients undergoing CABG (Table 15-4). In general, these trials have enrolled patients with stable angina and reversible myocardial perfusion defects who were not optimal candidates for percutaneous or surgical revascularization. Patients with a history of cancer, retinopathy, low ejection fraction (<20–25%), or recent unstable angina, myocardial infarction, or revascularization have been excluded. In three trials, the growth factor has been given as an adjunct to CABG. Although the initial results are encouraging in regard to both safety and efficacy, the number of patients enrolled in placebo-controlled trials remains small.

15.2.1. VEGF Protein Therapy

In the initial phase I $VEGF_{165}$ protein dose-escalation trial, 15 patients received two 10-min intracoronary infusions of 5, 17, 50, or 167 ng/kg/min into each of two coronary distributions for a total of 20 min (Henry et al., in press). A significant decrease in blood pressure occurred with the 167 ng/kg/min dose, therefore the maximum tolerated dose was identified as 50 ng/kg/min. On the basis of myocardial perfusion imaging, no significant change was seen in the summed stress score at day 60, but there was a significant improvement in the summed rest score in the high-dose VEGF group at 14.7 versus 10.7 (p < 0.05). Five of the six patients receiving the higher doses demonstrated improvement in both stress and resting perfusion in two segments (Hendel, 2000a). All seven patients

TABLE 15-3. Clinical Trials with VEGFs in Myocardial Ischemia

Growth factor	Protocol	Results
VEGF$_{165}$ protein	IC for 20 min 5 to 167 ng/kg/min $n = 15$ (no placebo)	Angina: 13 of 15 improved Nuclear perfusion: decrease in summed rest score, no change in summed stress score Angiographic: collateral density increased in 7 of 7
VEGF$_{165}$ protein	IV for 1–4 h 17–100 ng/kg/min $n = 28$ (no placebo)	Nuclear perfusion: improved by 2 grades in 40% of rest defects, 20% of stress defects Angiographic: 38% increased collaterals
VEGF$_{165}$ protein	IC (20 min) + IV (4 h on days 3, 6, 9) Placebo, 17 ng/kg/min, 50 ng/kg/min $n = 178$ (63 placebo, 56 low dose, 59 high dose)	Improvements in angina and exercise time in all 3 groups at day 60, but no difference versus placebo Angina: significant improvement at day 120 in high-dose versus placebo ($P = 0.05$) Nuclear perfusion: no difference at day 60 Exercise time: 24-s improvement from baseline in placebo versus 48 s with high-dose VEGF at day 120 ($P = 0.15$)
Naked DNA-VEGF$_{165}$	IM via thoracotomy 125, 250, 500 μg $n = 30$ (no placebo)	Increase in serum VEGF levels Angina: 28 of 30 improved by 2 classes Nuclear perfusion: improvement in summed stress and summed rest scores Exercise time: 170-s improvement from baseline at day 180
Naked DNA-VEGF-2	IM via minithoracotomy 200, 800, 2,000 μg $n = 30$ (no placebo)	Angina: 2 class reduction in 40%, 60%, 70% at 4, 8, and 12 weeks Nuclear perfusion: 47% of stress and 63% rest scans improved in higher doses Exercise time: 126 second improvement from baseline at 12 weeks
Naked DNA-VEGF-2	IM via percutaneous 200, 800 μg $n = $ ongoing with placebo	Trial in progress
Adenovirus-VEGF$_{121}$	A) IM with CABG B) IM via minithoracotomy C) IM via video-assisted thoracoscopy 4×10^8–4×10^{10} vpu $n = 16$ (A), 6 (B), 10 (C) (no placebo)	Trend to improvements in angina class and exercise time at 6 months in 6 patients in group B
VEGF-A local delivery	Intra-arterial using dispatch A) Adenovirus VEGF-A (1–2×10^{10} vpu) B) Plasmid/liposome VEGF-A (200 μg) C) Placebo $n = $ ongoing in CAD and PVD	Trial in progress to prevent restenosis Temporary fever, increased C-reactive protein and liver function tests in some patients

CABG = coronary artery bypass graft; IC = intracoronary; IM = intramyocardial; IV = intravenous; VEGF = vascular endothelial growth factor; vpu = viral particle unit.

TABLE 15-4. Clinical Trials with FGF in Myocardial Ischemia

Growth Factor	Protocol	Results
FGF-1 protein	IM in combination with CABG 0.01 mg/kg $n = 40$ (20 placebo)	Significant improvement in digital subtraction angiography at 12 weeks and 3 years ($P < 0.005$) At 3 years improved angina and fewer medications in treatment group
FGF-2 protein	Perivascular beads in conjunction with CABG $n = 24$ (8-placebo, 8 10µg, 8 100µg)	Angina: 14/15 angina-free in treatment group vs. 4/7 in placebo group at 16 months Nuclear: Significant improvement in target defect size in 100µg/kg group
FGF-2 protein	IC for 20 min 0.33–48 µg/kg $n = 52$ (no placebo) IV 18–36 µg/kg $n = 14$ (no placebo)	Angina: Significant improvement in SAQ ($P < 0.001$) Nuclear: Significant reduction in per segment reversibility score (rest > s tress) Exercise time: 99-s improvement at day 57 and 123 s at day 180
FGF-2 protein	IC for 20 min Placebo, 0.3, 3.0, or 30 µg/kg $n = 337$	Angina: Favorable trend in angina class at day 90 ($P = 0.09$) with significant improvement in SAQ ($P = 0.008$) 3 µg/kg vs. placebo Nuclear: No significant improvement at day 90 Exercise time: No significant improvement at day 90 (63 s in 3 µg/kg vs. 45 s in placebo) Day 180 results pending
Adenovirus FGF-4	IC 3.2×10^8 to 3.2×10^{10} vpu $n = 79$ (3:1 active:placebo)	Trial in progress

CABG = coronary artery bypass graft; IC = intracoronary; IM = intramyocardial; IV = intravenous; VEGF = vascular endothelial growth factor; vpu = viral particle unit.

with follow-up angiograms had a significant improvement in collateral density score. In addition, 13 of the 15 patients had a significant decrease in angina class ($P = 0.002$).

In a second phase I trial, 28 patients received escalating intravenous doses of VEGF$_{165}$ protein (17–100 ng/kg/min for 1–4 hours) (Henry and Abraham, 2000). Similar to the intracoronary trial, 50 ng/kg/min was identified as the maximally tolerated dose based on the decrease in systolic pressure at 100 ng/kg/min. Myocardial perfusion imaging improved in at least two segments by two perfusion grades in 54% of patients. As in the intracoronary trial, the improvement was more impressive in resting perfusion (40% of rest defects vs. 20% of stress defects improved). An improvement in ejection fraction from 39.8% to 47.8% ($P = 0.09$) was noted at day 60 in the 10 patients who began the study with left ventricular ejection frac-

tion <50%. A blinded angiographic assessment based on follow-up angiograms at day 60 demonstrated more collateral vessels in 38% of patients (Gibson et al., 1999). In both phase I trials VEGF$_{165}$ protein was well tolerated with no significant adverse events such as cancer, retinopathy, or angiographic evidence for progression of atherosclerotic disease.

The results of these trials led to the phase II Vascular Endothelial Growth Factor in Ischemia for Vascular Angiogenesis (VIVA) trial (Henry et al., 1999). A total of 178 patients were randomized to receive placebo or low-dose (17 ng/kg/min) or high-dose (50 ng/kg/min) VEGF$_{165}$ protein for 20 min intracoronary, followed by 4-h intravenous infusions of the same dose on days 3, 6, and 9. At day 60 all three groups had significant improvement in exercise time, quality of life, and angina class. In contrast, at day 120, there was a loss of benefit in exercise time, angina class, and quality of life scores in the placebo group, whereas the patients receiving high-dose VEGF$_{165}$ demonstrated an ongoing improvement in all three measures. This resulted in a significant improvement in angina class at 120 days in the high-dose VEGF group ($P = 0.0$) and a trend for improvement in exercise time with 24-s improvement over baseline in the placebo group versus 48-s improvement in the high-dose VEGF$_{165}$ group ($P = 0.15$). The drug was well tolerated with no significant adverse effects. In contrast, there were two deaths, three newly diagnosed cancers, and one worsening retinopathy in the placebo group. No significant improvement was seen in myocardial perfusion scans at day 60.

In a substudy of the trial, 106 patients at 13 sites agreed to remain blinded to treatment assignment for 1 year to determine the long-term effects of placebo as well as the long-term safety and efficacy of VEGF$_{165}$ protein (Henry et al., 2000). In regard to angina class, by 1 year the placebo group was no longer improved from baseline (mean angina class 2.8 ± 0.6 vs. 2.4 ± 1.6), whereas the patients treated with high-dose VEGF$_{165}$ protein continued to have a significant improvement from baseline (2.7 ± 0.8 vs. 1.9 ± 1.3; $P < 0.001$). The clinical events at 1 year are shown in Table 15-5. Although there was no significant difference in death or myocardial infarction in the three groups, there were fewer overall events in patients treated with VEGF$_{165}$, driven primarily by the need for less subsequent revascularization. Four patients in the placebo group had developed cancer by 1 year, compared with one patient who received low-dose VEGF$_{165}$ protein.

TABLE 15-5.   VIVA One-Year Clinical Events

% of Patients	Placebo	17	50
Death	5.3	3.1	0
MI	2.7	0	5.9
Revascularization	18.9	9.7	8.8
Cancer	10.5	2.9	0
Any Event	31.6	16.1	*11.8

* $P < 0.04$ high dose vs. placebo.

On the basis of the results of the VIVA trial, it appears that VEGF$_{165}$ protein is safe and well tolerated with no significant adverse effects when followed to 1 year. In addition, a significant improvement in angina was demonstrated at both 4 months and 1 year, with a trend for improvement in exercise time at 4 months in patients receiving high-dose VEGF$_{165}$ protein. Results of this trial have important implications for the design of future angiogenesis trials. For example, they clearly demonstrate the critical importance of a placebo group for the interpretation of positive results as well as the risk of potential complications of angiogenic therapy. This point is well illustrated by the four patients who developed cancer in the placebo group. The loss of the initial improvements noted in the placebo group as well as the ongoing improvement over time observed in the patients treated with VEGF$_{165}$ protein provide important lessons for the timing of end points for future trials.

15.2.2. VEGF Gene Therapy

15.2.2.1. VEGF$_{165}$

The initial results of direct intramyocardial injection of naked plasmid DNA encoding VEGF$_{165}$ during a mini-left anterior thoracotomy in five patients demonstrated improvements in angina, use of nitroglycerin, and dobutamine sestamibi nuclear imaging (Losordo et al., 1998). A total of 30 patients received 125, 250, or 500 µg ($n = 10$ for each dose group) in 4×2-cc-aliquot intramyocardial injections (Symes et al., 1999; Vale et al., 1999). The initial procedure was well tolerated with no perioperative ischemia, ventricular arrhythmia, or hemodynamic instability. Mean hospital stay was 3.9 days, and there was one late death related to severe pulmonary disease and prolonged intubation. Successful gene transfer was demonstrated by an increase in plasma VEGF protein levels from 26.9 ± 3.2 pg/ml at baseline to 82.8 ± 4.8 pg/ml at 14 days after treatment, with a return to baseline plasma VEGF levels by day 90. An improvement from 240 to 410 s ($P < 0.05$) was seen in exercise time. In addition, 28 of 30 patients improved by at least two angina classes at day 180. In 23 of 24 patients with follow-up myocardial perfusion imaging, the summed stress scores improved from 19.4 ± 3.7 to 15.9 ± 3.4 ($P = 0.025$) and the summed rest scores improved from 15.3 ± 3.5 to 11.7 ± 2.7 ($P = 0.028$). The investigators reported a reduction in ischemic myocardium as measured by left ventricular electromechanical (NOGA) mapping, from 6.45 ± 1.4 to $0.95 \pm 0.4\,cm^2$ (Vale et al., 2000a). Similar to the VIVA trial, patients continued to improve over time, with 33%, 44%, and 70% angina free at 2, 3, and 6 months, respectively.

15.2.2.2. VEGF-2

A similar phase I dose escalation study has been completed using naked DNA encoding VEGF-2 in 30 patients receiving 200, 800, or $2000\,\mu g$ ($n = 10$ for each dose group) via direct intramyocardial injection during a minithoracotomy (Isner, presented at ACC, 2000). The gene was well tolerated, with no significant adverse events related to study drug but one perioperative death from cardiac arrest. Overall, patients treated with the VEGF-2 gene had a 1.6-min improvement in exercise time at 8 weeks and 2.1 min at 12 weeks. The percentage of patients with a two-class reduction in angina was 40%, 60% and 70% at 4, 8, and 12 weeks respectively. As shown by myocardial perfusion imaging, the two higher doses had more improvement seen in both stress (47%) and rest imaging (63%) than did the 200-μg dose (38% for both stress and rest) (Hendel et al., 2000b). In an ongoing trial, an additional 25 patients have received direct intramyocardial injections of the plasmid for VEGF-2 via a percutaneous approach using the NOGA system (Vale et al., 2000b). Multicenter trials with placebo-controlled groups (double blind with the percutaneous approach) have begun for both methods of delivery.

15.2.2.3. VEGF$_{121}$

The early (Rosengart et al., 1999a) and 6-month (Rosengart et al., 1999b) results of direct intramyocardial injection of an adenovirus vector expressing VEGF$_{121}$ have been reported. Fifteen patients received escalating doses of virus [4×10^8 to 4×10^{10} particle units (pu)] as an adjunct to CABG, whereas six patients received the virus as sole therapy ($4 \times 10^{10}\,pu$) via a minithoracotomy. There were two postoperative deaths [anterior myocardial infarction (MI) related to graft closure and complications of an atheroembolic event in the ileocolic artery] and one late sudden death in the CABG group, with no significant perioperative complications or deaths in the sole-therapy treatment group. All six patients receiving the vector as sole therapy had an improvement in angina class and four of six had improvements in perfusion scans, but it is difficult to assess clinical improvement related to the growth factor in the patients who were bypassed. There was no increase in plasma VEGF levels, no hypotension, and no evidence of viral shedding from any site in any patient. An increase in neutralizing antibodies to adenovirus was noted in most patients but without evidence for systemic immune-related toxicity. An additional 10 patients received $4 \times 10^{10}\,pu$ via video-assisted epicardial injections using a minithoracotomy or thoracoscopy (Rosengart et al., 1999c). Multicenter, double-blind, placebo-controlled trials using a percutaneous approach have begun.

15.2.3. VEGF-A Local Delivery

An ongoing trial is randomizing patients to adenovirus VEGF-A, plasmid/liposome VEGF-A, or placebo via a local delivery catheter in conjunction with angioplasty to prevent restenosis. Preliminary data regarding safety show transient fever, increases in C-reactive protein, liver function tests, leukopenia, and thrombocytopenia in some patients. Efficacy results are not currently available (Ylä-Herttuala et al., 2000).

15.2.4. FGF Protein Therapy

15.2.4.1. FGF-1

The first human trial of myocardial angiogenesis utilized intramyocardial injection of FGF-1 protein as an adjunct to CABG

(Schumacher et al., 1998a, 1998b). All patients received an internal mammary artery (IMA) graft to the left anterior descending coronary artery (LAD) and had a stenosis in the distal LAD or its branches. The 40 patients were then randomized to an intramyocardial injection of heat-denatured FGF-1 versus FGF-1 (0.01 mg/kg) distal to the IMA insertion.

The procedure was well tolerated, with no deaths or perioperative myocardial infarctions. Because all patients were bypassed clinical improvement was not assessed, but follow-up digital subtraction angiography at 12 weeks demonstrated a significant improvement in quantitative gray value analysis of contrast medium accumulation ($P < 0.005$) consistent with growth of new collateral blood vessels in patients receiving FGF-1 protein.

The 3-year follow up on 33 patients demonstrated a consistent increase in vascular density by digital subtraction angiography ($P < 0.005$) (Stegmann et al., 2000). There were three deaths (2 cerebral ischemia, 1 unknown) in the FGF-1-treated group and four deaths (1 cerebral ischemia, 1 MI, and 1 unknown) in the control group. Patients treated with FGF-1 were more likely to have class I angina (94% vs. 75%) and were less likely to require antianginal medications. Finally, there was no evidence for uncontrolled or pathologic angiogenesis in the FGF-1-treated patients.

15.2.4.2. FGF-2

In a phase I dose escalation trial, 52 patients received a 20-min intracoronary (10 min each into 2 coronary distributions) infusion of FGF-2 (Laham et al., 2000). Doses ranged from 0.33 μg/kg to 48 μg/kg. Because of significant hypotension in two patients at 48 μg/kg, 36 μg/kg was determined to be the maximally tolerated dose. There were four deaths; three were cardiovascular, with two sudden and one following cardiac transplant after recent myocardial infarction. One patient died from a large cell lymphoma, and a second patient was diagnosed with metastatic adenocarcinoma over 1 year after treatment. Finally, four patients sustained MI.

Transient leukocytosis was frequently seen in half the patients at doses ≥24 μg/kg, and proteinuria occurred in 7.8% of patients.

A significant improvement was noted in the angina frequency domain of the Seattle Angina Questionnaire ($P < 0.001$). The mean exercise time improved from 510 ± 24 s at baseline to 609 ± 26 s at day 57 ($P < 0.001$) and 633 ± 24 s at day 180 ($P < 0.001$). Myocardial perfusion, as shown by magnetic resonance imaging of delayed contrast arrival, improved from 15.4 ± 0.8% at baseline to 5.6% ± 7.0% at day 57 and 4.9 ± 0.8% at day 180. Overall left ventricular function and target wall thickening were also improved by magnetic resonance imaging. In the same phase I study, the results (Udelson et al., 2000) of myocardial perfusion imaging were reported at baseline and 30, 60, and 180 days after FGF-2 protein administration in 45 patients receiving intracoronary infusions and 14 patients with intravenous infusions. A significant reduction in per-segment reversibility score was demonstrated: 1.7 ± 0.4 at baseline, 1.1 ± 0.6 at day 29, 1.2 ± 0.7 at day 57, and 1.1 ± 0.7 at day 180. The 37 patients with resting hypoperfusion had significant improvement shown by the per-segment rest perfusion score (1.5 ± 0.5 at baseline, 1.0 ± 0.8 at day 29, 1.0 ± 0.8 at day 57, and 1.1 ± 0.9 at day 180). In summary, there was an attenuation of stress-induced ischemia and a significant improvement in resting myocardial perfusion. Although the results were promising, the trial was a phase I dose-finding trial without a placebo group and data for exercise time and magnetic resonance perfusion were incomplete.

The FIRST trial (FGF-2 initiating revascularization support trial) is the largest double-blind placebo-controlled trial in the field of angiogenesis. Three hundred and thirty-seven patients were enrolled from October 1998 to October 1999. Patients were randomized into four groups for a 20-min intracoronary infusion of placebo or 0.3, 3.0, or 30 μg/kg of FGF-2. The primary end point was a change in exercise time from baseline to day 90. Secondary end points included exercise time at day 180, quality of life scores at both day 90 and day 180, and changes in nuclear perfusion at day 90 and day 180. The results from day 90 have been reported, but the results from day 180 are pending. There was no significant improvement in the primary end point, but there was a trend in the 3 μg/kg dose ($P = 0.22$) with a 63-a improvement compared to 45 a for the placebo group. In a post hoc analysis, patients who were >63 years old had significant improvement from 40s in the placebo group to nearly 80s in the 3 μg/kg group ($P = 0.056$), whereas there was no significant improvement in patients ≤63 years old. This was likely caused by high baseline exercise times in the healthier, young patients. Although all four groups had a significant improvement in angina class at day 30, there was no significant difference between groups ($P = 0.12$), but a strong trend for improvement was seen at day 90 ($P = 0.09$). In addition, there was improvement in the angina frequency domain of the Seattle Angina Questionnaire: $P = 0.057$ for the entire group and $P = 0.008$ for the 3 μg/kg group versus placebo. In another analysis, patients with angina frequency scores of >40 at baseline (more angina) had a significant improvement. In contrast, patients with angina frequency scores <40 (less angina) at baseline had no significant improvement. As with the VIVA trial, there were no significant safety concerns. By day 180, the number of deaths, MIs, and cancer (respectively 1, 5, 1 for placebo; 1, 2, 0 for 0.3 μg/kg; 3, 5, 1 for 3.0 μg/kg; and 1, 5, 1 for 30 μg/kg) were similar in each group.

While the final results of the FIRST trial are pending, it appears that the results of FIRST are similar to VIVA, with improvements in angina by both angina class and angina frequency and trends toward improvement in exercise time (comparisons of the two trials in Table 15-6). In summary, after the first two moderate sized placebo-controlled trials, therapy with two different angiogenic protein growth factors appears to be safe at least in the short term, with modest evidence for efficacy, especially in certain subgroups.

In a novel approach to therapeutic angiogenesis, Laham and colleagues inserted FGF-2 in sustained-release heparin-alginate

TABLE 15-6. VIVA—FIRST Comparisons

	VIVA		FIRST	
Patients	178		337	
TIME	D60	D120	D90	D180
ETT	NS	0.17	0.22	NA
Angina	NS	0.04	0.09	NA
SAQ	NS	0.06	0.057	NA
Nuclear	Neg D60 (Low summed rest)		Neg D90 (+ in bad ischemia)	
Safety	++		++	

microcapsules into the epicardial fat of ischemic and viable but ungraftable myocardium (Laham et al., 1999; Selke et al., 1998). Twenty-four patients were randomized to 10 μg of FGF-2 ($n = 8$), 100 μg of FGF-2 ($n = 8$), or placebo ($n = 8$).

There were two perioperative deaths, one in the control group due to graft closure and subsequent MI and the other in the 100 μg group due to failure to wean off bypass (preoperative EF of 20%). Two patients had Q-wave MIs in the target area of myocardium. One was in the control group, and the other in the 10 μg group. One patient in the 10 μg group had an MI in a nontarget area of the myocardium.

Clinical follow-up was available in the 22 surviving patients at an average of 16 months (±6.8). In the treatment groups, 14 of 15 patients were angina free, compared with 4 of 7 in the control group. Nuclear perfusion imaging is difficult to interpret because of a change in methods midway through the study, but it did show a statistically significant improvement in the 100 μg group (target area defect size $19.2 \pm 5.0\%$ to $9.1 \pm 5.9\%$; $P = 0.01$) compared with control patients ($20.7 \pm 3.7\%$ to $23.8 \pm 5.7\%$) or with patients in the 10 μg cohort ($19.2 \pm 5.0\%$ to $16.9 \pm 8.1\%$). In addition, the authors reported an improvement in collateral perfusion as measured by MRI in four patients.

15.2.5. FGF Gene Therapy

A phase I, randomized, double-blind, placebo-controlled, dose-escalation trial was performed using Ad5FGF-4. Seventy-nine patients were enrolled in a 3:1 active drug to placebo ratio using doses from 3.2×10^8 to 3.2×10^{10} viral particles, increasing by half-log increments. An initial press release reported an improvement in exercise treadmill time, but complete data have not been reported at this time.

15.3. FUTURE CHALLENGES

Although the results of these initial clinical trials suggest at least short-term safety and promising signs of efficacy, a large number of unanswered questions remain, including the relative safety and efficacy of protein versus gene therapy and the optimal dose, dosing schedule, and route of administration. It is unclear which angiogenic growth factor or combination will result in the most effective therapeutic angiogenesis. Likewise, the relative safety and efficacy of each growth factor may depend on the route of administration and protein versus gene therapy. Given the complex process of angiogenesis, it is perhaps naive to believe that a single dose of a particular growth factor will be uniformly effective. The synergistic effects of VEGF and FGF have been reported in animal models. In addition, angiopoietin-1, a ligand for the endothelial cell-specific Tie2 receptor, has been shown to promote VEGF-mediated angiogenesis, whereas angiopoietin-2 acts as a naturally occurring antagonist (Asahara et al., 1998). Inhibitors of angiogenesis such as metalloproteinase antagonists, soluble receptors, asymmetric dimethylarginine (ADMA), angiostatin, endostatin, and thrombospondin-I may influence the effectiveness of exogenous growth factors. Clinical factors such as age, diabetes, or use of medications (angiotensin-converting enzyme inhibitors, nitrates, heparin, etc) may also influence response to the growth factors. For example, in the phase I peripheral vascular disease trials with $VEGF_{165}$, young patients with Buerger disease have a significantly better response to angiogenic therapy than older patients with atherosclerotic disease (Isner et al., 1998), and several studies indi-

cate that diabetics may have impaired angiogenesis. It will be critical to closely analyze the results of the early clinical trials for insights into responders and nonresponders. In the future, it is likely that we will be able to identify a particular patient's defect in angiogenesis and target our therapeutic regimen to that need.

15.4. CONCLUSION

Therapeutic angiogenesis is an exciting new approach to myocardial revascularization. Preclinical studies and initial phase I results are encouraging, and the three randomized double-blind, placebo-controlled angiogenesis trials suggest modest clinical benefit with short-term safety. Although many questions remain unanswered, therapeutic angiogenesis has the potential to revolutionize our approach to patients with severe myocardial ischemia and limited treatment options.

References

Asahara T, Chen D, Takahashi T et al. Tie2 receptor ligands, angiopoietin-1 and angiopoietin-2, modulate VEGF-induced postnatal neovascularization. *Circ Res* 1998; 83: 342–343.

Ferrara N, Davis-Smyth T. The biology of vascular endothelial growth factor. *Endocrinol Rev* 1997; 18: 4–25.

Ferrara H. Vascular endothelial growth factor: molecular and biological aspects. *Curr Top Microbiol Immunol* 1999; 237: 1–30.

Gibson CM, Simons M, Giordano FJ et al. Magnitude and location of new angiographically apparent coronary collaterals following intravenous VEGF administration (abstract). *J Am Coll Cardiol* 1999; 33: 384A.

Giordano FJ. Angiogenesis: mechanisms, modulation and targeted imaging. *J Nucl Cardiol* 1999; 6: 664–671.

Hendel RC, Henry TD, Rocha-Singh K et al. Effect of intracoronary recombinant human vascular endothelial growth factor on myocardial perfusion: evidence for a dose-dependent effect. *Circulation* 2000a; 101: 118–121.

Hendel RC, Vale PR, Losordo DW et al. The effects of VEGF-2 gene therapy on rest and stress myocardial perfusion: results of serial SPECT imaging (abstract). *Circulation* 2000b; 102: II-769.

Henry TD. Therapeutic angiogenesis. *Br Med J* 1999; 318: 1536–1539.

Henry TD, Annex BH, Azrin MA et al. Final results of the VIVA trial of rhVEGF for human therapeutic angiogenesis (abstract). *Circulation* 1999; 100: I-476.

Henry TD, Abraham JA. Review of preclinical and clinical results with vascular endothelial growth factors for therapeutic angiogenesis. *Curr Interv Cardiol Rep* 2000; 2: 228–241.

Henry T, McKendall GR, Azrin MA et al., VIVA trial: One-year followup (abstract). *Circulation* 2000; 102: II-309.

Henry TD, Rocha-Singh K, Isner JM et al. Intracoronary administration of recombinant human vascular endothelial growth factor (rhVEGF) to patients with coronary artery disease. *Am Heart J.* In press.

Iruela-Arispe ML, Dvorak HF. Angiogenesis: a dynamic balance of stimulators and inhibitors. *Thromb Haemost* 1997; 78: 672–677.

Isner JM, Baumgartner I, Rauh G et al. Treatment of thromboangitis obliterans (Buerger's disease) by intramuscular gene transfer of vascular endothelial growth factor: preliminary clinical results. *J Vasc Surg* 1998; 28: 964–973.

Isner JM, Asahara T. Angiogenesis and vasculogenesis as therapeutic strategies for postnatal neovascularization. *J Clin Invest* 1999; 103: 1231–1236.

Laham RJ, Sellke FW, Edelman ER et al. Local perivascular delivery of basic fibroblast growth factor in patients undergoing coronary bypass surgery: results of a phase I randomized, double-blind, placebo-controlled trial. *Circulation* 1999; 100: 1865–1871.

Laham RJ, Rezaee M, Post M et al. Intrapericardial delivery of fibroblast growth factor-2 induces neovascularization in a porcine model of chronic myocardial ischemia. *J Pharmacol Exp Ther* 2000; 292: 795–802.

Losordo DW, Vale PR, Symes JF et al. Gene therapy for myocardial angiogenesis: initial clinical results with direct myocardial infarction of phVEGF$_{165}$ as sole therapy for myocardial ischemia. *Circulation* 1998; 98: 2800–2804.

Mukherjee D, Bhatt DL, Roe MT et al. Direct myocardial revascularization and angiogenesis—How many patients might be eligible? *Am J Cardiol* 1999; 84: 598–600.

Neufeld G, Cohen T, Gengrinovitch S et al. Vascular endothelial growth factor (VEGF) and its receptors. *FASEB J* 1999; 13: 9–22.

Rosengart T, Lee L, Patel S et al. Angiogenesis gene therapy: Phase I assessment of direct intramyocardial administration of an adenovirus vector expressing VEGF$_{121}$ cDNA to individuals with clinically significant severe coronary artery disease. *Circulation* 1999a; 100: 468–474.

Rosengart T, Lee LY, Patel SR et al. Six-month assessment of a phase I trial of angiogenic gene therapy for the treatment of coronary artery disease using direct intramyocardial administration of an adenovirus vector expressing the VEGF$_{121}$ cDNA. *Ann Surg* 1999b; 230: 466–472.

Rosengart T, Lee L, Port J et al. Video assisted epicardial delivery of angiogenic gene therapy to the human myocardium utilizing an adenovirus vector encoding for VEGF$_{121}$ (abstract). *Circulation* 1999c; 100: I-770.

Schumacher B, Pecher P, von Specht BU et al., Induction of neoangiogenesis in ischemic myocardium by human growth factors. First clinical results of a new treatment of coronary artery disease. *Circulation* 1998a; 97: 645–650.

Schumacher B, Pecher P, Stegmann T. The stimulation of neoangiogenesis in ischemic human heart by growth factor FGF: first clinical results. *J Cardiovasc Surg* 1998b; 39: 783–789.

Sellke FW, Wang SY, Friedman M et al. Basic FGF enhances endothelium-dependent relaxation of the collateral-perfused coronary microcirculation. *Am J Physiol* 1994; 267: H1303–H1311.

Selke FW, Laham, RJ, Edelman ER et al. Therapeutic angiogenesis with basic fibroblast growth factor: technique and early results. *Ann Thorac Surg* 1998; 65: 1540–1544.

Stegmann TJ, Hoppert T, Schlurmann W et al. First angiogenic treatment of coronary heart disease by FGF-1: long-term results after 3 years. *Cardiac and Vascular Regeneration* 2000; 1: 5–10.

Symes JF, Losordo DW, Vale PR et al. Gene therapy with vascular endothelial growth factor for inoperable coronary artery disease. *Ann Thorac Surg* 1999; 68: 830–837.

Udelson JE, Dilsizian V, Laham RJ et al. Therapeutic angiogenesis with recombinant fibroblast growth factor-2 improves stress and rest myocardial perfusion abnormalities in patients with severe symptomatic chronic coronary artery disease. *Circulation* 2000; 102: 1605–1610.

Vale PR, Losordo DW, Dunnington C et al. Direct myocardial infarction of phVEGF$_{165}$: results of complete patient cohort in phase I/II clinical trial (abstract). *Circulation* 1999; 100: I-477.

Vale PR, Losordo DW, Milliken CE et al. Left ventricular electromechanical mapping to assess efficacy of phVEGF$_{165}$ gene transfer for therapeutic angiogenesis in chronic myocardial ischemia. *Circulation* 2000a; 102: 965–974.

Vale PR, Losordo DW, Milliken CE et al. Randomized, placebo-controlled clinical study of percutaneous catheter-based left ventricular endocardial gene transfer of VEGF-2 for myocardial angiogenesis in patients with chronic myocardial ischemia (abstract). *Circulation* 2000b; 102: II-563.

Ware JA, Simons M. Angiogenesis in ischemic heart disease. Inducing the formation of new blood vessels—a novel approach to treating myocardial ischemia. *Nat Med* 1997; 3: 158–164.

Ylä-Herttuala S, Martin JF. Cardiovascular gene therapy. *Lancet* 2000; 355: 213–222.

Ylä-Herttuala S, Laitinen M, Virtanen AI et al. Safety of VEGF gene therapy with adenovirus and plasmid/liposome vectors in coronary and peripheral vascular disease patients (abstract). *Circulation* 2000; 102: II-34.

16

The Coronary Veins As an Alternative Access for Gene Transfer and Angiogenesis by Selective Pressure-Regulated Retroinfusion

Peter Boekstegers, M.D., Georges von Degenfeld, M.D., Wolfgang Franz, M.D., and Christian Kupatt, M.D.

Internal Medicine I, Klinikum Großhadern
Ludwig-Maximilians-University of Munich
Munich, Germany

SUMMARY

Selective retroinfusion was developed in 1990 to improve efficacy and feasibility of retrograde catheter approach and was found to be dependent on several factors, including pressure regulation of the retrograde flow.

As a consequence, retrograde blood flow has been adapted to the individual coronary venous system by using a pressure-regulated device for selective retroinfusion called Myoprotect®.

Selective pressure-regulated retroinfusion can target and enhance drug delivery to ischemic myocardium as well as enhance myocardial concentrations of β-blockers and calcium antagonists.

Retrograde administration into the vein may target the vessel segments most receptive and responsive to angiogenic growth factors.

As a result of this, pressure-regulated retroinfusion may target regional delivery of recombinant growth factors, DNA-carrying liposomes, or viral gene vectors encoding for angiogenic proteins.

Liposome-mediated DNA delivery by selective retroinfusion has been shown to be feasible, and therefore this strategy could be used for the delivery of angiogenic growth factors.

16.1. INTRODUCTION

Early work on catheter-based percutaneous retroperfusion of coronary veins was initiated by Meerbaum et al. (1976) and Mohl et al. (1984). It was focused on a nonselective treatment using a balloon catheter placed in the coronary sinus or the great cardiac vein. Although ECG-synchronized diastolic retroperfusion of the coronary sinus reached

Myocardial Revascularization: Novel Percutaneous Approaches, Edited by George S. Abela.
ISBN 0-471-36166-6 Copyright © 2002 Wiley-Liss, Inc.

clinical application between 1986 and 1991 (Boekstegers et al., 1990; Costantini et al., 1991; Kar et al., 1991; O'Byrne et al., 1991), its relatively low efficacy and complex procedure limited widespread clinical use.

As a consequence of the limited success of synchronized diastolic retroperfusion, selective retroinfusion was developed in 1990 (Boekstegers et al., 1994) with the aim of improving efficacy and feasibility of the retrograde catheter-based approach through the coronary veins. In experimental as well as clinical studies during the past 10 years, we learned that the efficacy of retroinfusion was clearly dependent on two factors.

First, selective catheterization of the vein draining the ischemic myocardium was necessary to facilitate and target retrograde delivery to the ischemic myocardium without affecting antegrade blood flow to nonischemic tissue at the same time (Boekstegers et al., 1998). Access to different myocardial regions was possible through the coronary veins (Fig. 16-1), as has been demonstrated in high-risk patients undergoing retroinfusion-supported stent implantation (Oh et al., 1992).

Second, pressure regulation of retrograde flow (Fig. 16-2) was a prerequisite to optimize efficacy by avoiding under- or overperfusion of the ischemic myocardium. Myocardial protection was found to be dependent on the individual venous anatomy, reflecting different venous capacities and the existence of arteriovenous and venovenous shunts as well as thebesian veins. Furthermore, the efficacy

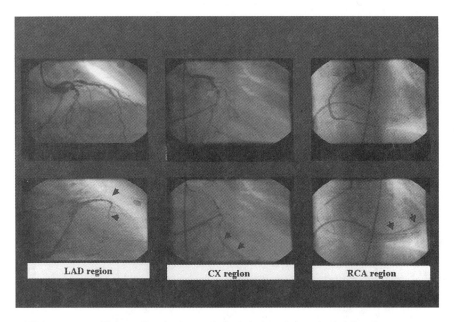

FIGURE 16-1. Selective catheterization and retroinfusion of the vein draining the ischemic region in three patients. Left upper panel: patient with a proximal stenosis of the left anterior descending (LAD) artery (red arrow), retroinfusion catheter placed in the anterior cardiac vein. Left lower panel: selective retroinfusion of the anterior cardiac vein (blue arrows) during balloon inflation in the proximal LAD artery. Middle upper panel: patient with an occluded LAD artery and a high grade stenosis of the circumflex (CX) artery (red arrow), retroinfusion catheter placed in the vein accompanying the CX artery. Right lower panel: selective retroinfusion of the CX vein (blue arrows) during balloon inflation in the CX artery. Right upper panel: patient with a high-grade stenosis of the right coronary artery (RCA) (red arrow), retroinfusion catheter placed in the vein accompanying the RCA. Right lower panel: selective retroinfusion of the vein accompanying the RCA (blue arrows) during balloon inflation in the RCA.

of retroinfusion was dependent on coronary venous pressure in studies with nonpulsatile (Giehrl et al., 1996) and pulsatile (Giehrl et al., 2000) retrograde flow (Fig. 16-3).

As a consequence, retrograde blood flow has been adapted to the individual coronary venous system by using a pressure-regulated device for selective retroinfusion (Myoprotect®).

The feasibility and high efficacy of selective pressure-regulated retroinfusion of the coronary veins (Myoprotect®) has been shown in a clinical pilot study during acute myocardial ischemia (Boekstegers et al., 1998). Despite complete occlusion of the artery, preservation of 70–80% of baseline flow and regional myocardial function was possible during a 10-min (Oh et al., 1992) to 1-h ischemic period. More recently, the Myoprotect® system has been successfully used in acute myocardial infarction and cardiogenic shock. Table 16-1 summarizes the clinical applications and sites of interventions in 258 patients treated by

selective pressure-regulated retroinfusion so far (Giehrl et al., 2000).

16.2. TARGETING OF REGIONAL DRUG DELIVERY TO ISCHEMIC MYOCARDIUM BY SELECTIVE RETROINFUSION

Regional drug delivery by selective pressure-regulated retroinfusion relies on the concept that tissue binding and myocardial concentrations of a drug can be substantially increased by prolonging contact time of the drug with the myocardium as a consequence of the delivery through the coronary veins. Indeed, angiographic studies in pigs and humans showed that pressure-regulated retroinfusion is able to prolong passage time of contrast agent by about 10-fold compared with antegrade delivery (Boekstegers et al., 2000) (Fig. 16-4). Selective retroinfusion of coronary veins enhances myocardial concentrations of β-blockers and calcium

TABLE 6-1.

| Age | 67 ± 10 years | |
Artery	Vein (selective retroinfusion)	Number of patients
LAD	Anterior cardiac vein	205
RCA	Right coronary vein	10
CX/Marginal	Circumflex/marginal vein	29
Main stem	Great cardiac vein	25
Acute MI	Anterior cardiac vein	5
Cardiogenic shock	Anterior cardiac vein	3

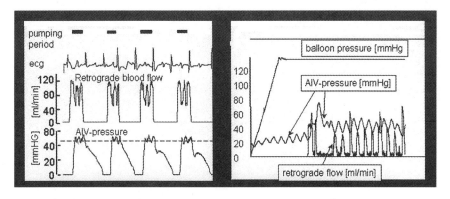

FIGURE 16-2. (Left) Selective pressure-regulated suction and retroinfusion triggered by the ECG. AIV = anterior cardiac vein. (Modified from Boekstegers et al., 1998). (Right) Continuous selective pressure-regulated retroinfusion without suction during balloon occlusion of the vein. (Modified from Boekstegers et al., 2000).

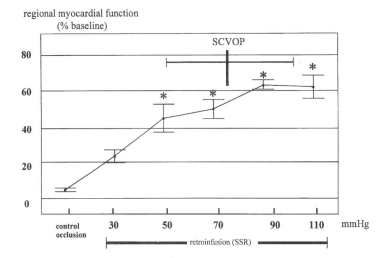

FIGURE 16-3. Pressure-dependent efficacy of selective retroinfusion. Regional myocardial function (subendocardial segment shortening in the ischemic region) during balloon occlusion of the LAD supported by selective pressure-regulated retroinfusion using different preset pressures in a randomized protocol. SSR = selective suction and retroinfusion; SCVOP = systolic coronary venous occlusion pressure. *$P < 0.001$ vs. control.

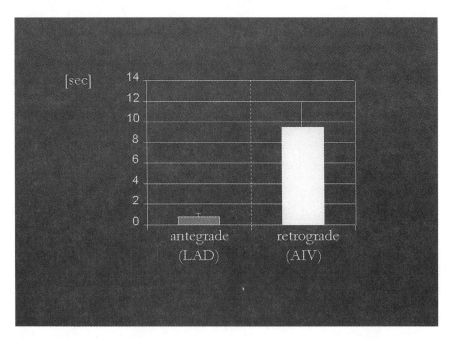

FIGURE 16-4. Comparison of the passage time of contrast agent between antegrade and retrograde delivery in pigs.

antagonists in ischemic myocardium, as has been shown previously by other groups (Haga et al., 1994; Hatori et al., 1991; Ryden et al., 1991). In addition, we could demonstrate that pressure-regulated retroinfusion was able to target dobutamine selectively to the ischemic myocardium without systemic effects (von Degenfeld et al., 1997). Similar results were obtained in patients undergoing retroinfusion-supported high-risk percutaneous transluminal coronary angioplasty (PTCA) showing inotropic effects of dobutamine in the targeted left anterior descending artery (LAD) region during ischemia (Boekstegers et al., 1998). Furthermore, regional delivery of an angiotensin-converting enzyme inhibitor during ischemia was well tolerated and attenuated regional leukocyte activation as determined by MAC-1 expression (Kupatt et al., 1999). From these observations we infer that selective pressure-regulated retroinfusion can target and enhance drug delivery to ischemic myocardium in patients, which is of increasing interest for gene transfer and therapeutic angiogenesis.

16.3. GENE TRANSFER TO ISCHEMIC MYOCARDIUM BY SELECTIVE RETROINFUSION

Previous attempts of percutaneous transluminal gene delivery (PTGD) included systemic intravenous and intra-arterial injections (Barr et al., 1997; Feldman et al., 1997; Steg et al., 1997). Direct delivery of adenoviral vectors into coronary arteries resulted in relatively low myocardial gene expression in a canine model (Feldman et al., 1997). For efficient gene transfer very high viral titers were required, carrying the worrisome risk of undesired effects in tissues other than the myocardium. An alternative catheter-based gene delivery device using pericardial application of adenoviral vectors limited systemic contamination. However, gene expression was restricted to the parietal and visceral pericardium (Barr et al., 1997; Lamping et al., 1997; March et al., 1999). Although some focal areas of the epicardium were reached after pretreatment with doxycyclin (March et al., 1999), the pericardial approach does not yet seem to be sufficient to provide myocardial gene expression with homogeneous transmural distribution.

Apparently, one of the major limitations of intravascular delivery for myocardial gene transfer in larger animals, in contrast to tissue culture systems (Giordano et al., 1997; Hajjar et al., 1997; Rothmann et al., 1996), is the short adhesion time of the adenoviral vectors with the endothelial cells and cardiomyocytes. Prolongation of the viral adhesion time, as shown by intramyocardial injections and local gene delivery into the wall of coronary arteries, substantially increased transfection and gene expression (French et al., 1994a, 1994b; Rothmann et al., 1996). To solve this limitation of intra-arterial gene delivery, we sought to develop a novel approach of percutaneous transluminal retrograde gene delivery (PTRGD) through the coronary veins.

Following the concept of regional drug delivery by selective retroinfusion, the efficacy and selectivity of PTRGD using continuous pressure-regulated retroinfusion (Fig. 16-2) was studied in pigs (Boekstegers et al., 2000). To optimize percutaneous transluminal adenoviral gene delivery, different approaches for antegrade intracoronary and retrograde coronary venous delivery were compared in four experimental groups in this study (Fig. 16-5).

Previous studies in larger animals using intracoronary delivery without ischemia and similar vector concentrations found negligible levels of gene expression (Magovern et al., 1996). To test whether ischemia can increase viral transfection, intracoronary delivery was performed during ischemia. Despite delivery with and without ischemia (groups A and B) an equally distributed but nonsignificant slight increase in luciferase activity resulted after 7 days [159 ± 156 vs. 50 ± 81 RLU/mg protein, LAD vs. circumflex artery (CX) region] (Fig. 16-6).

To test whether retrograde gene delivery can increase viral transfection, the viral vectors were applied through the coronary veins in groups C and D. In contrast to antegrade delivery during ischemia, continuous pressure-regulated retroinfusion into the anterior cardiac vein substantially increased mean reporter gene expression in the LAD region (23.425 ± 25.238 RLU/mg protein; $P < 0.001$) (group D, Fig. 16-6). Apparently, gene transfer was selectively targeted to the LAD region because luciferase activity was at background level in the CX region. In another series of experiments (group E), repeated

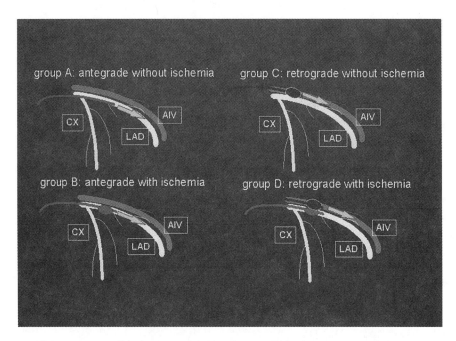

FIGURE 16-5.   Experimental groups for gene transfer by selective pressure-regulated retroinfusion. LAD = left anterior descending artery; CX = circumflex artery; AIV = anterior cardiac vein.

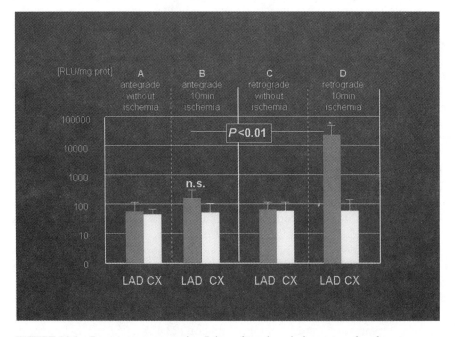

FIGURE 16-6.   Reporter gene expression 7 days after adenoviral gene transfer of 2.5×10^9 pfu Ad.rsv-Luc using antegrade or retrograde delivery with or without 10 min of ischemia. LAD = left anterior descending artery, CX = circumflex artery, n.s. = nonsignificant, p = P-value. (Modified from Boekstegers et al., 2000).

retrograde administration of the viral vectors during a second ischemic period approximately doubled luciferase activity (55.010 ± 40.926 RLU/mg protein) in the LAD region compared with the administration during a single ischemic period. Although there was still a gradient from the epicardial to the endocardial layers, reporter gene expression was also more equally distributed than after a single retrograde delivery (Fig. 16-7).

In summary, adenovirus-mediated reporter gene transfer was substantially increased by retrograde delivery through the coronary veins compared with antegrade delivery into the coronary artery (Fig. 16-6). After two retrograde treatments of 10 min, a fairly homogeneous distribution of gene transfer was observed, showing no difference between proximal and distal probes of the targeted LAD region (Fig. 16-7). Gene transfer to the endocardial probes was somewhat less pronounced but still at considerable levels of expression. Of note, gene transfer was targeted exclusively to the LAD region, and no adenoviral transfection was detected in the nontargeted CX region (by PCR technique). However, systemic contamination during PTRGD cannot be excluded because of the presence of venovenous and venoarterial shunts, although no transfection of noncardiac tissues was detected in this study.

16.4. IMPLICATIONS FOR THERAPEUTIC ANGIOGENESIS

Therapeutic angiogenesis is an emerging new option for the treatment of patients with severe symptomatic coronary artery disease who do not respond to conventional therapy such as balloon angioplasty and bypass surgery. Angiogenic growth factors such as fibroblast growth factor (FGF) and vascular endothelial growth factor (VEGF) have been shown to induce therapeutic angiogenesis in myocardial ischemia (Kornowski et al., 2000a). Growth factors can be applied by injection into the myocardium (Schumache et al., 1998) or by infusion into the coronary artery (Battler et al., 1993; Sharmini et al., 2000; Unger et al., 1993). However,

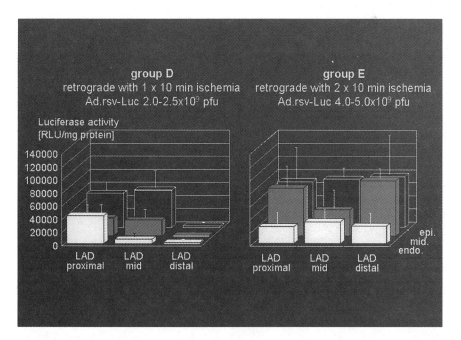

FIGURE 16-7. Distribution of reporter gene expression in the targeted LAD region 7 days after retrograde delivery during 1 × 10 min (group D) or 2 × 0 min of ischemia (group E) (Modified from Boekstegers et al., 2000).

intracoronary application has typically been successful only if delivery is prolonged (Battler et al., 1993; Unger et al., 1993). For example, functionally relevant angiogenesis was consistently induced by surgical implantation of a minipump (Unger et al., 1993) or microembolization with beads containing growth factors (Battler et al., 1993). Because these techniques are not suitable for patients, growth factors have been directly infused into the coronary artery (Lopez et al., 1998; Sharmini et al., 2000). The first placebo-controlled clinical trial, however, using intracoronary and intravenous delivery of recombinant VEGF-A$_{165}$ showed only weak evidence for efficacy (Henry et al., 1999; Henry et al., 2000). The short contact time with limited tissue binding of the growth factor might have been responsible for the lack of a clear efficiency. Sustained cellular production of angiogenic growth factors by gene transfer has been proposed to overcome these limitations (Giordano et al., 1996; Kornowski et al., 2000b; Mack et al., 1998; Magovern et al., 1997; Mühlhauser et al., 1995). The clinical usefulness of these approaches, however, has not yet been established (Lewis et al., 1997).

Selective catheterization of the coronary veins (Fig. 16-1) provides a unique intravascular access to ischemic myocardium that cannot be reached through severely diseased or occluded coronary arteries. Moreover, because capillary sprouting originates mainly from venules and capillaries, retrograde administration into the vein may target angiogenic growth factors to these vessel segments that are most receptive and responsive to them (Battegay et al., 1995; Folkman et al., 1992). Thus pressure-regulated retroinfusion may target regional delivery of recombinant growth factors, DNA-carrying liposomes, ·or viral gene vectors encoding for angiogenic proteins.

16.4.1. Retrograde Delivery of Angiogenic Growth Factors

To study retrograde delivery of angiogenic growth factors, pressure-regulated retroinfusion of recombinant FGF-2 into coronary veins was performed in a pig model of chronic myocardial ischemia (Fig. 16-8).

Chronic myocardial ischemia was induced for the first time by percutaneous implanta-

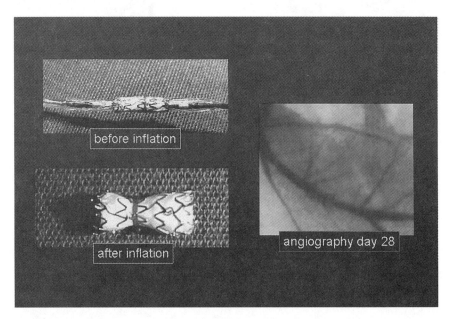

FIGURE 16-8. Reduction stent in a pig model: (A) and (B) reduction stent crimped on a PTCA-balloon (top) before and after inflation. (C) angiogram 28 days after implantation of a reduction stent.

tion of a reduction stent, which created an hourglass-shaped stenosis with an acute stenosis of about 70% (Fig. 16-8). The well-known ameroid constrictor model (Lopez et al., 1998; Unger et al., 1993) was not suitable for our studies because compression of the accompanying anterior cardiac vein would not have been avoidable. Immediately after implantation of the reduction stent in our studies, a highly reproducible degree of stenosis of about 70% was achieved, leading to severely compromised peak postischemic LAD blood flow. Moreover, progressive chronic ischemia was seen in this model, the stenosis increasing from about 70% to 90% 7 days after stent implantation. Similar to the ameroid constrictors (Lopez et al., 1998; Unger et al., 1993), the time point of complete closure of the coronary artery is not exactly defined after implantation of the reduction-stent. At follow-up after 28 days, 60% of the stents were occluded in both groups so that there was no difference between the treatment groups at either time point. Regarding the progression of the stenosis up to complete occlusion, this model seems to be fairly comparable to the ameroid constrictor. However, surgery was avoided using this less invasive and time-consuming

procedure that, in particular, did not hamper access to the coronary veins.

After selective retroinfusion of FGF-2 (day 7), the number of collaterals visible at postmortem angiography (day 28) was significantly increased (Fig. 16-9), showing a typical corkscrew shape and connecting large proximal vessels to the distal LAD. Although collateral blood flow in pigs is very low in the setting of acute ischemia (White et al., 1992), the development of angiographically visible collaterals has been described in case of severe chronic ischemia (Magovern et al., 1997). This process of arteriogenesis was clearly enhanced after retroinfusion of FGF-2 into the anterior cardiac vein (von Degenfeld et al., 2000) (Fig. 16-10). Histology also showed an increased capillary density in the targeted LAD-region 21 days after retroinfusion of FGF-2, with a significantly higher capillary-muscle fiber ratio in the ischemic LAD territory (von Degenfeld et al., 2000) (Fig. 16-11). Similar effects on angiogenesis have been described after prolonged coronary artery infusion using an osmotic minipump in a comparable pig model (Unger et al., 1993). Thus short-term treatment (30 min) by selective pressure-regulated retroinfusion of FGF-2 into the anterior cardiac vein may enhance

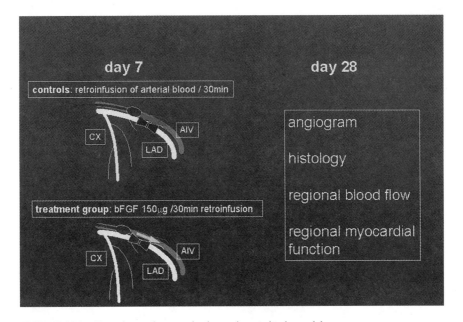

FIGURE 16-9. Experimental groups in the angiogenesis pig model.

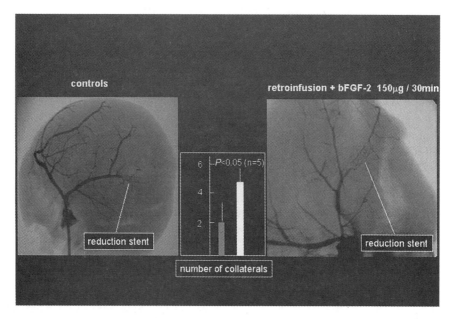

FIGURE 16-10.   Collateral development with (right panel) and without (left panel) retroinfusion of bFGF-2.

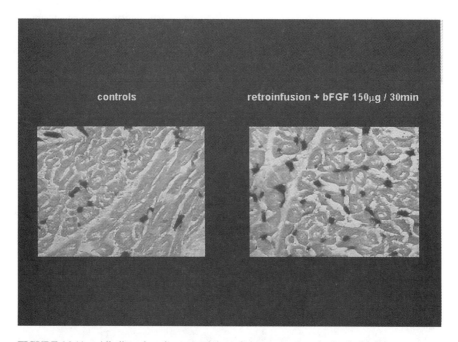

FIGURE 16-11.   Alkaline phosphatase staining of tissue samples obtained after 28 days of chronic myocardial ischemia (LAD area) in controls (left panel) and pigs treated by selective pressure-regulated retroinfusion of FGF-2 (right panel).

tissue binding of FGF-2 and lead to angiogenic effects similar to those of prolonged delivery through coronary arteries. Indeed, we were able to show that tissue binding of radioactively labeled basic fibroblast growth factor (bFGF) was substantially increased after retrograde delivery in a chronic pig model (von Degenfeld et al., 2000) (Figs. 16-12 and 16-13). Moreover, arteriogenesis and angiogenesis induced by selective pressure-regulated retroinfusion of bFGF-2 in the targeted LAD region was associated with functional improvement in the treated pigs. Regional myocardial function (sonomicrometry) as well as global left ventricular function was improved (von Degenfeld et al., 2000) (Fig. 16-14).

16.4.2. Retrograde Delivery of cDNA Encoding for Angiogenic Growth Factors by Liposome or Adenoviral Transfection

Catheter-based retrograde DNA delivery using liposomes has been studied so far in a chronic pig model of ischemia and reperfusion injury (Kupatt et al., 2000). Targeted delivery of nuclear factor (NF)-κB decoy oligonucleotide into ischemic myocardium aimed at inhibiting subacute endothelial activation. Selective retroinfusion of NF-κB decoy oligonucleotide immediately before reperfusion resulted in a subsequent downregulation of NF-κB activation as a key regulator of subacute endothelial activation. This inhibition of NF-κB activation was associated with a decrease in infarct size and a preservation of regional myocardial function 7 days after ischemia (Kupatt et al., 2000). Thus, liposome mediated DNA delivery by selective retroinfusion was shown to be feasible and functionally relevant. Therefore, this strategy may be also used for delivery of angiogenic growth factors.

Whether sustained production of growth factors can be induced by adenovirus-mediated PTRGD is currently being investigated using a third-generation adenovirus (Kochanek et al., 1996; Franz et al., 2000), which should reduce immunoresponse. As long as sufficient transfection and gene

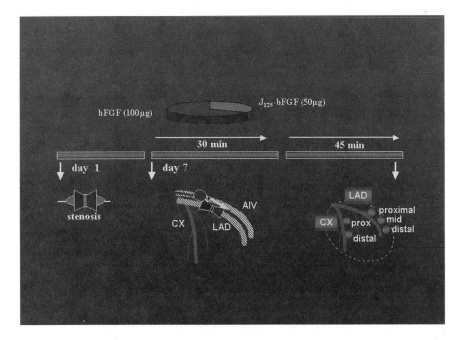

FIGURE 16-12. Experimental setting for the determination of tissue binding of bFGF-2. LAD = left anterior descending artery, CX = circumflex artery, AIV = anterior cardiac vein.

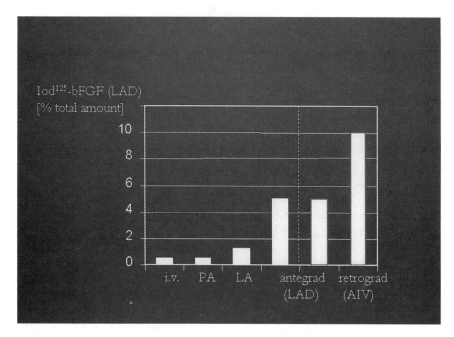

FIGURE 16-13. Comparison of bFGF-2 tissue binding between antegrade (Lazarous et al., 1997) and retrograde application. i.v. = intravenous; PA: pulmonary artery; LA = left atrium; LAD = left anterior descending artery; AIV = anterior cardiac vein.

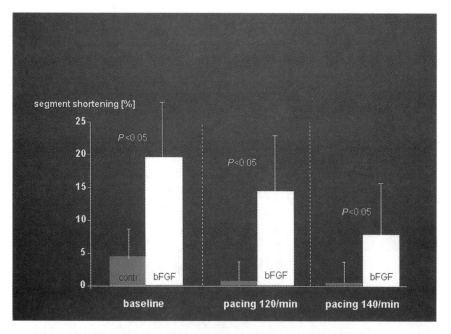

FIGURE 16-14. Regional myocardial function (subendocardial segment shortening) with and without atrial pacing. Contr = controls; bFGF = pigs treated by selective pressure-regulated retroinfusion of bFGF-2 after 7 days of chronic ischemia.

delivery into ischemic myocardium can be provided by PTRGD, this approach may overcome some of the present limitations of adenoviral gene transfer for angiogenesis.

REFERENCES

Barr E, Carroll J, Kalynych AM et al. Efficient catheter-mediated gene transfer into the heart using replication-deficient adenovirus. *Gene Ther* 1994; 1: 51–58.

Battegay EJ. Angiogenesis: mechanistic insights, neovascular diseases, and therapeutic prospects. *J Mol Med* 1995; 73: 333–346.

Battler A, Scheinowitz M, Hasdai D et al. Intracoronary injection of basic fibroblast growth factor enhances angiogenesis in infarcted swine myocardium. *J Am Coll Cardiol* 1993; 22: 2001–2006.

Boekstegers P, Diebold L, Weiss C. Selective ECG synchronized suction and retroinfusion of coronary veins: first results of studies in acute myocardial ischaemia in dogs. *Cardiovasc Res* 1990; 24: 456–464.

Boekstegers P, Peter W, von Degenfeld G et al. Preservation of regional myocardial function and myocardial oxygen tension during acute ischemia in pigs: comparison of selective synchronized suction and retroinfusion of coronary veins (SSR) to synchronized coronary venous retroperfusion (SRP). *J Am Coll Cardiol* 1994; 23: 459–469.

Boekstegers P, von Degenfeld G, Giehrl W et al. Selective suction and pressure-regulated retroinfusion: an effective and safe approach to retrograde protection against myocardial ischemia in patients undergoing normal and high risk percutaneous transluminal coronary angioplasty. *J Am Coll Cardiol* 1998; 31: 1525–1523.

Boekstegers P, Degenfeld G, Giehrl W et al. Myocardial gene transfer by selective pressure-regulated retroinfusion of coronary veins. *Gene Ther* 2000; 7: 232–240.

Costantini C, Sampoalesi A, Serra CM et al. Coronary venous retroperfusion support during high risk angioplasty in patients with unstable angina: preliminary experience. *J Am Coll Cardiol* 1991; 18: 283–292.

Feldman LJ, Steg G. Optimal techniques for arterial gene transfer. *Cardiovasc Res* 1997; 35: 391–404.

Folkman J, Shing Y. Angiogenesis. *J Biol Chem* 1992; 267: 10931–10934.

Franz WM, Müller OJ, Katus HA et al. Myocardial specific gene delivery. In: *Molecular Approaches to Heart Failure Therapy*, Hasenfuß G, Marban E (eds). Darmstadt: Steinkopf Verlag, pp. 126–143, 2000.

French BA, Mazur W, Geske RS et al. Direct in vivo gene transfer into porcine myocardium using replication-deficient adenoviral vectors. *Circulation* 1994a; 90: 2414–2424.

French BA, Mazur-W, Ali-NM et al. Percutaneous transluminal in vivo gene transfer by recombinant adenovirus in normal porcine coronary arteries, atherosclerotic arteries, and two models of coronary restenosis. *Circulation* 1994b; 90: 2402–2413.

Giehrl W, von Degenfeld G, Boekstegers P. Die druck-gesteuerte selektive Retroinfusion von Koronarvenen (SSR) erlaubt die Anpassung des Retroinfusionsdruckes an das individuelle Koronarvenensystem zur Optimierung der Myokardprotektion während koronarer Ischämie (abstract). *Z Kardiol* 1996; 85: 169.

Giehrl W, Von Degenfeld G, Molnar A et al. The coronary veins as an alternative access to ischaemic myocardium: experiences in 260 patients undergoing high risk PTCA (abstract). *Eur Heart J* 2000; 21: 162.

Giordano FJ, Ping P, McKirnan MD et al. Intracoronary gene transfer of fibroblast growth factor-5 increases blood flow and contractile function in an ischemic region of the heart. *Nat Med* 1996; 2: 534–539.

Giordano FJ, He H, McDonough P et al. Adenovirus-mediated gene transfer reconstitutes depressed sarcoplasmic reticulum Ca^{2+}-ATPase levels and shortens prolonged cardiac myocyte Ca^{2+} transients. *Circulation* 1997; 96: 400–403.

Haga Y, Uriuda Y, Bjorkman JA et al. Ischemic and nonischemic tissue concentrations of felodipine after coronary venous retroinfusion during myocardial ischemia and reperfusion: an experimental study in pigs. *J Cardiovasc Pharmacol* 1994; 24: 298–302.

Hajjar RJ, Kang JX, Gwathmey JK et al. Physiological effects of adenoviral gene transfer of sarcoplasmic reticulum calcium ATPase in isolated rat myocytes. *Circulation* 1997; 95: 423–429.

Hatori N, Sjoquist PO, Regardh C et al. Pharmacokinetic analysis of coronary sinus retroinfusion in pigs. Ischemic myocardial concentrations in the left circumflex arterial area using metoprolol as a tracer. *Cardiovasc Drugs Ther* 1991; 5: 1005–1010.

Henry TD, Annex BH, Azrin MA et al. Double-blind, placebo controlled trial of recombinant human vascular endothelial growth factor: the VIVA trial (abstract). *J Am Coll Cardiol* 1999; 33 (Suppl A): 383A.

Henry TD, McKendall GR, Azrin MA et al. VIVA Trial: one year follow up (abstract). *Circulation* 2000; 102 (Suppl): II-309.

Kar S, Drury JK, Hajduzki I et al. Synchronized coronary venous retroperfusion for support and salvage of ischemic myocardium during elective and failed angioplasty. *J Am Coll Cardiol* 1991; 18: 271–282.

Kochanek S, Clemens PR, Mitani K et al. Caskey. A new adenoviral vector: replacement of all viral coding sequences with 28 kb of DNA independently expressing both full length dystrophin and β-galactosidase. *Proc Natl Acad Sci USA* 1996; 93: 5731–5736.

Kornowski R, Fuchs S, Leon MB et al. Delivery strategies to achieve therapeutic myocardial angiogenesis. *Circulation* 2000a; 101: 454–458.

Kornowski R, Leon MB, Fuchs S et al. Electromagnetic guidance for catheter-based transendocardial injection: a platform for intramyocardial angiogenesis therapy. Results in normal and ischemic porcine models. *J Am Coll Cardiol* 2000b; 35: 1031–1039.

Kupatt C, Habazettl H, Gödecke A et al. TNFα trägt zur erhöhten subakuten Leukozytenadhäsion in der postischämischen Reperfusion bei (abstract). *Z F Kardiol* 1999; 88: 171.

Kupatt C, Wichels R, Molnar A et al. Regionally targeted NFκB decoy transfection by selective pressure-regulated retroinfusion improves cardiac function and diminishes infarct size 7 days after ischemia in pigs (abstract). *Circulation* 2000; 102: II-347.

Lamping KG, Rios CD, Chun JA et al. Intrapericardial administration of adenovirus for gene transfer. *Am J Physiol* 1997; 272: H310–H317.

Lazarous DF, Shou M, Stiber JA et al. Pharmacodynamics of basic fibroblast growth factor: Route of administration determines myocardial and systemic distribution. *Cardiovasc Res* 1997; 36: 78–85.

Lewis BS, Flugelman MY, Weisz A et al. Angiogenesis by gene therapy: a new horizon for myocardial revascularization? *Cardiovasc Res* 1997; 35: 490–497.

Lopez JJ, Laham RJ, Stamler A et al. VEGF administration in chronic myocardial ischemia in pigs. *Cardiovasc Res* 1998; 40: 272–281.

Mack CA, Patel SR, Schwarz EA et al. Biologic bypass. *J Thorac Cardiovasc Surg* 1998; 115: 168–177.

Magovern CJ, Mack CA, Zhang J et al. Direct in vivo gene transfer to canine myocardium using a replication-deficient adenovirus vector. *Ann Thorac Surg* 1996; 62: 425–433.

Magovern CJ, Mack CA, Zhang J et al. Regional angiogenesis induced in nonischemic tissue by an adenoviral vector expressing vascular endothelial growth factor. *Hum Gene Ther* 1997; 8: 215–227.

March KL, Woody M, Mehdi K et al. Efficient in vivo catheter-based pericardial gene transfer mediated by adenoviral vectors. *Clin Cardiol* 1999; 22: I23–I29.

Meerbaum S, Lang TW, Osher JV et al. Diastolic retroperfusion of acutely ischemic myocardium. *Am J Cardiol* 1976; 37: 588–589.

Mohl W, Glogar H, Mayr D et al. Reduction of infarct size induced by pressure-controlled intermittent coronary sinus occlusion. *Am J Cardiol* 1984; 53: 923–930.

Mühlhauser J, Merrill MJ, Pili R et al. VEGF165 expressed by a replication-deficient recombinant adenovirus vector induces angiogenesis *in vivo*. *Circ Res* 1995; 77: 1077–1086.

O'Byrne GT, Nienaber CA, Miyazki A et al. Positron emission tomography demonstrates that coronary sinus retroperfusion can restore regional myocardial perfusion and preserve metabolism. *J Am Coll Cardiol* 1991; 18: 257–270.

Oh BH, Volpini M, Kambayashi M et al. Myocardial function and transmural blood flow during coronary venous retroperfusion in pigs. *Circulation* 1992; 86: 1265–1279.

Rothmann T, Katus HA, Hartong R et al. Heart muscle-specific gene expression using replication defective recombinant adenovirus. *Gene Ther* 1996; 3: 919–926.

Ryden L, Tadokoro H, Sjoquist PO et al. Pharmacokinetic analysis of coronary venous retroinfusion: a comparison with anterograde coronary artery drug administration using metoprolol as a tracer. *J Am Coll Cardiol* 1991; 18: 603–612.

Schumacher B, Pecher P, Von Specht BU et al. Induction of neoangiogenesis in ischemic myocardium by human growth factors: first clinical results of a new treatment of coronary heart disease. *Circulation* 1998; 97: 645–650.

Rajanayagam MA, Shou M, Thirumurti V et al. Intracoronary basic fibroblast growth factor enhances myocardial collateral perfusion in dogs. *J Am Coll Cardiol* 2000; 35: 519–526.

Steg PG, Feldman LJ, Scoazec JY et al. Arterial gene transfer to rabbit endothelial and smooth muscle cells using percutaneous delivery of an adenoviral vector. *Circulation* 1994; 90: 1648–1656.

Unger EF, Banai S, Shou M et al. A model to assess interventions to improve collateral blood flow: Continuous administration of agents into the left coronary artery in dogs. *Cardiovasc Res* 1993; 27: 785–791.

Von Degenfeld G, Giehrl W, Boekstegers P. Targeting of dobutamine to ischemic myocardium without systemic effects by selective suction and pressure-regulated retroinfusion. *Cardiovasc Res* 1997; 35: 233–240.

Von Degenfeld G, Lebherz C, Raake P et al. Functionally relevant therapeutic angiogenesis by selective pressure-regulated retroinfusion of basic fibroblast growth factor into coronary veins in chronic myocardial ischemia in pigs (abstract). *Circulation* 2000; 102: II-310.

White FC, Carroll SM, Magnet A et al. Coronary collateral development in swine after coronary artery occlusion. *Circ Res* 1992; 71: 1490–1500.

17

Percutaneous Intrapericardial Drug Delivery for Myocardial Angiogenesis

Sergio Waxman, M.D.

Interventional Cardiology
University of Texas Medical Branch at Galveston
Galveston, Texas

SUMMARY

Percutaneous intrapericardial myocardial angiogenesis may be a potential alternative to laser and other forms of percutaneous revascularization.

Because of the natural barrier action of the pericardium, systemic absorption of drugs or biologic agents is considerably less than with intravascular routes. This allows for the use of smaller doses of such substances to obtain higher concentrations in the pericardial fluid, prolonging their time of action and increasing their cardiac specificity.

Studies have demonstrated the ability to induce functionally significant angiogenesis by intrapericardial use of cytokines. This offers an attractive route for efficient drug delivery and gene therapy.

Percutaneous methods for pericardial drug delivery are being explored and appear to be feasible and well tolerated.

Despite promising results, there are concerns regarding the limited penetration of pericardially delivered angiogenic cytokines into the deeper layers of myocardium and endocardium, where ischemia tends to be more severe.

Even though the localized delivery of therapeutic agents into the pericardial space appears to have advantages over other routes of administration, the long-term effects of peptides or genes injected into the pericardial space are unknown. Further studies are needed to evaluate this approach.

17.1. INTRODUCTION

The pericardium may have an important role in the regulation of various myocardial and coronary vascular processes (Spodick, 1999). The presence of elevated levels of angiogenic cytokines such as basic fibroblast growth factor (bFGF) and vascular endothelial growth factor (VEGF) in pericardial fluid of patients with unstable angina (Fujita et al., 1996) suggests that the pericardial milieu may be closely related with the underlying myocardium. Vasoactive substances such as atrial natriuretic peptide and endothelin-1 have also been found in high concentrations

Myocardial Revascularization: Novel Percutaneous Approaches, Edited by George S. Abela.
ISBN 0-471-36166-6   Copyright © 2002 Wiley-Liss, Inc.

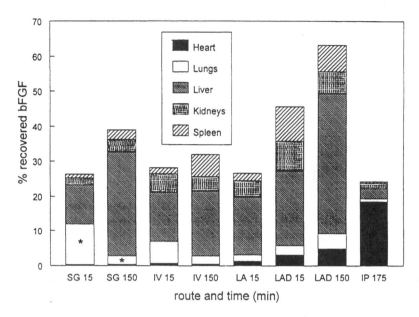

FIGURE 17-1. Comparison of 5 routes of administration on regional bFGF distribution: pulmonary artery (Swan-Ganz, SG), intravenous (IV), left atrium (LA), intracoronary (LAD), and intrapericardial (IP). Recovered bFGF is expressed as a percentage of the total recovered counts. ^{125}I activity was assessed 15 and 150 min after injection. The greatest proportion of bFGF was recovered from the liver, except with pericardial delivery, which was associated with the greatest myocardial uptake (up to 19% of the total injected dose). By comparison, intracoronary administration was associated with only 3–5% myocardial uptake. Thus pericardial delivery of bFGF was associated with the highest myocardial uptake and the lowest systemic levels, suggesting that this route may be effective for angiogenesis. Modified from Lazarous DF et al., *Cardiovasc Res* 1997; 36: 79, with permission from Elsevier Science.

in pericardial fluid (Horkay et al., 1995, 1998). It is unclear whether the presence of these biologically important agents in pericardial fluid may be the result of spillage into the pericardial space or whether they have a physiologic function in disease or normal states, regulating vascular tone, contractility, or development of collaterals. Whatever their true purpose, the concept of using the pericardial space as a drug depot seems a logical way of delivering pharmacologic agents to the myocardium and coronary vessels. One potential application of this route of delivery is induction of angiogenesis and collateral formation in myocardial ischemic tissue and is supported by experimental data in various animal models. Finally, a number of new methods to access the normal pericardial space are available to deliver these agents

safely and minimally invasively. Percutaneous intrapericardial myocardial angiogenesis is discussed in this chapter as a potential alternative to laser and other forms of percutaneous revascularization.

17.2. ADVANTAGES OF USING THE PERICARDIAL SPACE FOR DRUG DELIVERY

Intrapericardial delivery of therapeutic agents takes advantage of the pericardial sac as a reservoir where a drug or biologic agent will have a prolonged residence time and therefore direct exposure with epicardial myocardial and coronary tissue (Spodick, 2000). Because of the natural barrier action of the pericardium, absorption into the systemic circulation is considerably less than

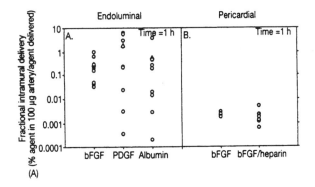

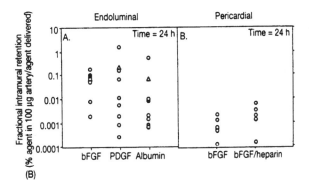

FIGURE 17-2. (A) Fractional intramural delivery (FID) expressed as a percentage of each infused agent found in arterial tissue 1 h after delivery. The left panel shows one value for each coronary artery harvested after endoluminal delivery of bFGF, PDGF, and albumin. The right panel shows one value for each coronary artery harvested after intrapericardial delivery of bFGF and bFGF/heparin. Endoluminal delivery results in greater variation in FID by several orders of magnitude compared with intrapericardial delivery, which is associated with more uniform uptake. (B) Fractional intramural retention (FIR) expressed as a percentage of each infused agent found in arterial tissue 24 h after delivery. As in (A), the left panel shows one value for each coronary artery harvested after endoluminal delivery and the right panel shows one value for each coronary artery harvested after intrapericardial delivery of the agents listed on the *x*-axis. Again, endoluminal delivery results in a substantially greater variability in FIR compared with intrapericardial delivery. The more uniform uptake seen with intrapericardial delivery can have the advantage of using smaller and more predictable doses of angiogenic agents. Modified from Stoll et al., *Clin Cardiol* 1999; 22: 1–13, with permission.

with intravascular routes of delivery. This enables the use of smaller doses of drugs, proteins, or other biologic substances while obtaining higher local concentrations in the pericardial fluid, prolonging the time of action of these agents and increasing their specificity to act on the target tissue while minimizing untoward systemic effects.

Evidence for the localizing advantage and barrier action of the pericardium with regard to potential angiogenic agents comes from a number of studies. Lazarous and colleagues evaluated regional uptake of ^{125}I labeled bFGF after administration via different routes (Lazarous et al., 1997). Pericardial administration was associated with the highest myocardial uptake (19% at 150 min) and was far more effective in achieving high cardiac tissue uptake than intracoronary or left atrial delivery (Fig. 17-1). Furthermore, uptake in extracardiac tissues such as lungs, liver, and spleen was minimal with intrapericardial injection compared with other routes of delivery. There was a striking transmural gradient with epimyocardial concentration one order of magnitude greater than that of mid- or endocardium, suggesting also that transmural penetration is not uniform and may depend on molecule size or transport mechanisms. Stoll et al. (Stoll et al., 1999) determined that, although intracoronary delivery of bFGF results in a wide range of intramural coronary arterial retention with 33,000-fold variability, pericardial administration has much more uniform intramural concentrations with 10–15-fold variability, which can translate into more accurate and smaller dosing of agents (Fig. 17-2). Redistribution rates were also lower with pericardial delivery (22 h) compared with endoluminal delivery (7 h), again suggesting prolongation of the residence time of an agent after pericardial delivery and therefore increased myocardial and coronary arterial exposure.

These pharmacokinetic properties of drugs administered in the pericardial space may be of clinical benefit. Our group (Waxman et al., 1999) demonstrated that nitroglycerin delivered intrapericardially is associated with more prolonged and marked coronary vasodilation compared with same-dose intracoronary administration (Fig. 17-3). Furthermore, the effects of the pericardial drug were devoid of hypotension, which was observed with the intracoronary route, supporting the idea that potential adverse effects of angiogenic agents may be reduced when they are administered intrapericardially.

A pivotal study with ample implications for human gene therapy was performed by March and colleagues (March et al., 1999). They instilled adenoviral vectors into the pericardial space of dogs, obtaining efficient gene transfer that was mainly localized to the pericardial mesothelium with very little transduction of extracardiac tissues and demonstrating the possibility of pericardial gene transfer as an approach to sustained-release protein delivery (Fig. 17-4). This method can provide the means to generate sufficiently

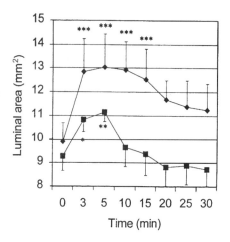

FIGURE 17-3. Comparison of the effects of intrapericardial (diamonds) and intracoronary (squares) nitroglycerin on left anterior descending coronary artery luminal area as assessed by intravascular ultrasound. The asterisks indicate significance with respect to baseline value (***$P < 0.001$, **$P < 0.01$, *$P < 0.05$). The curves were statistically different using 2-way analysis of variance ($P = 0.03$). Intrapericardial nitroglycerin resulted in greater and more prolonged luminal area dilation compared with intracoronary administration, suggesting that pericardial delivery may potentiate the effects of some agents on the myocardium and coronary arterial wall. In addition, intracoronary, but not intrapericardial, delivery was associated with transient hypotension (not shown). Modified from Waxman et al., *J Am Coll Cardiol* 1999; 33: 2075, with permission from the American College of Cardiology.

high concentrations of desired gene products, that is, an angiogenic protein or signal that can then diffuse into the epicardial region to potentially produce a therapeutic biologic effect.

17.3. STUDIES OF ANGIOGENESIS USING PERICARDIAL DELIVERY

A number of studies have demonstrated the use of various growth factors to induce angiogenesis in chronic myocardial ischemia. Delivery has been achieved through intracoronary, left atrial, and, more recently, direct intramyocardial injection of these factors with various degrees of success. Delivery of these compounds into the pericardial space has also been performed with promising

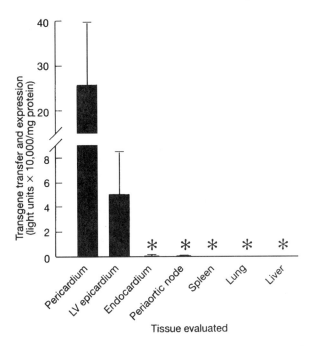

FIGURE 17-4.   Cardiac and extracardiac distribution of luciferase expression after intrapericardial adenovirus vector delivery. Tissue sampling was performed from numerous sites to evaluate systemic vector distribution and gene expression after intrapericardial installation. Luciferase activity is given as relative light units/mg tissue protein (RLU/mg) normalized per 10^7 pfu administered. Asterisks indicate a mean luminometry of <1,000 RLU/mg. Gene transfer and expression was highest in the parietal pericardium and epicardium and markedly reduced by 500- to 1,000-fold in endocardial and noncardiac tissues. Intrapericardial gene transfer is thus highly localized and could be used to produce angiogenic cytokines to obtain a therapeutic effect. Modified from March et al., *Clin Cardiol* 1999; 22: I–26, with permission from Clinical Cardiology Publishing Company, Inc.

results in animal models. Landau et al. studied the effects of continuous intrapericardial delivery of bFGF using an osmotic pump in a rabbit model of angiotensin II-induced left ventricular hypertrophy and ischemia (Landau et al., 1995). Intrapericardial bFGF was associated with a highly localized angiogenic effect compared with control animals. Uchida and colleagues (Uchida et al., 1995) demonstrated in a canine model of myocardial infarction that a single intrapericardial injection of bFGF and heparin sulfate is associated with significant angiogenesis in the infarcted area (up to 10-fold compared with controls) and myocardial salvage as assessed by ventricular function and infarct weight (Fig. 17-5). The reason for using heparin sulfate is that it acts as a carrier for

bFGF, facilitating its diffusion by competing with its binding to surrounding matrix structures and protecting it from proteolytic degradation. This combination was superior to administration of bFGF alone. Uchida et al. noted, however, that the vascular number was larger in the subepicardial than in the subendocardial infarcted areas, suggesting that ways to enhance diffusion across the entire myocardial wall may be needed to obtain a transmural effect. Trying to emulate a model of ischemia that most resembles progressive atherosclerosis, Laham et al. used a porcine model of chronic ischemia with an ameroid occluder in the left circumflex artery and studied the effect of a single intrapericardial injection of bFGF. Treatment resulted in a significant increase in angiographic

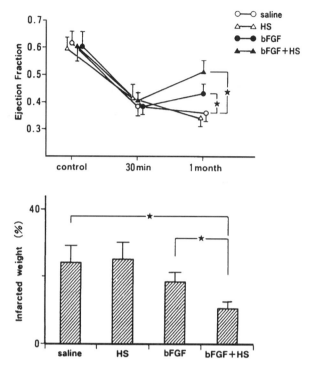

FIGURE 17-5. (A) Ejection fraction (EF) of left ventricle before, 30 min after, and 1 month after myocardial infarction and a single intrapericardial injection of bFGF plus heparin sulfate (bFGF+HS), bFGF alone (bFGF), heparin sulfate alone (HS), or control (saline) in a canine model of infarction after coronary embolization. EF was similarly decreased in all groups at 30 min. One month later, however, EF in the bFGF+HS group was significantly larger than in the control and HS groups but not different from that of the bFGF group. *$P < 0.05$. (B) Percentage of infarcted weight/left ventricular weight in the same groups at 1 month. Relative infarct size was the smallest in the bFGF+HS group. Intrapericardial bFGF effectively achieves myocardial salvage and localized angiogenesis in the infarcted area. Modified from Uchida et al., *Am Heart J*, 1995; 130: 1184, with permission.

collaterals, regional myocardial blood flow, myocardial function in the ischemic territory, collateral extent, and myocardial vascularity compared with controls (Laham et al., 2000). Intrapericardial bFGF treatment was also associated with improved endothelium-dependent vasodilatation in the affected region (Laham et al., 1998). These studies demonstrate the ability to induce functionally significant angiogenesis by intrapericardial use of cytokines and offer an attractive drug delivery method that may indeed possess some of the advantages mentioned above.

The intrapericardial approach may also be an effective way of delivering gene therapy.

Instead of delivering a peptide, Lazarous et al. administered a replication-deficient adenovirus carrying the cDNA for AdCMV.VEGF165 intrapericardially in a canine model of progressive coronary occlusion (Lazarous et al., 1999). Pericardial delivery resulted in sustained (8–14 days) pericardial transgene expression with VEGF levels peaking 3 days after infection (>200 ng/ml) and decreasing thereafter. There was no detectable increase in serum VEGF level (Fig. 17-6). Transfection efficiency was again extensive in the pericardium and epicardium and minimal in midmyocardium and endocardium. Despite successful induction of sus-

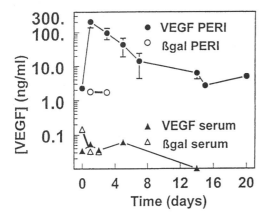

FIGURE 17-6. Pericardial and serum VEGF levels from 6 animals that underwent intrapericardial adenovirus-mediated gene transfer (3 AdCMV.VEGF treated and 3 AdRSV.β-gal treated). Transgene expression was evident 24 h after viral infection, with a measurable increase in VEGF persisting for 14 days. Pretreatment VEGF levels were negligible in both virus-treated groups. The VEGF concentration in pericardial fluid peaked on day 3 in AdCMV. VEGF-treated dogs (>200 ng/dl). VEGF levels diminished to ~15 ng/ml by day 8 and tapered off gradually thereafter. VEGF levels were not elevated in AdRSV.β-gal-treated animals. Serum VEGF concentrations remained at pretreatment levels in all groups. Intrapericardial gene transfer is capable of sustaining localized cytokine expression without an increase in systemic levels. Modified from Lazarous et al., *Cardiovasc Res* 1999; 44: 299, with permission.

tained VEGF expression in the pericardium, maximal collateral perfusion did not differ from that of controls. Although angiogenesis did not occur in this study, it demonstrates the ability to use the pericardium to produce cytokines or other signaling-agents that could be effective in achieving localized myocardial revascularization while avoiding systemic levels that may have potentially deleterious effects. Whether transfection can be successfully achieved deeper in the myocardium or whether it is even desirable remains to be determined.

17.4. PERCUTANEOUS METHODS FOR PERICARDIAL DRUG DELIVERY

Non-thoracotomy access to the pericardial space has been restricted to patients with pericardial effusions large enough for a needle or catheter to be inserted safely and reserved for specific treatment or diagnosis of such conditions. Recently, a number of percutaneous methods to access the normal pericardial space have emerged, and they appear to be feasible and well tolerated. Some of these rely on a transvenous route, whereas others use a subxiphoid approach. Although they are in different stages of development, these methods are discussed here in their present form.

March et al. described a percutaneous approach in large animals using a hollow, helix-tipped catheter positioned transmurally across the right ventricular wall (March et al., 1999). Injection of a mixture of saline and contrast was necessary to confirm position of the catheter tip in the pericardial space (Fig. 17-7). They described no significant bleeding or electrocardiographic changes up to 3 days after the procedure.

Uchida et al. used a thin needle-tipped catheter to inject bFGF through the right atrial wall into the pericardial space of dogs (Uchida et al., 1995). Their technique required the use of contrast material to confirm position of the needle in the pericardial space. Verrier and Waxman described the transatrial method for pericardial access (Verrier et al., 1998, Waxman et al., 2000), in which a guiding catheter is advanced into the right atrial appendage and a wire is used to pierce the atrial wall and advanced into the pericardial space (Fig. 17-8). The wire confirms adequate position in the pericardial space as it conforms to the contour of the heart and secures the point of entry into the pericardial space. A number of catheters can then be introduced over the wire for sampling of pericardial fluid or drug delivery. This method takes advantage of the orientation of the right atrial appendage, directing the wire tangentially to the heart and minimizing the risk of coronary and myocardial laceration. The safety and feasibility of this system have been demonstrated in the porcine model under normal conditions (Waxman et al., 2000) and in the presence of aspirin therapy and experimental pulmonary hypertension

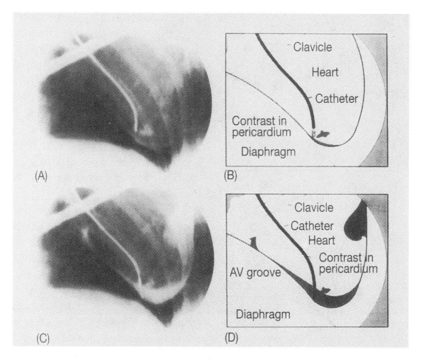

FIGURE 17-7.   Fluoroscopic image and corresponding drawing of a percutaneous intrapericardial delivery procedure using a transventricular approach. The cardiac silhouette is seen from a right anterior oblique projection. A specialized helix catheter has been positioned transmurally in the right ventricular wall, and contrast has been injected through the catheter to confirm pericardial loculation. Modified from March et al., *Clin Cardiol* 1999; 22: I–26, with permission from Clinical Cardiology Publishing Company, Inc.

(Pulerwitz et al., 2000), achieving pericardial access consistently in 3–5 min. Thus transvenous methods appear promising and safe for drug delivery. However, because these approaches involve penetration through myocardial tissue, alternative means to access the pericardial space may be required if large catheters are to be used.

Sosa and colleagues used a subxiphoid technique to access the normal pericardial space of patients to perform epicardial mapping and ablation (Sosa et al., 1998, 1999). They used a blunt epidural needle advanced under fluoroscopy toward the cardiac silhouette. When a slight negative pressure is felt, contrast medium is injected to corroborate position within the pericardial space and a guidewire is inserted through the hollow needle. A catheter can then follow the wire into the pericardial space. In their series, hemopericardium requiring drainage developed in 1 of 10 patients and 3 other patients developed minimal retrosternal discomfort and pericardial friction rub. A similar method was used by Laham et al. in pigs, but in this method the needle is connected to pressurized saline. As the needle is advanced and it enters the pericardial space, flow of saline suggests entry into the low-pressure space (Laham et al., 1999). Although the subxiphoid approach is feasible in the absence of pericardial effusion, the risk of myocardial or coronary laceration cannot be ignored and may be higher than when the procedure is performed in the presence of a sizable effusion.

Seferovic and Macris reported their experience with a device for accessing the pericardial space that is undergoing feasi-

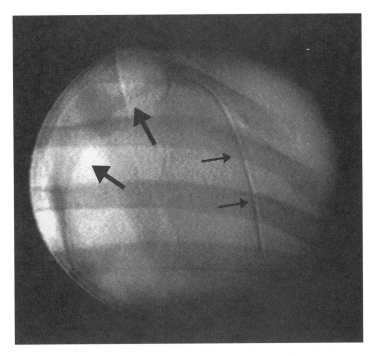

FIGURE 17-8. Fluoroscopic image of the heart in shallow right anterior oblique projection demonstrating the presence of an intrapericardial drug delivery catheter using the percutaneous transatrial technique. The image shows an 8 Fr guiding catheter (large arrows) in the right atrium and a 0.038-in. infusion guidewire (small arrows) inside the pericardial space. The infusion guidewire mounted on a 0.014-in. wire (not shown) exits through the right atrial appendage and conforms to the contour of the heart, confirming its position within the pericardial space. Modified from Waxman et al., *Cathet Cardiovasc Interv* 2000; 49: 473. Reprinted by permission of Wiley-Liss, Inc., a subsidiary of John Wiley & Sons, Inc.

bility testing in humans (Macris et al., 1999; Seferovic et al., 1999). The procedure requires accessing the mediastinal space through a subxiphoid incision with a blunt cannula. A guidewire and dilator-introducer sheath are inserted, through which the device is introduced to capture the pericardium by applying vacuum (Fig. 17-9). The pericardium is punctured and a guidewire advanced into the pericardial space, over which catheters can be exchanged. Variable results have been obtained in these studies, mainly limited to difficult access in obese patients, pain at the access site, and mild transient fever.

Whatever approach is used, pericardial access technology is in its early stages of development, and it is likely that improvement in design and materials will lead to wider acceptance of this route of drug delivery.

17.5. CURRENT LIMITATIONS OF INTRAPERICARDIAL DRUG DELIVERY FOR MYOCARDIAL ANGIOGENESIS

Despite promising initial results of intrapericardial drug delivery, a number of limitations must be addressed. Concerns exist regarding the limited penetration of pericardially delivered angiogenic cytokines into the deeper layers of myocardium and endocardium, where ischemia tends to be more severe. This may require use of technologies aimed at increasing diffusion gradients, such as iontophoretic delivery systems (Avitall et al.,

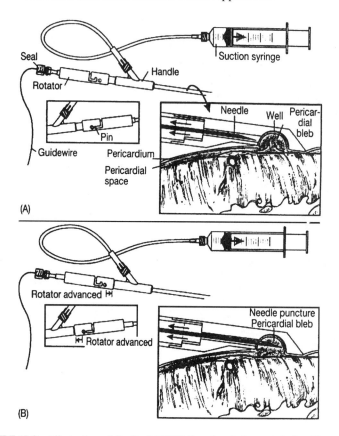

FIGURE 17-9.   Illustration of the PerDUCER® pericardial access device (Comedicus Inc., Columbia Heights, MN.) showing its handle, suction syringe, and cross section (close-up) of tip, pericardium, and myocardium during capture of the pericardium with suction (A) and pericardial puncture with the hollow needle (B). The device is introduced in the anterior mediastinal space through a subxiphoid incision. Modified from Macris and Igo, *Clin Cardiol* 1999; 22: I–37, with permission from Clinical Cardiology Publishing Company, Inc.

1992), or use of smaller molecules. Further understanding of the pharmacokinetics of pericardially delivered drugs will be required to address this issue.

The optimal angiogenic agent and the dosing regimen that is needed are unknown, and whether a sustained effect can be achieved with single versus multiple injections needs to be investigated further. If repeated administration is required, chronic pump delivery systems or polymer technology may be used and developed to circumvent this limitation.

It also remains to be determined whether functional angiogenesis can best be achieved by administration of the protein itself or by gene delivery or manipulation and whether feedback mechanisms will be required to turn the angiogenic signals "on and off" to prevent potential adverse effects.

Finally, although localized delivery of agents in the pericardial space appears to have some theoretical advantages over alternative routes, the long-term effects of peptides or genes injected into the pericardial space are unknown. Whether the supposed advantages of this route as an ideal method for revascularization will hold true remains a matter of speculation until further studies are performed.

17.6. SUMMARY

The pericardial space offers an attractive and effective route of delivering cytokines and genetic material to the heart for the purpose of myocardial angiogenesis and vascular modulation. The possibility of localizing delivery of these agents to the target sites while minimizing systemic adverse effects constitutes one of the main advantages of this route of delivery. New percutaneous methods to access the normal pericardial space are now available and will likely facilitate the exploration of this route for drug delivery. Although initial results appear promising, extensive research addressing the issues of myocardial penetration, pharmacokinetics, ideal agents, and optimal dosing is required.

References

Avitall B, Hare J, Zander G et al. Iontophoretic transmyocardial drug delivery. A novel approach to antiarrhythmic drug therapy. *Circulation* 1992; 85: 1582–1593.

Fujita M, Ikemoto M, Kishishita M et al. Elevated basic fibroblast growth factor in pericardial fluid of patients with unstable angina. *Circulation* 1996; 94: 610–613.

Horkay F, Laine M, Szokodi I et al. Human pericardial fluid contains the highest amount of endothelin-1 of all mammalian biologic fluids thus far tested. *J Cardiovasc Pharmacol* 1995; 26 (Suppl III): S-502–S-504.

Horkay F, Szokoki I, Lasxlo S et al. Presence of immunoreactive endothelin-1 and atrial natriuretic peptide in human pericardial fluid. *Life Sci* 1998; 62: 267–274.

Laham RJ, Simons M, Tofukuji M et al. Modulation of myocardial perfusion and vascular reactivity by pericardial basic fibroblast growth factor: insight into ischemia-induced reduction in endothelium-dependent vasodilatation. *J Thorac Cardiovasc Surg* 1998; 116: 1022–1028.

Laham RJ, Simons M, Hung D. Subxyphoid access of the normal pericardium: a novel drug delivery technique. *Cathet Cardiovasc Interv* 1999; 47: 109–111.

Laham RJ, Rezaee M, Post M et al. Intrapericardial delivery of fibroblast growth factor-2 induces neovascularization in a porcine model of chronic myocardial ischemia. *J Pharmacol Exp Ther* 2000; 292: 795–802.

Landau C, Jacobs AK, Haudenschild CC. Intrapericardial basic fibroblast growth factor induces myocardial angiogenesis in a rabbit model of chronic ischemia. *Am Heart J* 1995; 129: 924–931.

Lazarous DF, Shou M, Stiber J et al. Pharmacodynamics of basic fibroblast growth factor: route of administration determines myocardial and systemic distribution. *Cardiovasc Res* 1997; 36: 78–85.

Lazarous DF, Shou M, Stiber JA et al. Adenoviral-mediated gene transfer induces sustained pericardial VEGF expression in dogs: effect on myocardial angiogenesis. *Cardiovasc Res* 1999; 44: 294–302.

Macris MP, Igo SR. Minimally invasive access of the normal pericardium: initial clinical experience with a novel device. *Clin Cardiol* 1999; 22 (Suppl I): I-36–I-39.

March K, Woody M, Mehdi K et al. Efficient in vivo catheter-based pericardial gene transfer medicated by adenoviral vectors. *Clin Cardiol* 1999: 22 (Suppl 1) I-23–I-29.

Pulerwitz T, Waxman S, Rowe K et al. Transatrial access to the normal pericardial space for local cardiac therapy: preclinical safety testing with aspirin and pulmonary artery hypertension. *J Interv Cardiol*. In press.

Seferovic PM, Ristic AD, Maksimovic R et al. Initial clinical experience with PerDUCER device: promising new tool in the diagnosis and treatment of pericardial disease. *Clin Cardiol* 1999; 22 (Suppl I): I-30–I-35.

Sosa E, Scanavacca M, D'Avila A et al. Endocardial and epicardial ablation guided by nonsurgical transthoracic epicardial mapping to treat recurrent ventricular tachycardia. *J Cardiovasc Electrophysiol* 1998; 9: 229–239.

Sosa E, Scanavacca M, d'Avila A. Different ways of approaching the normal pericardial space. *Circulation* 1999; 100: E-115–E-116.

Spodick DH. Microphysiology of the pericardium in relation to intrapericardial therapeutics and diagnostics. *Clin Cardiol* 1999; 22 (Suppl I): I-2–I-3.

Spodick DH. Intrapericardial therapeutics and diagnostics. *Am J Cardiol* 2000; 85: 1012–1014.

Stoll H, Carlson K, Keefer L et al. Pharmacokinetics and consistency of pericardial delivery directed to coronary arteries: direct comparison with endoluminal delivery. *Clin Cardiol* 1999; 22 (Suppl I): I-10–I-16.

Uchida Y, Yanagisawa-Miwa A, Nakamura F et al. Angiogenic therapy of acute myocardial infarction by intrapericardial injection of basic fibroblast growth factor and heparin sulfate: an experimental study. *Am Heart J* 1995; 130: 1182–1188.

Verrier RL, Waxman S, Lovett EG et al. Transatrial access to the normal pericardial space: a novel approach for diagnostic sampling, pericardiocentesis, and therapeutic intervention. *Circulation* 1998; 98: 2331–2333.

Waxman S, Moreno R, Rowe K et al. Persistent primary coronary dilation induced by transatrial delivery of nitroglycerin into the pericardial space: a novel approach for local cardiac drug delivery. *J Am Coll Cardiol* 1999; 33: 2073–2077.

Waxman S, Pulerwitz T, Quist W et al. Preclinical safety testing of percutaneous transatrial access to the normal pericardial space for local cardiac drug delivery and diagnostic sampling. *Cathet Cardiovasc Interv* 2000; 49: 472–477.

18

Cell Transplantation: Its Application in the Treatment of Cardiac Dysfunction and Its Effect on Angiogenesis

Mu Yao, M.D., Ph.D., and Robert A. Kloner, M.D., Ph.D.

Heart Institute, Good Samaritan Hospital
Los Angeles, California
University of Southern California
Division of Cardiology
Los Angeles, California

SUMMARY

Several studies with experimental animals have shown that cell implantation into the myocardium results in improved cardiac function and therefore potentially might be effective in the treatment of ischemic heart disease.

To replace damaged myocardium, it would be ideal to implant cardiomyocytes because they have the same unique electrophysiological, structural, and contractile properties.

Results from several studies have indicated that fetal and neonatal cardiomyocytes, but not adult cardiomyocytes, can survive and develop into cardiac tissue after transplantation into both normal and damaged myocardium.

Because of the ability of skeletal muscle to repair itself after injury, interest has been raised in testing the possibility that damaged myocardium can be repaired by implantation of skeletal muscle cells (cellular cardiomyoplasty).

One of the obstacles to cell transplantation is the insufficient number of donor cells. This has resulted in the search for alternative sources of donor cells, including embryonic stem cells, which are capable of both proliferation and differentiation.

Studies have shown that implanted myocytes are separated from host myocardium by scar tissue, and therefore it is unlikely that the implanted cells contribute to host myocardial contraction. However, they may reduce wall stress by increasing wall thickness and diastolic compliance by formation of new tissue with elastic properties in the scar.

Myocardial Revascularization: Novel Percutaneous Approaches, Edited by George S. Abela.
ISBN 0-471-36166-6 Copyright © 2002 Wiley-Liss, Inc.

18.1. INTRODUCTION

A variety of myocardial insults (e.g., myocardial infarction) can lead to loss of cardiomyocytes, the cellular component for cardiac contraction. Although mitosis was reported in both normal and diseased adult myocardium (Anversa and Kajstura, 1998), myocardial infarction inevitably results in nonfunctional scar tissue in the affected myocardium. Adult cardiomyocytes thus have a limited ability to proliferate, and consequently lost cells cannot be adequately replaced by the regeneration of remaining cardiac muscle cells. Accordingly, myocyte loss will result in an overload on the remaining, surviving myocardium, which then undergoes hypertrophy. However, long-term hypertrophy can induce deleterious cellular changes including myofibrillar loss (Maron, 1975) and apoptosis of the myocytes (Diez et al., 1997; Shizukuda al., 1998; Wang et al., 1998). These changes result in additional overload on the remaining viable muscle cells. If this vicious cycle persists, cardiac function gradually deteriorates and, eventually, overt heart failure may occur. Theoretically, heart failure could be cured or minimized by implantation of viable muscle cells into the area of the lesion. In the last decade, numerous studies in which different types of muscle cells were transplanted into experimentally injured myocardium have been carried out to test this hypothesis. The purpose of this chapter is to review the experimental studies that have implanted cardiomyocytes, skeletal muscle cells, and stem cells into the myocardium and to review their effects on cardiac function and angiogenesis.

18.2. IS IT FEASIBLE TO IMPLANT CELLS INTO MYOCARDIUM?

18.2.1. Cardiomyocytes

Logically, it would be ideal to implant cardiomyocytes to replace damaged myocardium, because they have their unique electrophysiological, structural, and contractile properties. In a pioneering study performed by Soonpaa et al., fetal cardiomyocytes were isolated from transgenic mice carrying a fusion gene of the α-cardiac myosin heavy chain promoter and a modified β-galactosidase (β-gal) reporter (nLAC). The nLAC reporter carried an SV40 nuclear transport signal, resulting in nuclear accumulation of β-gal activity in targeted cells. The isolated cells (1×10^4 to 10×10^4) were implanted into the left ventricles of syngeneic nontransgenic recipients by direct intramyocardial injection. The grafts were examined 19 days after implantation and found in 11 of 19 recipients. The grafted cells containing β-gal activity were shown to juxtapose to the host myocytes. By electron microscopy, the implanted cells were identified by nuclear crystalloid deposit as a result of formation of X-gal reaction product. At many sites, nascent intercalated disks were detected between engrafted cells and the host myocytes. ECG recording showed that there were no adverse electrocardiographic effects of intracardiac grafts on the host myocardium (Soonpaa et al., 1994).

Leor et al. cultured tissue chunks from fetal human ventricles or fetal rat ventricles and transplanted four to six contracting fragments into cardiac scar tissue of experimental myocardial infarctions in rats. Either electron microscopy or antibody against α-smooth muscle actin (present in fetal but not in adult cardiomyocytes) was used to detect engrafted tissue. In the first group, tissue fragments of cultured human fetal ventricles were injected into 7- to 24-day-old scars. The animals in this group were treated with cyclosporin A to prevent graft rejection. The grafts were found in 6 of 11 rats 7 days after transplantation. In four of four rats the grafts were detected 14 days after transplantation. In the second group, fragments of cultured fetal rat ventricles were injected into 9- to 17-day-old scars of rats. Grafted cardiomyocytes were detected in one of two rats at 8 days, one of two rats at 14 days, one of one rat at 32 days, and two of two rats at 65 days after transplantation. In the infarcted area where saline was injected, positive staining for α-smooth muscle actin was only found within the vasculature (Leor et al., 1996).

Scorsin et al. transplanted fetal rat cardiomyocytes (6×10^6) into the left ventricles of both normal rats ($n = 10$) and rats with infarction ($n = 10$). In the infarcted hearts, cells were placed along the peri-infarct border zone. Control rats ($n = 6$) were only injected with culture medium. Two days later the hearts were collected for morphologic analysis. Grafted fetal myocytes were found in the host myocardium of all noninfarcted animals and at the border zone in 50% of the rats with infarction. On H&E staining, the implanted cells appeared to be small and round and their nuclei were darkly stained with a high ratio of nucleus to cytoplasm. The histologic immunostaining with antibody against sarcomeric α-actinin confirmed the fetal nature of these cells by demonstrating a loose myofibrillar organization that was similar to the pattern of the myocytes grown in culture (Scorsin et al., 1996).

Koh et al. implanted fetal cardiomyocytes (1×10^4 to 1×10^5) from transgenic mice with MHC-nLAC reporter into dystrophic mdx mice ($n = 44$). The latter were non-transgenic and thus did not express β-gal activity. The donor myocytes were identified in 60% of recipient mice by both β-gal activity and dystrophin in the host myocardium, where these markers were absent. Ultrastructural examination revealed the formation of intercalated discs consisting of fascia adherens, desmosomes, and gap junctions between donor and host myocytes. Subsequently, they transplanted fetal canine cardiomyocytes into the hearts of three dogs with canine X-linked muscular dystrophy. The recipient dogs received cyclosporine to suppress immunorejection. The donor myocytes were identified by positive immunoreactivity of dystrophin. In all these dogs, the implanted myocytes could be found between 2.5 and 10 weeks after implantation. Confocal microscopy detected the presence of connexin 43 between donor and host myocardium. The results showed that dystrophin could be used to follow up the graft in both small and large mammals under these experimental conditions (Koh et al., 1995).

In a study performed by Li et al. fetal rat cardiomyocytes were transfected with plasmid containing the β-gal reporter gene and injected into myocardial scar ($54 \pm 11 \, mm^2$) that were formed 4 weeks after cryoinjury in rats. Cell culture medium was injected into the scar tissue of control animals. Four weeks after implantation, grafted cardiomyocytes had formed cardiac tissue ($20.7 \pm 6.9 \, mm^2$) that stained positively for β-galactosidase activity in the scar ($90.4 \pm 25.0 \, mm^2$). These cardiomyocytes formed sarcomeres and were connected with each other by junctions composed of desmosomes and fascia adherens. However, the connection between implanted and host myocytes were not described. At 20 weeks after transplantation, the graft size ($6 \pm 6 \, mm^2$; $n = 7$) was smaller ($P = 0.007$) than at 4 weeks, and the scar ($162 \pm 46 \, mm^2$; $n = 7$) was larger ($P = 0.005$). Lymphocytes were observed around cardiac tissue formed by transplanted cells throughout the period of study despite administration of cyclosporin A. The authors postulated that the decrease in size of the graft over time may have resulted from host rejection (Li et al., 1997).

Gojo et al. transfected murine fetal cardiomyocytes with replication-defective recombinant adenovirus carrying the β-gal reporter gene and transplanted these myocytes (5×10^5 to 1×10^6) into the hearts of syngeneic recipients. The expression of β-gal activity in the grafted cells was detected by both histochemical and electron microscopic analysis 7 days to 12 weeks after transplantation. Implanted cardiomyocytes were found to be aligned along the layers of the host myocardium. Electron microscopic examination revealed formation of desmosomes and gap junctions between engrafted and host cardiomyocytes, indicating that it is possible for the implanted myocytes to form functional syncytia with native myocytes (Gojo et al., 1997).

Matsushita et al. transplanted rat neonatal cardiomyocytes into the border zone of 18 rats with 10-day-old myocardial infarctions. Grafted neonatal cardiomyocytes (1×10^6) were detected with antibody against α-smooth muscle actin within 7 days after transplantation. Connexin 43, desmoplakin and cadherin were localized not only between grafted cardiomyocytes but also between grafted and native myocytes. Semiquantitative analysis showed increase in the density of all three junctional proteins as time advanced from 4 to 7 days after transplantation (Matsushita et al., 1999).

In the study done by Reinecke et al. an aliquot of 5×10^5 adult, 4×10^6 neonatal, or 2×10^6 fetal rat cardiomyocytes was grafted into normal myocardium, acutely cryoinjured myocardium, or granulation tissue that formed 6 days after cryoinjury. Adult cardiomyocytes were not able to survive under any of these circumstances, whereas fetal and neonatal cardiomyocytes formed viable grafts under all conditions. The adherens junction protein N-cadherin was distributed circumferentially at day 1 but began to organize into intercalated disklike structures by day 6. The gap junction protein connexin 43 followed a similar but delayed pattern relative to N-cadherin. During 2–8 weeks after transplantation, there was progressive increase in the size of implanted myocytes with formation of mature intercalated disks. In most cases, grafts were separated from the host myocardium by scar tissue, although the formation of adherens and gap junctions between implanted cells and host cardiomyocytes was sometimes detected. Therefore, grafted fetal and neonatal cardiomyocytes form new and mature myocardium with the capacity to couple with injured host myocardium. Undoubtedly, a better approach is required to reduce the amount of intervening scar tissue that separates the graft from host myocardium (Reinecke et al., 1999).

Watanabe et al. examined the feasibility of transplanting either HL-1 cells, which are derived from an atrial cell line of the mouse (Claycomb et al., 1998), or fetal or neonatal pig cardiomyocytes into hearts with myocardial infarctions in large mammals. The myocardial infarction was induced by placing an embolization coil in the distal portion of the left anterior descending artery in Yorkshire pigs. Four to five weeks after infarction, an aliquot (1×10^6) of these cells was grafted into both the center of the infarcted area and noninfarcted myocardium. The recipient animals were treated with immunosuppression therapy to prevent graft rejection. At 4–5 weeks after implantation, formation of grafts in normal myocardium was found with HL-1 cells (44%) and with fetal pig cardiomyocytes (27%) but not with neonatal myocytes at injection sites. Electron microscopic analysis demonstrated that fetal cardiomyocytes and native myocardium were coupled with adherens-type junctions and gap junctions. However, neither of these cell preparations was found in the infarcted area (Watanabe et al., 1998).

In our own preliminary studies, 1×10^6 to 2×10^6 cardiomyocytes (Fig. 18-1) isolated from fetal Fisher rats were implanted into normal hearts of adult rats. Histologic examination of these adult hearts 1 week after implantation showed that grafts were formed from the implanted cells and were readily distinguished from host myocardium by their features. The transplanted cells appeared small in size with basophilic cytoplasm. In longitudinal profile, these fetal cells were found to form myotubes with some degree of striation, although the new myofibers were thinner than host muscle cells (Fig. 18-2). Immunohistochemistry showed the grafts were positive for antibodies against α-slow skeletal myosin heavy chain and α-sarcomeric actin.

Thus the results from the majority of studies described above demonstrate that fetal and neonatal, but not adult cardiomyocytes, can survive and develop into cardiac tissue after transplantation into both normal and damaged myocardium. Furthermore, coupling between implanted cells and host cardiomyocytes was detected in several of these studies. This coupling is a prerequisite for the transplanted cardiomyocytes to play a role in cardiac contraction.

18.2.2. Skeletal Muscle Cells

Skeletal muscle has been introduced in the treatment of cardiac dysfunction. In the surgical procedure of so called dynamic cardiomyoplasty, the diseased hearts are

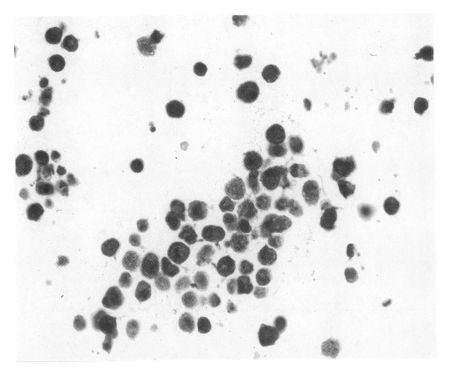

FIGURE 18-1. This photomicrograph illustrates a sample of cells to be transplanted into normal rat myocardium. They were isolated from ventricular tissue of fetal rat and then cultured for 2 days. Note their round shape and lack of cellular process.

wrapped with autologous latissimus dorsi muscle. Two weeks after placement, the muscle flap is conditioned by progressive electrical stimulation, allowing it to become fatigue resistant. The muscle is then stimulated electrically in synchrony with each cardiac contraction to augment ventricular function (Chachques et al., 1988). The chronic electrical stimulation of fast-twitch skeletal muscle induces the expression of an isoform of myosin with characteristics similar to those of adult ventricular muscle. Electron microscopy revealed preserved myofibrillar structure and an increased number of mitochondria in these stimulated skeletal muscles (Chachques et al., 1988). Upregulation of the isoforms of sarcoplasmic reticulum proteins that are expressed in slow muscle by chronic stimulation also was reported (Hu et al., 1995). The observed plasticity may explain why skeletal muscle can be used in assisting cardiac performance.

Unlike cardiac muscle, skeletal muscle is able to repair itself after injury because it contains satellite cells, quiescent precursor cells, which are located between the mature muscle fiber and its sheath of external lamina. These cells are activated when muscle is injured or stressed and migrate into damaged areas, where they enter the cell cycle and produce myoblasts that will fuse with each other or into damaged myofibers, thus generating new myotubes (Campion, 1984). These biological properties have raised an enormous interest in testing the possibility that damaged myocardium can be repaired by implantation of skeletal muscle cells or "cellular cardiomyoplasty."

Koh et al. introduced C2C12 cells (4×10^4 to 1×10^5), a myoblast line derived from adult mouse satellite cells, into ventricular myocardium of syngeneic mice. In all of the recipient animals ($n = 13$), implanted cells were found to develop into grafts in the host

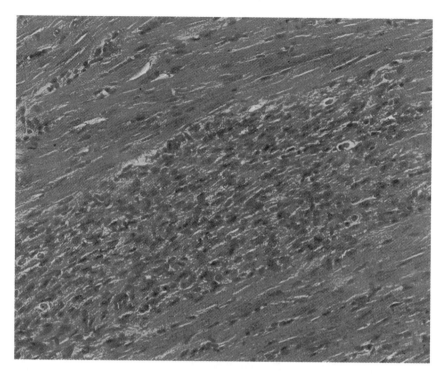

FIGURE 18-2. This photomicrograph demonstrates a 7-day-old graft (in the middle of the micrograph) that is readily distinguishable from host myocardium. The implanted cells have begun to differentiate and therefore appear totally different from those cells that are displayed in Figure 18-1. Note that the grafted cells have elongated but they are thinner than host muscle fibers, indicating that more time is required for them to develop into functional mature myocardium.

myocardium and were present for as long as 3 months. The implanted cells could be labeled with antibody against myosin heavy chain (MY-32), suggesting that differentiation had been initiated within the graft. By electron microscopy, the differentiated cells in the graft demonstrated abundant mitochondria localized between well-developed myofibrils with prominent Z bands. In the less-differentiated cells, some features of satellite cells, such as large nuclei with obvious heterochromatin, and a limited number of mitochondria were found. Thymidine uptake assay indicated that all the implanted cells were virtually withdrawn from the cell cycle by 14 days after implantation. ECG recording did not show overt arrhythmia in the recipient animals (Koh et al., 1993).

Comparable results with C2C12 cells were obtained in another study. Robinson et al. injected C2C12 cells containing β-gal reporter gene into left ventricular cavities of mice. Initially, the injected cells were entrapped in myocardial capillaries, but at 1 week the myoblasts were mainly present in the myocardial interstitium instead of the myocardial capillary bed. The cells underwent myogenic development, characterized by the expression of a fast-twitch skeletal muscle sarcoendoplasmic reticulum calcium ATPase (SERCA1) and formation of myofilaments. Four months later these cells began to express a slow-twitch/cardiac protein, phospholamban, which is normally not expressed by C2C12 cells in vitro. At the regions of close apposition between implanted cells and native cardiomyocytes, structures resembling desmosomes, fascia adherens junctions, and gap

junctions were detected. Connexin 43 was localized to some of the interfaces between implanted cells and host cardiomyocytes. The results suggest that the engrafting can also be achieved by arterial delivery and that the microenvironment in the myocardium may alter the phenotype of skeletal muscle-derived cells (Robinson et al., 1996).

Murry et al. transplanted neonatal skeletal muscle cells (3×10^6) into cryoinjured myocardium either immediately or 1 week after induction of injury. With either approach, multinucleated myotubes were formed by 3 days after implantation. Immunohistochemical staining revealed both embryonic and fast fiber myosin heavy chains in the myotubes. By 2 weeks, β-myosin heavy chain, a phenotype of slow fiber, appeared in the graft that was formed by myocytes that had been transplanted into 1-week-old scar tissue. In contrast, this isoform did not appear in the cells that were engrafted immediately after injury to 7 weeks after implantation. Two weeks after transplantation, the myoblast grafts could contract when they were stimulated ex vivo and were able to exhibit a cardiac-like performance, alternating tetanic contraction and relaxation for at least 6 min (Murry et al., 1996).

In a study performed by Chiu et al., canine skeletal satellite cells were isolated, cultured, labeled with either tritiated thymidine or β-gal reporter gene, and transplanted (5×10^6 to 7.5×10^6) autologously into acutely cryoinjured myocardium. In an experiment with thymidine-labeled cells, the specimens were harvested 4 to 18 weeks thereafter. Histologic examination revealed the presence of striated muscles with centrally located nuclei and intercalated discs in 5 of 17 samples where grafts were found. Tritiated thymidine radioactivity was not identified clearly, probably because of a dilutional effect of cell replication. X-gal staining of specimens that were collected 4–6 weeks later found β-gal activity in the cells at the implant site, confirming the originality of implanted cells (Chiu et al., 1995).

In another study, satellite cells were isolated from the skeletal muscle of adult rats and labeled with 4′,6-diamidino-2-phenylindole, which binds to DNA and to tubulin to form a fluorescent complex. The labeled cells (1×10^6) were implanted into the left ventricles of recipient rats. and the specimens were collected 1 and 4 weeks thereafter. Labeled cells were found in 4 of 24 samples. Fluorescent microscopy showed a progressive differentiation of implanted myoblasts into fully developed striated muscle fibers (Dorfman et al., 1998).

Atkins et al. transplanted autologous skeletal myoblasts (7×10^6) from adult New Zealand White rabbits into the cryoinjured area of left ventricles either at the time of injury ($n = 6$) or 1 week later ($n = 12$). The hearts were collected and examined 2 weeks after implantation. In 13 of these recipients, histologic examination revealed structures resembling skeletal muscle, which covered up to 75% of the central lesion. However, the newly formed myotubes were inevitably surrounded by inflammatory cells and scar tissue. Immunohistochemistry and visual examination demonstrated two populations of striated cells in the area of the lesion. Multinucleated cells were observed within the central area of the lesion and were confirmed to be of skeletal muscle origin by immunohistochemical labeling of myogenin, a skeletal muscle-specific transcription factor. At the periphery of the lesion, small clusters of myogenin-negative cells were visualized, and they appeared to be immature cardiomyocytes in terms of centrally located nuclei and striations (Atkins et al., 1999a).

These data suggest that skeletal myoblasts can also be used to replace lost myocardium in damaged areas of the heart. The significance of these findings is that (1) implanted skeletal muscle cells can survive in the damaged myocardium, and some of them can take on a cardiac-like phenotype; (2) skeletal muscle is able to regenerate itself on injury, and this property would limit the impact of any further injury to the implanted site; and (3) the application of autologous skeletal muscle could avoid troublesome immunosuppressive therapy.

18.2.3. Stem Cells

The insufficient number of donor cells that can be collected by current standard techniques serves as one of the obstacles to the clinical application of cell transplantation. Therefore, alternative sources of donor cells have been sought. One of these is the embryonic stem (ES) cell. The advantage of using ES cells is that they are capable of proliferating as well as differentiating. In a study by Klug et al., a fusion gene consisting of the α-cardiac myosin heavy chain promoter and a cDNA encoding aminoglycoside phosphotransferase was transfected into murine ES cells, which are derived from the inner cell mass of blastocysts. They are pluripotent and able to differentiate into a variety of cell lineages in vitro. After in vitro differentiation, ES-derived cardiomyocytes expressed aminoglycoside phosphotransferase through the operation of α-cardiac myosin heavy chain promoter and became resistant to G418 (an aminoglycoside antibiotic), which is inactivated by their aminoglycoside phosphotransferase. The nonmyocytes that did not express aminoglycoside phosphotransferase were eliminated by G418 (an inhibitor of both prokaryotes and eukaryotes). Consequently, the selection with G418 (200 μg/ml) yielded a pure population of cardiomyocytes (99.6%) that were shown to be highly differentiated by immunocytological and ultrastructural examination. To test whether these cardiomyocytes were able to form intracardiac grafts, about 1×10^4 cells were implanted into each adult dystrophic mouse heart. In six of eight recipients, the graft was found by immunostaining for dystrophin and PCR analysis with primers specific for the myosin heavy chain-aminoglycoside phosphotransferase transgene. The presence of ES-derived cardiomyocytes was detected for as long as 7 weeks after implantation (Klug et al., 1996). These results showed that a genetic manipulation facilitated the selection of cardiomyocytes among the differentiating ES cells. The data suggested that ES cells can be a potential source of cardiomyocytes for the purpose of transplantation.

IS IT POSSIBLE TO IMPROVE CARDIAC FUNCTION BY IMPLANTATION OF MYOCYTES?

Li et al. produced left ventricular damage in the rat by cryoinjury and transplanted fetal rat cardiomyocytes into 4-week-old scars. Four weeks after transplantation, cardiac function was assayed in vitro using a Langendorff apparatus. Systolic and developed pressures were greater in hearts receiving cell implants compared with control hearts that were injected with culture medium only. The transplanted cardiomyocytes formed cardiac tissue within the myocardial scar (Li et al., 1996).

Scorsin et al. implanted fetal rat cardiomyocytes (6×10^6) of both sexes into the infarcted area of 23 female rats after 45 min of ischemia and 30-min reperfusion. In 10 control animals, only culture medium was injected. One month after transplantation, left ventricular function was assessed by echocardiography and myocardium was examined by fluorescent in situ hybridization (FISH) to detect Y chromosome by taking advantage of the fact that about 50% of implanted cells were male. The ejection fraction and cardiac output were significantly higher in the transplanted group than in the control group ($P < 0.02$ and $P < 0.02$). The improvement in left ventricular function was associated with the detection of the Y chromosome signal, indicating that functional improvement resulted from cell transplantation (Scorsin et al., 1997).

This group also compared the effects of fetal cardiomyocyte and skeletal myoblast implantation on left ventricular function after infarction in the rat. Fetal cardiomyocytes or neonatal skeletal myoblasts were injected into 1-week-old infarctions. In control animals, only culture medium was injected. Left ventricular function was assessed by echocardiography immediately before implantation and 1 month thereafter. In rats in which fetal cardiomyocytes were transplanted, the left ventricular ejection fraction increased from $39.3 \pm 3.9\%$ to $45 \pm 3.4\%$. Transplantation of neonatal myoblasts achieved a comparable

result in the rats with ejection fraction increasing from $40.4 \pm 3.6\%$ to $47.3 \pm 4.4\%$. In contrast, the ejection fraction decreased in control animals from $40.6 \pm 4\%$ to $36.7 \pm 2.7\%$. These results showed that transplantation of skeletal myoblasts was as effective as fetal cardiomyocytes for improving left ventricular function after myocardial infarction (Scorsin et al., 2000).

To determine the possible mechanisms by which cell transplantation may improve heart function, Sakai et al. injected fetal cardiomyocytes, enteric smooth muscle cells, and skin fibroblasts into 4-week-old myocardial scar areas in the rat (cardiomyocytes, $n = 13$; smooth muscle cells, $n = 10$; skin fibroblasts $n = 10$). Each recipient animal was implanted with 4×10^6 cells of one type, whereas the controls ($n = 15$) were injected with culture medium only. At 4 weeks of transplantation, the hearts were isolated and left ventricular function was evaluated in a Langendorff apparatus. At an end-diastolic volume of 0.2 ml, developed pressures in the hearts transplanted with cardiomyocytes (using the value obtained from controls as baselines) were significantly greater than the hearts transplanted with smooth muscle cells and skin fibroblasts (cardiomyocytes, $134 \pm 22\%$ of control; smooth muscle cells, $108 \pm 14\%$ of control; skin fibroblasts, $106 \pm 17\%$ of control), The improvements were also observed in $+dP/dt$ (max) (cardiomyocytes, $119 \pm 37\%$ of control; smooth muscle cells, $98 \pm 18\%$ of control; skin fibroblasts, $92 \pm 11\%$ of control; $P = 0.0001$) and in $-dP/dt$ (max) (cardiomyocytes, $126 \pm 29\%$ of control; smooth muscle cells, $108 \pm 19\%$ of control; skin fibroblasts, $99 \pm 16\%$ of control). Histologic examination showed that all transplanted cell types formed tissue within the myocardial scar. These results demonstrated that the degree of improvement in ventricular function was determined by the contractile and elastic properties of transplanted cells (Sakai et al., 1999).

Taylor et al. tested whether skeletal myoblast transplantation was capable of improving cardiac performance after myocardial injury. In their study, 17 rabbits were subjected to myocardial cryoinjury. One week later 1×10^7 autologous skeletal myoblasts were injected into the cryoinjured area in 12 of the animals. The remaining five animals received medium injection only as controls. In 7 of 12 animals, structures resembling striated skeletal myotubes were found by histology 3–6 weeks after implantation. The largest graft occupied 75% of the lesion area but did extend to or beyond the border of the lesion. The implanted cells were elongated, and their nuclei were stained positive for myogenin, which is specific to skeletal muscle cells. Electron microscopic examination revealed that structures resembling skeletal myotubes observed by histology consisted of single mononucleated myocytes that were connected to each other by intercalated discs. In five of these seven rabbits in which implantation was successful, preload recruitable stroke work slope was significantly increased compared with control animals. The trend for functional improvement was seen in the other two rabbits (Taylor et al., 1999). In another study under similar experimental conditions, diastolic properties of cryoinjured hearts were improved in the rabbit after implantation of autologous skeletal myoblasts (Atkins et al., 1999b).

Tomita et al. evaluated the effect of autologous bone marrow cells (BMCs) on cardiac function because the pluripotential progenitor cells in bone marrow have the capacity to differentiate into various types of cells, including muscle cells. In their study, the cells collected from the bone marrow of adult rats were cultured and treated with 5-azacytidine (10 mM), TGF-β1 (10 ng/ml), or insulin (1 nM). Only BMCs cultured with 5-azacytidine formed myotubes that stained positively for troponin I and myosin heavy chain. At 3 weeks after cryoinjury, 1×10^6 fresh BMCs, cultured BMCs, or 5-azacytidine-treated BMCs or medium as control were transplanted into the scar area of the left ventricular free wall. Cardiac-like muscle cells with myosin heavy chain and troponin I were observed in all three groups of rats transplanted with cells 5 weeks after implantation. However, only implantation of

5-azacytidine-treated BMCs resulted in smaller scar and larger wall thickness in the cryoinjured area. Consistently, the hearts transplanted with these cells had greater systolic and developed pressures than those in the control group. These results showed that BMCs could be differentiated into cardiac-like muscle cells with the treatment of 5-azacytidine in culture and that such cells were able to improve myocardial function. The treated BMCs may represent an additional source of donor cells to replace damaged cardiomyocytes (Tomita et al., 1999).

These data demonstrate that it may be practical to implant myocytes to improve cardiac dysfunction. However, it has not been shown consistently that implanted cells can develop cellular contact with host cardiomyocytes around damaged myocardium. The results from most studies also found that implanted cells were separated from the native myocardium by scar tissue. In addition, although cells may improve global left ventricular function, it is not clear whether they perform spontaneous contraction and relaxation within a graft, or whether improved function is related to passive or elastic properties of the implants.

18.4. ANGIOGENESIS

Some investigators have reported that implantation of cardiomyocytes is associated with an increased number of arterioles and venules in the graft (Li et al., 1997; Watanabe et al., 1998). Using immunohistochemical staining, Li et al. labeled factor VIII-related antigen of vascular endothelial cells in the grafts. The positive cells were counted under the light microscope. At 4 weeks of implantation, more arterioles and venules were found ($P < 0.01$) in the cardiomyocyte grafts (1.2 ± 0.6 vessel/0.8 mm^2; $n = 14$) than in the control scar tissue (0.1 ± 0.1 vessels/0.8 mm^2; $n = 14$). Interestingly, a comparable result was also achieved with implantation of BMCs (Tomita et al., 1999).

The growth factors that are involved in angiogenesis include fibroblast growth factors (FGFs), vascular endothelial growth factor

(VEGF) and insulin growth factors (IGFs). Cardiomyocytes have been documented to express both acidic FGF (Engelmann et al., 1993; Speir et al., 1992; Zhao et al., 1994) and basic FGF (Casscells et al., 1990; Fischer et al., 1997; Speir et al., 1992), VEGF (Gao et al., 2000), and both IGF-I (Brink et al., 1999; Kluge et al., 1995; Suzuki et al., 1999) and IGF-II (Kluge et al., 1995). Therefore, the association of cardiomyocyte implantation with angiogenesis in the graft indicates that implanted cardiomyocytes may release their angiogenic factors, which in turn facilitate formation of new vasculature.

FGF-1, also called acidic FGF, is a 140-amino acid peptide (Esch et al., 1985). FGF-2 or basic FGF has 146 amino acids (Abraham et al., 1986). These two FGFs are encoded by two different genes but have a 55% amino acid sequence homology (Gospodarowicz et al., 1989). Of note, it has been reported that FGF-2 can not only promote angiogenesis but also can acutely reduce myocardial infarct size (Miyataka et al., 1998; Uchida et al., 1995; Yanagisawa-Miwa et al., 1992). Under the condition of ischemia-reperfusion, myocardial protection has also been reported to be conferred by administration of FGF-1 (Cuevas et al., 1997; Htun et al., 1998) and FGF-2 (Horrigan et al., 1996; Padua et al., 1995).

Insulin growth factors I and II are polypeptides with 70 and 67 amino acids, respectively, and they have 62% amino acid homology (Humbel, 1990). These two growth factors are encoded by two separate genes located on two different chromosomes (Tricoli et al., 1984). In a murine model of ischemia-reperfusion injury, it was demonstrated that administration of IGF-I 1 hour before ischemia could attenuate myocardial injury as evidenced by reduction in creatine kinase loss and incidence of myocyte apoptosis as well as neutrophil accumulation in the ischemic area (Buerke et al., 1995). Delivery of IGF-II into the infarct area was also shown to improve wall motion in injured segments (Battler et al., 1995).

Because angiogenesis and collateral remodeling take a few days to accomplish (Schaper et al., 1990) and the time window for viability for most cardiomyocytes is limited to a few hours of severe ischemia (Reimer and Jennings, 1979), it is difficult to conceive that acute beneficial effects conferred by these growth factors on ischemic myocardium are due to an angiogenic mechanism. Therefore, these growth factors may have direct effects on the myocytes to prevent them from cell death due to ischemic injury. It will be interesting to determine whether the reported beneficial effects of angiogenic growth factors can be harnessed and applied to cell transplantation technology by coimplantation of myocytes and the cells that can specifically secrete these growth factors.

18.5. SUMMARY

The literature reviewed above demonstrates that it is feasible to transplant cardiac muscle cells (fetal and neonatal) or skeletal muscle-derived cells such as satellite cells or stem cells. Several studies showed that cell implantation into myocardium resulted in an improvement in cardiac function in experimental animals. Therefore, cell transplantation could potentially be effective in the treatment of heart failure, especially that due to ischemia. Use of autologous cells (either skeletal myoblast or myocytes derived from bone marrow stem cells) is advantageous because their sources are relatively abundant and the problems of immunosuppression can be avoided. The mechanism underlying the improvement of cardiac performance by cell implantation is complicated. Because implanted myocytes are reported to be separated from host myocardium by scar tissue in most studies, it is unlikely that implanted cells can contribute directly to the host myocardial contraction. However, it is possible that these cells can reduce wall stress by increasing wall thickness and increasing diastolic compliance by formation of new tissue with elastic properties in the scar (Sakai et al., 1999). We believe that the new myocardium formed from implanted cells may at least absorb to some degree the mechanical overload imposed on noninjured myocardium and thus delay or prevent the processes of cellular degeneration and cell death in noninjured areas with a result of limiting progressive ventricular dilation and worsening of ventricular function. Angiogenesis associated with cardiomyocyte implantation also may play a protective role, and therefore implantation of specific type of cells that secrete angiogenic growth factors may maximize the salutary effects of cell transplantation on the myocardium.

18.6. OPENED QUESTIONS

Despite numerous studies that have been carried out in this field, several important questions still need to be answered. They include (1) whether cell transplantation can modulate the molecular and cellular events involved in the pathophysiology of heart failure, such as sympathetic overshoot, augmentation of both the circulating and cardiac renin-angiotensin system, and apoptosis in the myocardium, with a result of reversing ventricular remodeling; (2) whether the combination of cell transplantation plus medical treatment such as ACE inhibitors and β-blockers can achieve better results in improvement of cardiac function; (3) whether cell transplantation is also effective in the treatment of heart diseases in which myocardium is globally inflicted such as dilated cardiomyopathy; (4) whether it is possible for the implanted skeletal muscle cells to regenerate in response to any further injury in the implanted area; and (5) whether it is feasible to use implanted cells that have been modified genetically as a platform to deliver angiogeneic and cardioprotective growth factors to the diseased heart. Certainly, many more studies are needed to test these hypotheses and to answer these questions.

ACKNOWLEDGMENT

The authors' work is supported in part by NHLBI Grant R01-HL-61488.

References

Abraham JA, Mergia A, Whang JL et al. Nucleotide sequence of a bovine clone encoding the angiogenic protein, basic fibroblast growth factor. *Science* 1986; 233: 545–548.

Anversa P, Kajstura J. Ventricular myocytes are not terminally differentiated in the adult mammalian heart. *Circ Res* 1998; 83: 1–14.

Atkins BZ, Hueman MT, Meuchel J et al. Cellular cardiomyoplasty improves diastolic properties of injured heart. *J Surg Res* 1999a; 85: 234–242.

Atkins BZ, Lewis CW, Kraus WE et al. Intracardiac transplantation of skeletal myoblasts yields two populations of striated cells *in situ. Ann Thorac Surg* 1999b; 67: 124–129.

Battler A, Hasdai D, Goldberg I et al. Exogenous insulin-like growth factor II enhances post-infarction regional myocardial function in swine. *Eur Heart J* 1995; 16: 1851–1859.

Brink M, Chrast J, Price SR et al. Angiotensin II stimulates gene expression of cardiac insulin-like growth factor I and its receptor through effects on blood pressure and food intake. *Hypertension* 1999; 34: 1053–1059.

Buerke M, Murohara T, Skurk C et al. Cardioprotective effect of insulin-like growth factor I in myocardial ischemia followed by reperfusion. *Proc Natl Acad Sci USA* 1995; 92: 8031–8035.

Campion DR. The muscle satellite cell: a review. *Int Rev Cytol* 1984; 87: 225–251.

Casscells W, Speir E, Sasse J et al. Isolation, characterization, and localization of heparin-binding growth factors in the heart. *J Clin Invest* 1990; 85: 433–441.

Chachques JC, Grandjean P, Schwartz K et al. Effect of latissimus dorsi dynamic cardiomyoplasty on ventricular function. *Circulation* 1988; 78 (*Suppl*): III-203–III-216.

Chiu RC, Zibaitis A, Kao RL. Cellular cardiomyoplasty: myocardial regeneration with satellite cell implantation. *Ann Thorac Surg* 1995; 60: 12–18.

Claycomb WC, Lanson NA Jr, Stallworth BS et al. HL-1 cells: a cardiac muscle cell line that contracts and retains phenotypic characteristics of the adult cardiomyocyte. *Proc Natl Acad Sci USA* 1998; 95: 2979–2984

Cuevas P, Reimers D, Carceller F et al. Fibroblast growth factor-1 prevents myocardial apoptosis triggered by ischemia reperfusion injury. *Eur J Med Res* 1997; 2: 465–468.

Diez J, Panizo A, Hernandez M et al. Cardiomyocyte apoptosis and cardiac angiotensin-converting enzyme in spontaneously hypertensive rats. *Hypertension* 1997; 30: 1029–1034.

Dorfman J, Duong M, Zibaitis A et al. Myocardial tissue engineering with autologous myoblast implantation. *J Thorac Cardiovasc Surg* 1998; 116: 744–751.

Engelmann GL, Dionne CA, Jaye MC. Acidic fibroblast growth factor and heart development. Role in myocyte proliferation and capillary angiogenesis. *Circ Res* 1993; 72: 7–19.

Esch F, Ueno N, Baird A et al. Primary structure of bovine brain acidic fibroblast growth factor (FGF). *Biochem Biophys Res Commun* 1985; 133: 554–562.

Fischer TA, Ungureanu-Longrois D, Singh K et al. Regulation of bFGF expression and ANG II secretion in cardiac myocytes and microvascular endothelial cells. *Am J Physiol* 1997; 272: H958–H968.

Gao M, Shirato H, Miyasaka K et al. Induction of growth factors in rat cardiac tissue by X irradiation. *Radiat Res* 2000; 153: 540–547.

Gospodarowicz D. Fibroblast growth factor. *Crit Rev Oncog* 1989; 1: 1–26.

Gojo S, Kitamura S, Hatano O et al. Transplantation of genetically marked cardiac muscle cells. *J Thorac Cardiovasc Surg* 1997; 113: 10–18.

Hu P, Yin C, Zhang KM et al. Transcriptional regulation of phospholamban gene and translational regulation of SERCA2 gene produces coordinate expression of these two sarcoplasmic reticulum proteins during skeletal muscle phenotype switching. *J Biol Chem* 1995; 270: 11619–11622.

Horrigan MC, MacIsaac AI, Nicolini FA et al. Reduction in myocardial infarct size by basic fibroblast growth factor after temporary coronary occlusion in a canine model. *Circulation* 1996; 94: 1927–1933.

Htun P, Ito WD, Hoefer IE et al. Intramyocardial infusion of FGF-1 mimics ischemic preconditioning in pig myocardium. *J Mol Cell Cardiol* 1998; 30: 867–877.

Humbel RE. Insulin-like growth factors I and II. *Eur J Biochem* 1990; 190: 445–462.

Klug MG, Soonpaa MH, Koh GY et al. Genetically selected cardiomyocytes from differentiating embryonic stem cells form stable intracardiac grafts. *J Clin Invest* 1996; 98: 216–224.

Kluge A, Zimmermann R, Munkel B et al. Insulin-like growth factor I is involved in inflammation linked angiogenic processes after microembolisation in porcine heart. *Cardiovasc Res* 1995; 29: 407–415.

Koh GY, Klug MG, Soonpaa MH et al. Differentiation and long-term survival of C2C12 myoblast grafts in heart. *J Clin Invest* 1993; 92: 1548–1554.

Koh GY, Soonpaa MH, Klug MG et al. Stable fetal cardiomyocyte grafts in the hearts of dystrophic mice and dogs. *J Clin Invest* 1995; 96: 2034–2042.

Leor J, Patterson M, Quinones MJ et al. Transplantation of fetal myocardial tissue into the infarcted myocardium of rat. A potential method for repair of infarcted myocardium? *Circulation* 1996; 94 (*Suppl*): II-332–II-326.

Li RK, Jia ZQ, Weisel RD et al. Cardiomyocyte transplantation improves heart function. *Ann Thorac Surg* 1996; 62: 654–661.

Li RK, Mickle DA, Weisel RD et al. Natural history of fetal rat cardiomyocytes transplanted into adult rat myocardial scar tissue. *Circulation* 1997; 96 (*Suppl*): II-179–II-187.

Maron BJ, Ferrans VJ, Jones M. The spectrum of degenerative changes in hypertrophied human cardiac muscle cells: an ultrastructural study. *Recent Adv Stud Cardiac Struct Metab* 1975; 8: 447–466.

Matsushita T, Oyamada M, Kurata H et al. Formation of cell junctions between grafted and host cardiomyocytes at the border zone of rat myocardial infarction. *Circulation* 1999; 100 (*Suppl*): II-262–II-268.

Miyataka M, Ishikawa K, Katori R. Basic fibroblast growth factor increased regional myocardial blood flow and limited infarct size of acutely infarcted myocardium in dogs. *Angiology* 1998; 49: 381–390.

Murry CE, Wiseman RW, Schwartz SM et al. Skeletal myoblast transplantation for repair of myocardial necrosis. *J Clin Invest* 1996; 98: 2512–2523.

Padua RR, Sethi R, Dhalla NS et al. Basic fibroblast growth factor is cardioprotective in ischemia-reperfusion injury. *Mol Cell Biochem* 1995; 143: 129–135.

Reimer KA, Jennings RB. The "wavefront phenomenon" of myocardial ischemic cell death. II. Transmural progression of necrosis within the framework of ischemic bed size (myocardium at risk) and collateral flow. *Lab Invest* 1979; 40: 633–644.

Reinecke H, Zhang M, Bartosek T et al. Survival, integration, and differentiation of cardiomyocyte grafts: a study in normal and injured rat hearts. *Circulation* 1999; 100: 193–202.

Robinson SW, Cho PW, Levitsky HI et al. Arterial delivery of genetically labeled skeletal myoblasts to the murine heart: long-term survival and phenotypic modification of implanted myoblasts. *Cell Transplant* 1996; 5: 77–91.

Sakai T, Li RK, Weisel RD et al. Fetal cell transplantation: a comparison of three cell types. *J Thorac Cardiovasc Surg* 1999; 118: 715–725.

Schaper W, Sharma HS, Quinkler W et al. Molecular biologic concepts of coronary anastomoses. *J Am Coll Cardiol* 1990; 15: 513–518.

Scorsin M, Marotte F, Sabri A et al. Can grafted cardiomyocytes colonize peri-infarct myocardial areas? *Circulation* 1996; 94 (*Suppl*): II-337–II-340.

Scorsin M, Hagege AA, Marotte F et al. Does transplantation of cardiomyocytes improve function of infracted myocardium? *Circulation* 1997; 96 (*Suppl*): II-188–II-193.

Scorsin M, Hagege A, Vilquin JT et al. Comparison of the effects of fetal cardiomyocyte and skeletal myoblast transplantation on postinfarction left ventricular function. *J Thorac Cardiovasc Surg* 2000; 119: 1169–1175.

Shizukuda Y, Buttrick PM, Geenen DL et al. β-Adrenergic stimulation causes cardiocyte apoptosis: influence of tachycardia and hypertrophy. *Am J Physiol* 1998; 275: H961–H968.

Soonpaa MH, Koh GY, Klug MG et al. Formation of nascent intercalated disks between grafted fetal cardiomyocytes and host myocardium. *Science* 1994; 264: 98–101.

Speir E, Tanner V, Gonzalez AM et al. Acidic and basic fibroblast growth factors in adult rat heart myocytes. Localization, regulation in culture, and effects on DNA synthesis. *Circ Res* 1992; 71: 251–259.

Suzuki J, Ohno I, Nawata J et al. Overexpression of insulin-like growth factor-I in hearts of rats with isoproterenol-induced cardiac hypertrophy. *J Cardiovasc Pharmacol* 1999; 34: 635–644.

Taylor DA, Atkins BZ, Hungspreugs P et al. Regenerating functional myocardium: improved performance after skeletal myoblast transplantation. *Nat Med* 1998; 4: 929–933.

Tomita S, Li RK, Weisel RD et al. Autologous transplantation of bone marrow cells improves damaged heart function. *Circulation* 1999; 100 (*Suppl*): II-247–II-256.

Tricoli JV, Rall LB, Scott J et al. Localization of insulin-like growth factor genes to human chromosomes 11 and 12. *Nature* 1984; 310: 784–786.

Uchida Y, Yanagisawa-Miwa A, Nakamura F et al. Angiogenic therapy of acute myocardial infarction by intrapericardial injection of basic fibroblast growth factor and heparin sulfate: an experimental study. *Am Heart J* 1995; 130: 1182–1188.

Wang Y, Huang S, Sah VP et al. Cardiac muscle cell hypertrophy and apoptosis induced by distinct members of the p38 mitogen-activated protein kinase family. *J Biol Chem* 1998; 273: 2161–2168.

Watanabe E, Smith DM Jr, Delcarpio JB et al. Cardiomyocyte transplantation in a porcine myocardial infarction model. *Cell Transplant* 1998; 7: 239–246.

Yanagisawa-Miwa A, Uchida Y, Nakamura F et al. Salvage of infarcted myocardium by angiogenic action of basic fibroblast growth factor. *Science* 1992; 257: 1401–1403.

Zhao XM, Yeoh TK, Frist WH et al. Induction of acidic fibroblast growth factor and full-length platelet-derived growth factor expression in human cardiac allografts. Analysis by PCR, in situ hybridization, and immunohistochemistry. *Circulation* 1994; 90: 677–685.

19

Percutaneous Myocardial Revascularization: Financial Potential and Market Acceptance

Terry Woodward, Ph.D., M.B.A.

Ontario Teachers' Pension Plan
Venture Capital, Toronto
Ontario, Canada

and

George S. Abela, M.D., M.Sc., M.B.A.

Department of Medicine
Division of Cardiology
Michigan State University
East Lansing, Michigan

and

Nancy Briefs, M.B.A.

Percardia, Inc.
Merrimack, New Hampshire

SUMMARY

CABG and PTCA are the two most common methods of myocardial revascularization, with PTCA having a higher initial success rate and lower initial costs than CABG. However, studies indicate that PTCA procedures are more likely to be repeated and may not have lower long-term costs, and that some groups derive more benefit from CABG.

For groups of patients not amenable to either PTCA or CABG, minimally invasive techniques such as TMR may be effective treatment. Some estimates have concluded that between 100,000 and 450,000 patients worldwide would be eligible for such alternative procedures.

With an estimated U.S. market for alternative revascularization of 100,000–200,000 patients, market potential may exceed 5–10 billion dollars, especially with market

Myocardial Revascularization: Novel Percutaneous Approaches, Edited by George S. Abela.
ISBN 0-471-36166-6   Copyright © 2002 Wiley-Liss, Inc.

penetration into patient groups such as diabetics.

Several issues must be addressed before wide acceptance of TMR/PMR is possible, including retraining of interventional cardiologists to perform alternative revascularization, a clear definition of the mechanism of benefit, and assessment of the placebo effect.

There is clearly a substantial market for direct myocardial revascularization procedures in terms of both unmet patient need and a solid financial market. With PTCA market penetration slowing, it is likely that alternative revascularization strategies will be reexamined to improve treatment for cardiac patients in the future.

19.1. BACKGROUND

The American Heart Association (AHA) (2001) has reported that more than 60 million persons (or nearly 30% of the adult population) in the United States have one or more types of cardiovascular disease (CVD), including:

High blood pressure	50.0 million
Coronary heart disease	12.4 million
Myocardial infarction	7.3 million
Angina pectoris	6.4 million
Stroke	4.5 million
Congenital cardiovascular defects	1.0 million
Congestive heart failure	4.7 million

CVD is and has been the leading killer in the United States for the past 100 years, claiming 40.6% (949,619 people/year) of all deaths, and is the direct cause or contributing cause of death in approximately 70% (1.4 million/year) of all deaths (AHA, 2001). In fact CVD, claims more lives each year than the next six leading causes of death combined, including all cancers. The AHA has estimated that CVD costs Americans nearly $300 billion/year, with over $180 billion/year in direct costs (AHA, 2001). Global costs of CVD may exceed half a trillion dollars annually.

19.2. MYOCARDIAL REVASCULARIZATION

Coronary artery bypass graft (CABG) and percutaneous transluminal coronary angioplasty (PTCA) are the two most common methods for myocardial revascularization. Although more than 1 million CABG and PTCA procedures are performed every year in the U.S., a significant group of patients are not candidates for bypass surgery or angioplasty and other patients, such as diabetics, experience only modest relief from angina pectoris and increase in life expectancy from PTCA or CABG. Direct myocardial revascularization using laser transmyocardial revascularization (PMR or TMR) or other approaches (described in this monograph) constitute the only alternative for patients who can no longer be treated using angioplasty and bypass surgery. Usually these are patients with diffuse vascular disease, as is often seen in the diabetic patient. Also, they include patients that may be at high risk for bypass surgery because of comorbid conditions such as severe lung disease, metastatic cancer, or a severely calcified aorta (Muskerjee et al., 1999). Furthermore, patients who have had several CABG procedures may no longer have veins or internal mammary arteries suitable as bypass grafts. The number of patients that have had repeat revascularization procedures is expanding as patients with coronary artery disease are living longer because of improved supportive and medical care.

19.2.1. Current Revascularization Strategies, Costs, and Limitations

In 1998, 553,000 CABG procedures were performed on 336,000 patients and 539,000 PTCA procedures were performed. The first PTCA procedure was performed in 1977, the number of procedures increased to over 100,000 by 1987 and to 370,000 by 1993. PTCA continues to gain market share, but growth has slowed over the past 5 years (AHA, 1993, 2001; Fry, 1990). PTCA has increased market penetration because it is less invasive, it has a higher initial success rate, and initial costs are lower when compared to CABG. However, restenosis occurs in 20–40% of patients treated with PTCA within the first 6 months, and 70% of patients with multivessel disease have incomplete revascularization (Faxon, 1997). The use of coronary stents has reduced the incidence of arterial restenosis after PTCA. Restenosis rates with stents have been estimated to range from 16% when no other risk factors are present to 60% with risk factors such as diabetes (Kastrati et al., 1997). Additionally, PTCA procedures are more likely to be repeated than CABG. Several studies were conducted in the past 5–10 years to assess the costs and quality of life after CABG and PTCA procedures including the randomized treatment of angina (RITA) trial, the Emory Angioplasty versus Surgery Trial (EAST), and the Bypass Angioplasty Revascularization Investigation (BARI) trial (Hlatky et al., 1997; Schulper et al., 1994; Weintraub et al., 1995). The largest of these trials, the BARI trial, has demonstrated that initial mean costs of PTCA and CABG procedures were $21,113 versus $32,347, respectively. However, after 5 years the total medical cost of PTCA was similar to CABG, $56,225 versus $58,889, respectively. The BARI trial and the EAST trial concluded that PTCA may not have lower costs than CABG after 3–5 years.

Importantly, CABG may be more effective than PTCA in certain patient subgroups. For example, diabetic patients treated by CABG had significantly better 5-year survival than PTCA: 19.4% versus 34.5% deaths in CABG and PTCA, respectively (Pocock et al., 1995). CABG may also be more effective in patients with hypertension, multivessel disease, and severe vessel blockage. Unfortunately, these data demonstrate that patients with a worse prognosis are less likely to benefit from the less invasive PTCA procedure (Fudge, 2001). Therefore, there are significant groups of patients who are not effectively treated by PTCA and have high immediate mortality risks associated with the invasive CABG procedure. Minimally invasive techniques described in this monograft, including trans-

myocardial revascularization, may be effective in treating many of these patients.

19.3. MARKET SIZE OF ALTERNATIVE REVASCULARIZATION STRATEGIES

Mukherjee and colleagues (Mukherjee et al., 1999) examined how many patients may be eligible for direct myocardial revascularization procedures. In this study, patients were deemed ineligible for PTCA if they had chronic total occlusion with unfavorable morphologic features, multiple restenosis, diffuse disease, and severely degenerated saphenous vein graft. Ineligibility for CABG included poor targets, lack of conduits, and severe comorbidities. Under the most rigorous of the FDA-approved alternative revascularization strategy protocols, approximately 12% of the 500 patients in the study were not eligible for PTCA or CABG, whereas more than 1/3 of these rejected patients were suitable for alternative revascularization strategies. The authors estimate that more liberal criteria would permit inclusion of nearly three times as many patients for alternative revascularization strategies. This study concluded that 100,000–200,000 patients/year in the U.S. may be eligible for alternative revascularization methods. Ahern (1999) estimated that between 300,000 and 450,000 patients worldwide are eligible for these alternative procedures.

Fifteen years ago, PTCA had little to no market, but with increased usage, refinements and improvements to the procedure increased effectiveness and market acceptance. It is likely that with increased usage, refinement and improvements will develop in TMR and other alternative revascularization therapies that could significantly increase these estimates. Others have reported that TMR and PMR are safe and effective therapy for severe angina pectoris secondary to end-stage coronary artery disease and may be effective as a stand-alone treatment or as an adjunctive with PTCA or CABG (Ahern, 1999; Allen and Shaar, 2000; Hughes, 1999; Leon et al.,

2000; Nordrehaug et al., 2001; Oesterle et al., 2000).

In addition to patients that are not eligible for CABG or PTCA, many patient groups are not effectively treated by these procedures and may represent future market targets for PMR or TMR and alternative revascularization techniques. For instance, approximately 20% of patients who undergo myocardial revascularization are diabetic (Weintraub et al., 1998). As discussed above, diabetic patients respond better to CABG than PTCA, especially if they have multivessel disease. In addition, CABG patients are less likely to experience nonfatal heart attacks or nonfatal cardiac events (Weintraub et al., 1998). Diabetic patients are also nearly two times as likely to have restenosis after PTCA with coronary stent placement than nondiabetic patients (Kastrati et al., 1997). Irrespective of current treatment options, diabetic patients face a three times greater risk of dying from heart disease than non-diabetics. Therefore, diabetics represent a significant group of patients that develop CVD and are not effectively treated by CABG or PTCA. Diabetic patients may be candidates for alternative revascularization procedures.

Comparing patients that are currently eligible for alternative revascularization procedures with all patients that have CVD, there are only slightly more diabetics in the pool of patients eligible for alternative revascularization (Mukherjee et al., 1999). Using more liberal criteria for alternative revascularization strategies could significantly increase the percentage of diabetics that are treatable.

Similar to angioplasty, more liberal criteria for usage of alternative revascularization techniques may occur as the techniques are more widely used because 1) the mechanism of action of these procedures will be better understood, 2) increased usage should result in advances in technology and skill of physician using techniques, and 3) if these techniques are found to be safe in advanced diseased patients these alternative revascularization strategies may be beneficial in treating patients with earlier disease progression.

The approximate market for diabetic patients alone, assuming equal distribution among procedures, is 110,000 patients/year for the PTCA procedure (539,000 × 1.03 increase in population since 1998 ×20% diabetics) and 114,000 procedures/year for CABG (553,000 × 1.03 increase in population ×20% diabetics) (U.S. Census Bureau, 2001). The initial procedural costs for PTCA were estimated to be $21,113 in 1994; adjusted for inflation costs would be approximately $25,000/procedure in 2001. Inflation-adjusted CABG direct procedural costs are approximately $38,000. Using the BARI study, inflation adjusted 5-year costs would be approximately $66,350 and $69,500 for PTCA and CABG, respectively. Table 19-1 estimates the current direct costs associated with treating the diabetic population. Coincidentally, the number of diabetic patients used in this example is very similar to estimates for the number of patients that may currently be eligible for alternative revascularization studies in the U.S.

Using the estimates of Mukherjee and

TABLE 19-1.   Estimated Direct Costs of Treatment of Diabetic Patients

	PTCA # Proc	PTCA Costs/proc	CABG # Proc	CABG Costs/proc	TOTAL Costs*
Hospital		$18,500		$25,840	$4.981
Professional		$6,500		$12,160	$2.101
Total	110,000	$25,000	114,000	$38,000	$7.083
5-yr Hospital		$49,763		$47,260	$10.862
5-yr Professional		$16,587		$22,240	$4.360
Total	110,000	$66,350	114,000	$69,500	$15.222

* Total costs are in billions of U.S. dollars.

colleagues (Mukherjee et al., 1999) for the number of patients that are currently eligible in the U.S. for alternative revascularization procedures (100,000–200,000 patients), direct costs of current procedures would be approximately 3–6 billion dollars ($7.083 billion × 100,000 or 200,000 patients in the eligible pool/224,000 diabetic patients), whereas procedural annual costs could be 6.5–13 billion dollars. Additionally, continuous development of alternative revascularization procedures should increase market penetration into other patient groups such as diabetics. A small market penetration in the diabetic market could result in significant revenues because direct annual costs exceed 7 billion dollars, whereas procedural annual costs may exceed $15 billion. It is expected that the manufacturer's income would equal 20% of this market, leading to a 3 billion dollar market.

19.4. PHYSICIAN ACCEPTANCE OF PERCUTANEOUS MYOCARDIAL REVASCULARIZATION

The use of laser and other approaches to "drill" channels into the myocardium has not been a very appealing concept to many interventional cardiologists. A major skepticism from cardiologists relates to a lack of a well-established mechanism of action to explain the improvement reported by direct myocardial reperfusion. This is despite the many studies demonstrating improvement including a recent multicenter report (Oesterle et al., 2000). A recent report has refuted many previous studies (Leon et al., 2000). This study, which determined that randomized placebo was not different in relieving angina pectoris from DMR, has fueled the skepticism of many physicians (Leon et al., 2000). Thus a major element in the acceptance of direct myocardial revascularization is the clear definition of the mechanism of benefit. It is somewhat ironic that the exact mechanism of PTCA was not well understood for a long time while PTCA made major inroads into clinical application. The original concept of the mechanism described as a "footprint in

the snow" to simulate how the balloon compressed the plaque is now recognized to be a more complex mechanism resulting in stretching the artery at the site of least resistance, often where the plaque is less dense. Yet the lack of accurate mechanism of action with regard to PTCA did not seem to deter the treating cardiologist. Also, it took a long time for the restenosis response to deter many from treating lesions that were not hemodynamically limiting. Nevertheless, a recent study conducted in a randomized placebo and double-blinded fashion demonstrated a major significant improvement in PMR compared to placebo (Nordrehaug et al., 2001). This emphasizes the importance of the type of system being used and that generalization of systems is a potentially flawed approach.

Several other more subtle issues concerning acceptance are that 1) the interventional cardiologist could perform several cases of standard procedure (i.e., PTCA and/or stents) in the time it would take to perform a direct myocardial revascularization treatment and 2) the interventional cardiologist must be retrained to understand and perform alternative revascularization strategies. The reimbursement of PTCA and PMR are at least for now equivalent, thereby providing incentive for the performance of the quicker PTCA procedure. Thus acceptance of a new technology is slow and often laden with a struggle. Similar to PTCA market acceptance, alternative revascularization strategies will be slow to gain physician acceptance but will increase treatment options and should result in better therapies for more CVD patients.

19.5. CONCLUSION

Clearly, there is a substantial market for direct myocardial revascularization procedures, both in terms of an unmet patient need and a solid financial market. A major concern regarding physician and thus widespread PMR acceptance is confidence in the procedure. Physician acceptance should grow with a more detailed understanding mechanism of action. However, physician acceptance is more likely to be driven by proven and reproducible treatment success in specific patient classes. For example, if extensive clinical data from a multicenter trial indicated that PMR were found to relieve angina or extend life more in insulin-dependent diabetics than existing CABG or PTCA procedures, AHA and physician approval would likely follow. Skeptical concerns are legitimate in ensuring that this technology does provide the benefits that it claims. However, an over-zealous skepticism could clearly destroy a potentially useful tool that may help many patients. Because PTCA market penetrance is starting to slow, it is likely that alternative revascularization strategies will be reexamined to continually improve treatments for CVD patients. Certainly the patient volume and need are present.

References

AHA (American Heart Association). *Heart and Stroke Facts.* Dallas, TX, AHA, 1993.

AHA (American Heart Association). *Heart and Stroke Statistical Update.* AHA, Dallas, TX, 2001.

Ahern JE. Transmyocardial revascularization: an industry perspective. *J Inv Cardiol* 1999; 11: 192–194.

Allen KB, Shaar CJ. Transmyocardial laser revascularizations: surgical experience overview. *Semin Interv Cardiol* 2000; 5: 75–81.

Faxon DP. Myocardial revascularization in 1997: angioplasty versus bypass surgery. *Am Family Phys* 1997; 56: 1409–1418.

Fry SM. Market trends and business considerations. In: *Lasers in Cardiovascular Medicine and Surgery: Fundamentals and Techniques*, GS Abela ed., Kluwer, New York, 1990; 449–457.

Fudge TL. Bypass surgery or angioplasty: what determines the choice? Cardiovascular Institute of the South 2001:
http://www.cardio.com/articles/balloon.html.

Hlatky MA, Rogers WJ, Johnstone I et al. Medical care costs and quality of life after randomization to coronary angioplasty or coronary bypass surgery. Bypass angioplasty revascularization investigation (BARI) investigators. *N Engl J Med* 1997; 336: 92–99.

Hughes GC, Abdel-aleem S, Biswas SS et al. Transmyocardial laser revascularization: experimental and clinical results. *Can J Cardiol* 1999; 15: 797–806.

Kastrati A, Schomig A, Elezi S et al. Predictive factors of restenosis after coronary stent placement. *J Am Coll Cardiol* 1997; 30: 1428–1436.

Leon MB, Baim DS, Moses JW et al. A randomized blinded clinical trial comparing percutaneous laser myocardial revascularization (using Biosense LV Mapping) vs. placebo in patients with refractory coronary ischemia. *Circulation* 2000; 102: II–565.

Mukherjee D, Bhatt DL, Roe MT et al. Direct myocardial revascularization and angiogenesis—how many patients might be eligible? *Am J Cardiol* 1999; 84: 598–600.

Nordrehaug JE, Salem M, Rotevatn S et al. Blinded evaluation of laser (PTMR) intervention electively for angina pectoris (BELIEF). American College of Cardiology, Orlando, FL, March 19, 2001.

Oesterle SN, Sanborn TA, Ali N, et al., Percutaneous transmyocardial laser revascularization for severe angina: the PACIFIC randomized trial. *Lancet* 2000; 356: 1705–1710.

Pocock SJ, Henderson RA, Rickards AF et al. Meta-analysis of randomised trials comparing coronary angioplasty with bypass surgery. *Lancet* 1995; 346: 1184–1189.

Schulper MJ, Seed P, Henderson RA et al. Health service costs of coronary angioplasty and coronary artery bypass surgery: the randomised intervention treatment of angina (RITA) trial. *Lancet* 1994; 344: 927–930.

U.S. Census Bureau. 2001: http://www.census.gov.

Weintraub WS, Mauldin PD, Becker E et al. A comparison of the costs of and quality of life after coronary angioplasty or coronary surgery for multivessel coronary artery disease. Results from the Emory angioplasty versus surgery trial (EAST). *Circulation* 1995; 92: 2831–2840.

Weintraub WS, Stein B, Kosinski A et al. Outcome of coronary bypass surgery versus coronary angioplasty in diabetic patients with multivessel coronary artery disease. *J Am Coll Cardiol* 1998; 31: 10–19.

Glossary

Angiogenesis Sprouting of capillaries in an area of myocardium depleted of its blood supply. These originate from cells that are pre-existing in the region.

Argon laser A laser using a lasing medium of Ar^+ ions. Principal wavelengths emitted include 488 and 514 nm.

BELIEF (Blinded Evaluation of Laser Intervention Electively For Angina Pectoris) Norwegian study comparing PTMR to placebo in a double-blinded placebo trial.

BrdU A technique of labeling to identify new cell growth by incorporation of bromodeoxyuridine (BrdU) into the newly formed cell nuclear DNA.

Carbon dioxide laser A laser using CO_2 gas as the lasing medium. This radiation is emitted in the infrared region of 10,600 nm.

CABG Coronary artery bypass graft surgery.

CCS Canadian Cardiovascular Society classification of angina severity, grades I–IV.

Cryo- A method of tissue freezing that results in necrosis.

DIRECT (DMR in Regeneration of Endomyocardial Channels Trial) Study evaluating DMR for angina relief in a double-blinded placebo trial.

DMR (Direct Myocardial Revascularization) A noncontact laser catheter system that uses a navigational guidance with NOGA to create myocardial channels.

EMM Electromechanical mapping using the NOGA system.

Er:YAG laser A laser using erbium ion doped with aluminum-garnet crystal. The radiation is emitted at 2,940 nm.

Excimer laser A laser using a medium of excited homopolar or heteropolar dimers. Excimer lasers produce high-energy photons in the ultraviolet range (i.e., XeCl, 308 nm).

Fluence Energy deposited per unit area (i.e., joules/cm^2).

Ho:YAG laser A laser using holmium ion doped with aluminum-garnet crystal. The radiation is emitted at 2,100 nm.

Joule The unit of energy measure equivalent to one watt-second.

Laser An acronym for "light amplification by stimulated emission of radiation." This is a coherent light that was predicted by Albert Einstein's theory of light.

Nd:YAG laser A laser using neodymium ion doped with yttrium aluminum-garnet crystal. The radiation is emitted at 1,060 nm.

NOGA Navigational system to guide catheters using real time computer simulation of catheter tip localization. This is used with DMR and gene delivery to specific locations in the left ventricular wall.

Optical fiber   A wave guide, usually of glass or plastic. These are cylindrical and have a clad cover. They are usually very flexible.

PACIFIC (Potential Angina Class Improvement From Intramyocardial Channels) Prospective randomized trial comparing PTMR with medial treatment.

Percutaneous   The route of entry into the arterial or venous circulation by penetrating the skin overlying the vessel and then using catheters to advance various devices to the heart or other sites in the vascular tree.

PTCA   Percutaneous transluminal coronary angioplasty.

Percutaneous Transmyocardial Revascularization (PMR or PTMR) A technique of creating channels in the ventricle via a percutaneous route that is intented to only penetrate partially through the myocardial wall. The purpose is to enhance blood flow to ischemic myocardium. This is performed using a laser delivered via a fiberoptic catheter system.

Radio Frequency (RF) Electromagnetic waves used typically in radio and television transmission. These can be delivered at a tissue site to cause thermal injury.

Revascularization Any method used to bring blood supply to heart muscle that has been severely deprived of its native supply.

SPECT (Single-photon emission tomography) SPECT allows reconstruction of planar images in three dimensions by the triangulation of defects. This enhances sensitivity and specificity of nuclear myocardial scintigraphy.

Transmyocardial revascularization (TMR) A technique of creating channels in the ventricular muscle to enhance direct perfusion of the myocardium from the ventricular cavity. This procedure is performed from the outer myocardium into the ventricular chamber. This can be performed by using laser energy or mechanical devices. However, the common usage implies the use by laser, as in this text.

Ultrasound (US) energy Very high-frequency ultrasound energy can cause cavitation and bubble formation when local energy buildup exceeds $1,500\,W/cm^2$. This can lead to tissue destruction.

Vasculogenesis The synthesis of new arteries.

VEGF   Vascular endothelium growth factor; used to enhance angiogenesis.

Vineberg, Arthur (1903–1988)   Surgeon and chief of cardiac surgery at the Royal Victoria Hospital (1935–1965) and Associate Professor of Surgery at McGill University, Montreal, Canada. He is well known for the Vineberg operation.

Vineberg operation Implantation of the internal mammary artery into the ventricular myocardium to enhance blood flow to ischemic myocardium.

INDEX